ADVANCES IN
IMMUNOLOGY

AID FOR IMMUNOGLOBULIN DIVERSITY

VOLUME 94

Associate Editors

K. Frank Austen
Division of Rheumatology
Immunology & Allergy
Harvard Medical School, Boston, Massachusetts

Tasuku Honjo
Graduate School of Medicine and
Faculty of Medicine, Kyoto University
Kyoto, Japan

Fritz Melchers
Department of Cell Biology
University of Basel
Basel, Switzerland

Jonathan W. Uhr
Department of Microbiology &
Internal Medicine
University of Texas, Dallas, Texas

Emil R. Unanue
Department of Pathology & Immunology
Washington University
St. Louis, Missouri

ADVANCES IN IMMUNOLOGY

AID FOR IMMUNOGLOBULIN DIVERSITY

VOLUME 94

Edited By

Frederick W. Alt
CBRI Institute for Biomedical Research
Howard Hughes Medical Institute
Children's Hospital Boston
Boston, Massachusetts

Tasuku Honjo
Graduate School of Medicine
and Faculty of Medicine
Kyoto University
Kyoto, Japan

Series Editor

Frederick W. Alt
CBRI Institute for Biomedical Research
Howard Hughes Medical Institute
Children's Hospital Boston
Boston, Massachusetts

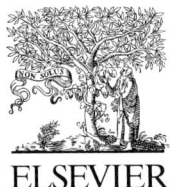
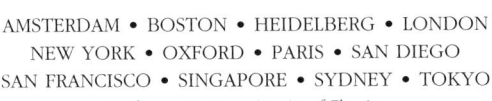
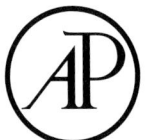

AMSTERDAM • BOSTON • HEIDELBERG • LONDON
NEW YORK • OXFORD • PARIS • SAN DIEGO
SAN FRANCISCO • SINGAPORE • SYDNEY • TOKYO
Academic Press is an imprint of Elsevier

Elsevier Academic Press
525 B Street, Suite 1900, San Diego, California 92101-4495, USA
84 Theobald's Road, London WC1X 8RR, UK

This book is printed on acid-free paper. ∞

Copyright © 2007, Elsevier Inc. All Rights Reserved.

No part of this publication may be reproduced or transmitted in any form or by any means, electronic or mechanical, including photocopy, recording, or any information storage and retrieval system, without permission in writing from the Publisher.

The appearance of the code at the bottom of the first page of a chapter in this book indicates the Publisher's consent that copies of the chapter may be made for personal or internal use of specific clients. This consent is given on the condition, however, that the copier pay the stated per copy fee through the Copyright Clearance Center, Inc. (www.copyright.com), for copying beyond that permitted by Sections 107 or 108 of the U.S. Copyright Law. This consent does not extend to other kinds of copying, such as copying for general distribution, for advertising or promotional purposes, for creating new collective works, or for resale.
Copy fees for pre-2007 chapters are as shown on the title pages. If no fee code appears on the title page, the copy fee is the same as for current chapters.
0065-2776/2007 $35.00

Permissions may be sought directly from Elsevier's Science & Technology Rights Department in Oxford, UK: phone: (+44) 1865 843830, fax: (+44) 1865 853333, E-mail: permissions@elsevier.com. You may also complete your request on-line via the Elsevier homepage (http://elsevier.com), by selecting "Support & Contact" then "Copyright and Permission" and then "Obtaining Permissions."

For all information on all Elsevier Academic Press publications
visit our Web site at www.books.elsevier.com

ISBN-13: 978-0-12-373706-9
ISBN-10: 0-12-373706-0

PRINTED IN THE UNITED STATES OF AMERICA
07 08 09 10 9 8 7 6 5 4 3 2 1

**Working together to grow
libraries in developing countries**

www.elsevier.com | www.bookaid.org | www.sabre.org

ELSEVIER   BOOK AID International   Sabre Foundation

Contents

Contributors ix
Preface xiii

Discovery of Activation-Induced Cytidine Deaminase, the Engraver of Antibody Memory

Masamichi Muramatsu, Hitoshi Nagaoka, Reiko Shinkura, Nasim A. Begum, and Tasuku Honjo

	Abstract.	1
1.	Introduction	2
2.	Identification of AID as a Key Molecule in CSR and SHM.	4
3.	AID Is the Only B-Cell-Specific Factor Required for Both CSR and SHM	8
4.	Functional Domains of AID	11
5.	AID Is Involved in a DNA Cleavage Step.	14
6.	Major Hypotheses for the Action of AID	16
7.	Critical Examination of the DNA Deamination Model.	19
8.	Evidence for a Novel Function of UNG in CSR	24
9.	Conclusion	28
	References	29

DNA Deamination in Immunity: AID in the Context of Its APOBEC Relatives

Silvestro G. Conticello, Marc-Andre Langlois, Zizhen Yang, and Michael S. Neuberger

	Abstract.	37
1.	Introduction	38

2. AID: The DNA Deaminase Trigger for
   Antibody Diversification 38
3. The Zn-Dependent Deaminase Superfamily 39
4. Timeline of AID/APOBEC Evolution 48
5. APOBEC1: An RNA-Editing Enzyme That Can Also
   Act on DNA 49
6. APOBEC2: A Muscle-Specific Family Member of Unknown
   Function/Activity 50
7. APOBEC4: A Distant or Ancestral Member of
   the AID/APOBEC Family 51
8. APOBEC3s: DNA Deaminases Active
   in Viral Restriction 52
9. Conclusion 63
   References 63

The Role of Activation-Induced Deaminase in Antibody Diversification and Chromosome Translocations

Almudena Ramiro, Bernardo Reina San-Martin, Kevin McBride, Mila Jankovic, Vasco Barreto, André Nussenzweig, and Michel C. Nussenzweig

   Abstract 75
1. Introduction 76
2. Events Preceding the DNA Lesion 77
3. The DNA Lesion 78
4. DNA Damage Detection and Resolution During CSR 85
5. AID and Lymphomagenic Lesions 93
6. Conclusions and Perspectives 96
   References 96

Targeting of AID-Mediated Sequence Diversification by *cis*-Acting Determinants

Shu Yuan Yang and David G. Schatz

   Abstract 109
1. Introduction 109
2. The Link Between Transcription and AID-Mediated
   Sequence Diversification 111
3. Other *cis*-Acting Determinants Involved in
   the Targeting of AID 116

4. Future Outlook.. 120
References 120

AID-Initiated Purposeful Mutations in Immunoglobulin Genes

Myron F. Goodman, Matthew D. Scharff, and Floyd E. Romesberg

Abstract... 127
1. Introduction 128
2. Biochemical Basis of C Deamination
   by APOBEC Enzymes 132
3. How and Why Might AID-Specific Mutations
   Be Targeted?... 141
4. Selection of AID-Induced Mutations
   During Ab Maturation 143
References 149

Evolution of the Immunoglobulin Heavy Chain Class Switch Recombination Mechanism

Jayanta Chaudhuri, Uttiya Basu, Ali Zarrin, Catherine Yan, Sonia Franco, Thomas Perlot, Bao Vuong, Jing Wang, Ryan T. Phan, Abhishek Datta, John Manis, and Frederick W. Alt

Abstract... 157
1. Overview of Genetic Alterations in B Lymphocytes 158
2. Activation-Induced Cytidine Deaminase 162
3. Role of Germ Line Transcription and Switch Regions in CSR.... 169
4. Posttranscriptional Regulation of AID.................... 180
5. Mechanisms Involved in Synapsis of AID Initiated DSBs in
   Widely Separated S Regions 184
6. General DNA Repair Systems in the Joining Phase of CSR...... 189
7. Evolution of CSR 197
References 198

Beyond SHM and CSR: AID and Related Cytidine Deaminases in the Host Response to Viral Infection

Brad R. Rosenberg and F. Nina Papavasiliou

Abstract... 215
1. Introduction 215

2. Evolution of the AID/APOBEC Cytidine
   Deaminase Family 216
3. APOBEC3: A Subfamily of Antiviral
   Cytidine Deaminases 217
4. AID in the Host Response to Viral Infection 229
5. Concluding Remarks.. 235
   References 237

Role of AID in Tumorigenesis

Il-mi Okazaki, Ai Kotani, and Tasuku Honjo

Abstract... 245
1. Introduction 246
2. AID Transgenic Mouse Models 247
3. Role of AID in Chromosomal Translocation and
   Subsequent Lymphomagenesis.................................. 249
4. AID Expression in Human B-Cell Malignancies.............. 252
5. Mechanism of AID Expression in
   Normal and Malignant B Cells................................. 259
6. AID Expression in Normal and Malignant
   Nonlymphoid Cells.. 263
7. Concluding Remarks.. 265
   References 265

Pathophysiology of B-Cell Intrinsic Immunoglobulin Class Switch Recombination Deficiencies

Anne Durandy, Nadine Taubenheim, Sophie Peron, and Alain Fischer

Abstract... 275
1. Introduction 276
2. Ig-CSR Deficiency Type 1 Caused by Activation-Induced
   Cytidine Deaminase Deficiency................................. 279
3. Ig-CSR Deficiency Type 2 Caused by UNG Deficiency 289
4. Molecularly Undefined Ig-CSR Deficiency
   with Normal SHM 292
5. Concluding Remarks.. 296
   References 298

Index.. 307
Contents of Recent Volumes 317

Contributors

Numbers in parentheses indicate the pages on which the authors' contributions begin.

Frederick W. Alt (157), The Howard Hughes Medical Institute, The Children's Hospital, The CBR Institute for Biomedical Research and Department of Genetics, Harvard Medical School, Boston, Massachusetts

Vasco Barreto (75), Laboratory of Molecular Immunology, The Rockefeller University, New York, New York

Uttiya Basu (157), The Howard Hughes Medical Institute, The Children's Hospital, The CBR Institute for Biomedical Research and Department of Genetics, Harvard Medical School, Boston, Massachusetts

Nasim A. Begum (1), Department of Immunology and Genomic Medicine and 21 Century COE Formation, Graduate School of Medicine, Kyoto University, Kyoto, Japan

Jayanta Chaudhuri (157), Immunology Program, Memorial Sloan Kettering Cancer Center, New York, New York

Silvestro G. Conticello (37), Medical Research Council Laboratory of Molecular Biology, Cambridge CB2 2QH, United Kingdom

Abhishek Datta (157), The Howard Hughes Medical Institute, The Children's Hospital, The CBR Institute for Biomedical Research and Department of Genetics, Harvard Medical School, Boston, Massachusetts

Anne Durandy (275), Inserm, U768, Paris F-75015, France; Univ René Descartes-Paris 5, F-75006, France; Assistance Publique Hôpitaux de Paris, Hôpital Necker-Enfants Malades, 149 rue de Sèvres 75015 Paris, France

Alain Fischer (275), Inserm, U768, Paris F-75015, France; Univ René Descartes-Paris 5, F-75006, France; Assistance Publique Hôpitaux de Paris and Unité d'immunologie et Hématologie Pédiatrique, Hôpital Necker-Enfants Malades, 149 rue de Sèvres 75015 Paris, France

Sonia Franco (157), The Howard Hughes Medical Institute, The Children's Hospital, The CBR Institute for Biomedical Research and Department of Genetics, Harvard Medical School, Boston, Massachusetts

Myron F. Goodman (127), Department of Biological Sciences and Department of Chemistry, University of Southern California, Los Angeles, California

Tasuku Honjo (1, 245), Department of Immunology and Genomic Medicine, Graduate School of Medicine, Kyoto University, Kyoto, Japan

Mila Jankovic (75), Laboratory of Molecular Immunology, The Rockefeller University, New York, New York

Ai Kotani (245), Department of Immunology and Genomic Medicine, Graduate School of Medicine, Kyoto University, Kyoto, Japan

Marc-Andre Langlois (37), Medical Research Council Laboratory of Molecular Biology, Cambridge CB2 2QH, United Kingdom

John Manis (157), Joint Program in Transfusin Medicine, Department of Pathology, Children's Hospital, Harvard Medical School, Boston, Massachusetts

Kevin McBride (75), Laboratory of Molecular Immunology, The Rockefeller University, New York, New York

Masamichi Muramatsu (1), Department of Immunology and Genomic Medicine and 21 Century COE Formation, Graduate School of Medicine, Kyoto University, Kyoto, Japan

Hitoshi Nagaoka (1), Department of Immunology and Genomic Medicine, Graduate School of Medicine, Kyoto University, Kyoto, Japan

Michael S. Neuberger (37), Medical Research Council Laboratory of Molecular Biology, Cambridge CB2 2QH, United Kingdom

André Nussenzweig (75), Experimental Immunology Branch, National Cancer Institute, National Institutes of Health, Bethesda, Maryland

Michel C. Nussenzweig (75), Laboratory of Molecular Immunology, The Rockefeller University, New York, New York; Howard Hughes Medical Institute, Maryland

Il-mi Okazaki (245), Department of Immunology and Genomic Medicine, Graduate School of Medicine, Kyoto University, Kyoto, Japan

F. Nina Papavasiliou (215), Laboratory of Lymphocyte Biology, The Rockefeller University, New York, New York

Thomas Perlot (157), The Howard Hughes Medical Institute, The Children's Hospital, The CBR Institute for Biomedical Research and Department of Genetics, Harvard Medical School, Boston, Massachusetts

Sophie Peron (275), Inserm, U768, Paris F-75015, France; Univ René Descartes-Paris 5, Paris F-75006, France; Hôpital Necker-Enfants Malades, 149 rue de Sèvres 75015 Paris, France

Ryan T. Phan (157), The Howard Hughes Medical Institute, The Children's Hospital, The CBR Institute for Biomedical Research and Department of Genetics, Harvard Medical School, Boston, Massachusetts

CONTRIBUTORS

Almudena Ramiro (75), DNA Hypermutation and Cancer Group, Spanish National Cancer Center (CNIO), Melchor Fernandez Almagro, 3, 28029 Madrid, Spain

Bernardo Reina San-Martin (75), Institut de Génétique et de Biologie Moléculaire et Cellulaire, Département de, Pathologie Moléculaire, 1 rue Laurent Fries, 67404 Illkirch CEDEX, France

Floyd E. Romesberg (127), Department of Chemistry, The Scripps Research Institute, La Jolla, California

Brad R. Rosenberg (215), Laboratory of Lymphocyte Biology, The Rockefeller University, New York, New York

Matthew D. Scharff (127), Department of Cell Biology, Albert Einstein College of Medicine, Bronx, New York

David G. Schatz (109), Section of Immunology and Howard Hughes Medical Institute, Yale University School of Medicine, New Haven, Connecticut

Reiko Shinkura (1), Department of Immunology and Genomic Medicine, Graduate School of Medicine, Kyoto University, Kyoto, Japan

Nadine Taubenheim (275), Inserm, U768, Paris F-75015, France; Univ René Descartes-Paris 5, Paris F-75006, France; Hôpital Necker-Enfants Malades, 149 rue de Sèvres 75015 Paris, France

Bao Vuong (157), Immunology Program, Memorial Sloan Kettering Cancer Center, New York, New York

Jing Wang (157), The Howard Hughes Medical Institute, The Children's Hospital, The CBR Institute for Biomedical Research and Department of Genetics, Harvard Medical School, Boston, Massachusetts

Catherine Yan (157), The Howard Hughes Medical Institute, The Children's Hospital, The CBR Institute for Biomedical Research and Department of Genetics, Harvard Medical School, Boston, Massachusetts

Shu Yuan Yang (109), Section of Immunobiology, Yale University School of Medicine, New Haven, Connecticut

Zizhen Yang (37), Medical Research Council Laboratory of Molecular Biology, Cambridge CB2 2QH, United Kingdom

Ali Zarrin (157), The Howard Hughes Medical Institute, The Children's Hospital, The CBR Institute for Biomedical Research and Department of Genetics, Harvard Medical School, Boston, Massachusetts

Preface

This volume covers the exciting advances that have been made in our understanding of the generation of antibody diversity subsequent to the discovery of the activation-induced cytidine deaminase (AID). In this regard, the volume is organized into nine separate chapters, most of which focus on particular aspects of AID and the immunoglobulin gene diversification processes in which it functions. This short introductory overview summarizes some of the most relevant topics and points to particular chapters in which specific topics are covered. However, the reader is encouraged to go through all of the chapters to gain a complete understanding of this fascinating area of biology. In that regard, while individual chapters tend to focus on particular topics, they necessarily cover overlapping subject matter but often, given that this is still a developing field, from different viewpoints.

The AID protein is necessary and sufficient for the initiation of immunoglobluin heavy chain class switch recombination (CSR) and the initiation of somatic hypermutation (SHM) of immunoglobulin variable region exons. That one enzyme can induce the seemingly very different CSR and SHM mechanisms, and that this enzyme can also induce the process of gene conversion in chickens, was a very remarkable and unexpected finding. Moreover, the mechanism of SHM was considered by many as one of the last major frontiers of immunology, until the discovery that AID is the long sought mutator. Thus, the discovery of AID, about 7 years ago, revolutionized our understanding of the peripheral mechanism of immunoglobulin gene diversification and led to a huge body of additional work. The work that led to the discovery of AID is discussed in depth in Chapter 1 by Muramatsu *et al*. An in-depth review of CSR is presented in Chapter 6 by Chaudhuri *et al*. and a detailed introduction to SHM is presented in Chapter 4 by Yuan and Schatz.

AID is comprised of less than 200-amino acid residues and carries a cytidine deaminase motif. AID clearly is required to introduce DNA lesions into variable region exons and switch regions during SHM and CSR, respectively. However, many important questions remain concerning how AID leads to DNA cleavage. A long-debated question is the nature of the direct target of cytidine deamination *in vivo* by AID, DNA or RNA. AID is structurally related to APOBEC1, which is an RNA editing enzyme. However, biochemical studies have shown that purified AID deaminates cytidines on single-strand DNA. Considerations relevant to DNA versus RNA models for AID activity are presented in depth in Chapter 1 by Muramatsu et al. and in Chapter 6 by Chaudhuri et al.

There are many other important questions regarding the function and regulation of AID. A key question is how AID-initiated lesions lead to mutation of variable region DNA and DNA double strand breaks within switch regions. In this context, another major question is the identification of modifications or cofactors that might influence AID activity and potentially channel AID functions into SHM or CSR. An extremely important question is the nature of the mechanisms that normally target the activities of this potent mutator to immunoglobulin genes and not other genes. These general topics are discussed in Chapter 1 by Muramatsu et al., in Chapter 3 by Ramiro et al., and in Chapter 6 by Chaudhuri et al. AID biochemistry is a particular focus of Chapter 5 by Goodman et al. while issues related to AID targeting are a focus of Chapter 4 by Yuan and Schatz, which also describes gene conversion.

The nature of the mechanisms that join AID-initiated breaks in the context of CSR has been a major area of study. Several studies have shown that general DNA double strand break repair mechanisms are harnessed to join AID-dependent breaks in switch regions. This topic is a particular focus of Chapter 3 by Ramiro et al. and is also covered in depth in Chapter 6 by Chaudhuri et al. AID also has been demonstrated to be involved in the initiation of translocations that arise in the context of IgH CSR, including oncogenic translocations found in certain B-cell lymphomas. Chapter 3 also discusses this topic in depth. Transgenic studies have further indicated that AID expression can lead to other types of tumors, raising the question of how broadly AID might function to generate certain forms of human cancer. This topic is discussed in Chapter 8 by Okazaki et al.

AID deficiency causes a severe immune deficiency in humans that is called hyper IgM syndrome type II. This disease causes the absence of IgH isotypes other than IgM and absence of hypermutation and, thereby, results in severe susceptibility to bacterial infection. As there are other forms of hyper IgM type II not yet fully characterized, the question arises whether further studies of these deficiencies may reveal other functions for AID or potential cofactors. The pathophysiology of AID deficiency in humans is the subject of Chapter 9 by Durandy et al.

Finally, an important question is whether AID might have functions beyond somatic mutation and CSR. This possibility is supported by findings that molecules related to AID in HIV resistance and that AID is induced after infection by various viruses. This exciting new area of investigation is covered in Chapter 2 by Conticello *et al.* and in Chapter 7 by Rosenberg and Papavasiliou.

Frederick W. Alt
Tasuku Honjo

Discovery of Activation-Induced Cytidine Deaminase, the Engraver of Antibody Memory

Masamichi Muramatsu,*,† Hitoshi Nagaoka,* Reiko Shinkura,* Nasim A. Begum,*,† and Tasuku Honjo*

*Department of Immunology and Genomic Medicine, Graduate School of Medicine, Kyoto University, Kyoto, Japan
†21 Century COE Formation, Graduate School of Medicine, Kyoto University, Kyoto, Japan

Abstract	1
1. Introduction	2
2. Identification of AID as a Key Molecule in CSR and SHM	4
3. AID Is the Only B-Cell-Specific Factor Required for Both CSR and SHM	8
4. Functional Domains of AID	11
5. AID Is Involved in a DNA Cleavage Step	14
6. Major Hypotheses for the Action of AID	16
7. Critical Examination of the DNA Deamination Model	19
8. Evidence for a Novel Function of UNG in CSR	24
9. Conclusion	28
References	29

Abstract

Discovery of activation-induced cytidine deaminase (AID) paved a new path to unite two genetic alterations induced by antigen stimulation; class switch recombination (CSR) and somatic hypermutation (SHM). AID is now established to cleave specific target DNA and to serve as engraver of these genetic alterations. AID of a 198-residue protein has four important domains: nuclear localization signal and SHM-specific region at the N-terminus; the α-helical segment (residue 47–54) responsible for dimerization; catalytic domain (residues 56–94) shared by all the other cytidine deaminase family members; and nuclear export signal overlapping with class switch-specific domain at the C-terminus. Two alternative models have been proposed for the mode of AID action; whether AID directly attacks DNA or indirectly through RNA editing. Lines of evidence supporting RNA editing hypothesis include homology in various aspects with APOBEC1, a bona fide RNA editing enzyme as well as requirement of de novo protein synthesis for DNA cleavage by AID in CSR and SHM. This chapter critically evaluates DNA deamination hypothesis and describes evidence to indicate UNG is involved not in DNA cleavage but in DNA repair of CSR. In addition, UNG appears to have a noncanonical function through interaction with an HIV Vpr-like protein at the WXXF motif. Taken together, RNA editing hypothesis is gaining the ground.

1. Introduction

Modern immunology was initiated by the first vaccination trial against smallpox virus infection by Jenner in 1789. However, understanding of the molecular basis for this miraculous medical application of vaccination has to wait 110 years until Behring and Kitazato identified antibodies in sera. In essence, therefore, immune memory induced by vaccination depends on antibody memory.

Subsequently, antibody memory was found to consist of somatic hypermutation (SHM) and class switch recombination (CSR) (Fig. 1). A large number of people including C. Milstein, M. Cohn, and W. Weigert made enormous

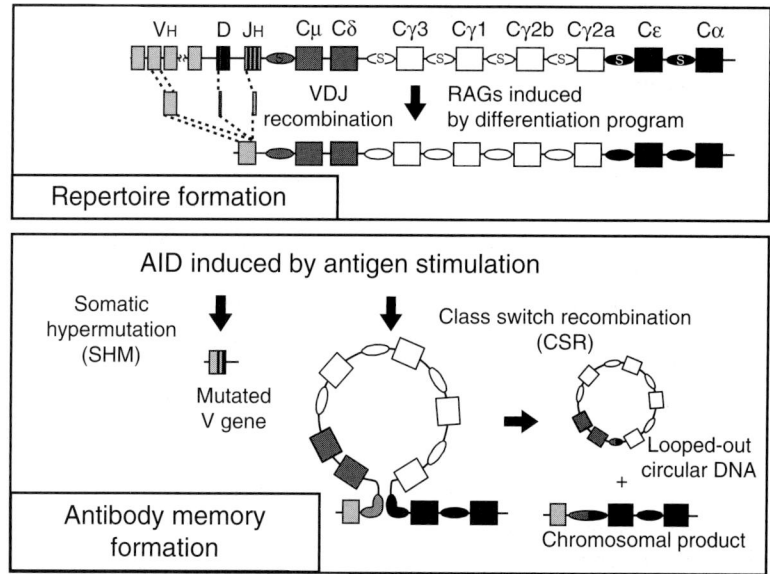

Figure 1 Antibody memory is engraved by AID. Three genetic alterations occur in the IgH locus. (Top) The first genetic alteration, VDJ recombination assembles V, D, and J gene segments to produce a single productive V exon in each B cell, generating V region repertoire in each individual. VDJ recombination that occurs in bone marrow on B-cell development is mediated by RAG-1 and RAG-2 recombinases that are expressed by differentiation program of B cells. (Bottom) After completion of VDJ recombination, B cells migrate to periphery. Stimulation by antigen induces AID in B cells resulting two additional genetic alterations. V genes are further diversified by SHM. CSR switches from Cμ to one of the downstream C genes. Intervening DNA segment is looped-out as a circular DNA. AID mediates SHM and CSR by inducing DNA strand breaks in V region and S regions, respectively. After selection of B cells with SHM and CSR by antigen, B-cell memory is registered on DNA.

contribution to demonstrate that SHM takes place by analysis of antibody proteins. Direct evidence for DNA modification of the immunoglobulin gene in SHM and CSR was obtained using recombinant DNA technology in 1970–1980. DNA sequence determination of the immunoglobulin gene structure first by Tonegawa (1983), followed by a number of groups, clearly demonstrated that point mutations take place in the variable (V) region gene. CSR takes place between two switch (S) regions, resulting in looping-out deletion of DNA segments between the V and constant (C) region of the heavy-chain gene to be expressed (Honjo et al., 2002). These findings clearly showed that immune memory is coined on DNA encoding immunoglobulins. These two molecular events, point mutations by SHM and DNA deletions by CSR, were considered to be regulated by totally different mechanisms until the discovery of activation-induced cytidine deaminase (AID) (Muramatsu et al., 1999), just another 100 years after the discovery of antibody. Functional analyses of AID have revealed an amazing observation that AID deficiency in mouse and human abolishes both CSR and SHM (Muramatsu et al., 2000; Revy et al., 2000). We now know that the vaccination induces AID in B cells, which prints the memory of vaccine on the immunoglobulin gene, giving rise to production of most efficient immunoglobulins for our defense.

AID is clearly shown to introduce DNA cleavage in the target DNA, namely the V region for SHM and the S region for CSR (Begum et al., 2004a; Dudley et al., 2002; Nagaoka et al., 2002; Petersen et al., 2001; Woo et al., 2003). However, the exact molecular mechanism by which AID introduces DNA cleavage is actively debated. Two hypotheses have been proposed: RNA editing and DNA deamination (Honjo et al., 2002; Neuberger et al., 2003). RNA editing hypothesis assumes that AID modifies bases on mRNA and generates new mRNA encoding endonuclease that cleaves DNA at the specific region. DNA deamination hypothesis predicts that AID itself modifies DNA bases and subsequent DNA repair mechanism introduces DNA cleavage.

AID is also shown to induce DNA cleavage in nonimmunoglobulin loci, which results in chromosomal translocation or aberrant mutations in oncogenes (Kotani et al., 2005; Okazaki et al., 2003; Ramiro et al., 2004). Therefore, AID, when aberrantly expressed, can cause tumor. This finding is beginning to open new fields in tumor biology.

In this chapter, we will describe historical perspective that led to the discovery of AID and its function. We will explain how two entirely different DNA alterations can be regulated by a single small molecule. The chapter also covers critical discussion of two opposing hypotheses, RNA editing and DNA deamination. We describe lines of evidence supporting RNA editing hypothesis. We then examine the real function of UNG, which is proposed to be involved in DNA cleavage in association with AID according to DNA deamination hypothesis.

We describe the evidence that UNG is involved in CSR by a novel function other than U removal. All these results suggest that AID cleaves DNA through the RNA editing mechanism.

2. Identification of AID as a Key Molecule in CSR and SHM

2.1. Cloning of AID

In the mid-1990s, Nakamura *et al.* established a useful B-cell line that precisely reproduces the CSR phenomenon observed *in vivo*. This cell line, mouse B-cell lymphoma line CH12F3-2 (Nakamura *et al.*, 1996), switches isotype very efficiently (up to 60%) from IgM to IgA on addition of stimulants (IL-4, TGFβ, and CD40 ligand) to the culture medium. Since CSR in this cell line is completely dependent on the addition of stimulants, Muramatsu *et al.* hypothesized the existence of inducible genes that execute CSR. To test this possibility, cycloheximide, a protein translation inhibitor, was applied to CH12F3-2 cells (Muramatsu *et al.*, 1999). Because surface IgA expression also depends on mRNA translation, CSR was assessed by PCR amplification of looped-out circular DNAs that are by-products of CSR. As predicted, the formation of looped-out circular DNA was completely blocked by cycloheximide addition during CSR stimulation. This result supported the idea that newly transcribed genes initiate CSR. Therefore, molecular cloning of the induced genes was attempted using the same cell line system. To isolate such genes, a cDNA library generated from CSR-stimulated CH12F3-2 cells was compared with one from nonstimulated CH12F3-2 cells.

Seven genes, including I-a, MDC, IFNγR, and four novel genes were identified as genes that were upregulated in response to stimulation (Muramatsu *et al.*, 1999). Among the seven genes, AID was considered the most interesting candidate due to its novelty and its spatiotemporal expression pattern (see below). A BLAST search revealed homology of AID (34% amino acid identity) with apolipoprotein B RNA editing catalytic component 1 (APOBEC1), the catalytic subunit of the apolipoprotein B (apoB) RNA editing enzyme. APOBEC1 deaminates the first base of a CAA codon corresponding to glutamine 2153 in apoB100. After deamination by APOBEC1, the CAA codon is converted to UAA, an in-frame stop codon, so that the resulting mRNA encodes a C-terminally truncated protein called apoB48. A cytidine deaminase motif is the most prominent structure in both AID and APOBEC1; thus, AID was expected to possess cytidine deaminase activity. GST-AID recombinant protein was prepared, and cytidine deaminase activity was assessed *in vitro*. As expected, GST-AID converted deoxycytidine to deoxyuridine as efficiently as APOBEC1 in a Zn chelator- and deaminase inhibitor-sensitive manner.

Thus, structural similarity and enzymatic activity indicated that AID is a novel member of the cytidine deaminase superfamily (Muramatsu et al., 1999).

AID expression at the transcriptional level was extensively investigated in the first report of AID (Muramatsu et al., 1999). Northern blot analysis showed that AID was predominantly expressed in lymph nodes and weakly expressed in spleen, but no detectable expression was observed in other organs such as lung, thymus, kidney, and liver. RT-PCR of mRNA from different lymphoid organs revealed that AID expression is tightly correlated with the existence of germinal centers in which CSR and SHM occur. A possible correlation between AID expression and germinal centers was further investigated by active immunization of protein antigens. It is well established that immunization with sheep red blood cells (SRBC) induces germinal centers in mouse spleen (Fu et al., 1998; Mackay et al., 1997). Indeed, germinal center formation visualized by peanut agglutinin (PNA) staining was observed in spleen only after immunization with SRBC. Combination of serial sections and PNA staining with *in situ* hybridization with an AID probe indicated exact colocalization of AID expression with germinal centers.

Next, to determine which cells are responsible for AID expression, spleen cells from SRBC-immunized mice were separated according to B- or T-cell surface markers. RT-PCR using the fractionated spleen cells indicated that B cells express AID transcripts. Consistent with the expression pattern observed *in vivo*, AID expression was induced in spleen B cells *in vitro* when they were activated by CSR stimulants such as LPS and IL-4. Taken together, these results indicate that AID is specifically induced in B cells when activated by antigen stimulation *in vivo* or by CSR stimulants *in vitro*.

Elucidation of the physiological function of AID was not accomplished until 2000. However, the initial study by Muramatsu et al. (1999) revealed two important features of AID: (1) AID is a novel gene that shares common structural and enzymatic properties with the RNA editing enzyme APOBEC1 and (2) its expression is spatially and temporally correlated with CSR.

2.2. Disruption of AID Results in Loss of CSR and SHM

To establish the functional relationship between AID and CSR, stable transfectants of AID controlled by the tetracycline promoter were established in CH12F3-2 cells. When AID expression was induced by removal of tetracycline from the culture medium, some of the cells began to express surface IgA (Muramatsu et al., 2000). This result was not observed in mock transfectants, demonstrating the specificity of the experimental system. This was the first indication of functional involvement of AID in CSR.

Subsequently, AID was disrupted in mice by the standard gene targeting method. As expected by the physiological expression pattern of AID *in vivo*, AID-deficient mice were born according to Mendel's laws, and their growth and appearance were indistinguishable from that of littermate controls. There were no gross defects in immune cell populations such as T cells, B cells, macrophages, and granulocytes as assessed by surface markers. The first phenotype that was found to be different from littermate controls was Ig levels in serum (Muramatsu *et al.*, 2000). Levels of all Ig isotypes produced after CSR were much lower in AID-deficient mice than in control mice, whereas the IgM level was comparable or even higher than in control mice. Residual IgGs detected in sera of AID-deficient mice were not observed in AID-deficient offspring of AID-deficient mothers, indicating that the residual IgGs detected in the early phase of the study were derived from the AID-proficient mother through placental transmission.

To determine why AID-deficient mice cannot produce CSR-dependent Ig's, a detailed analysis was performed. When mice were immunized with NP-CGG, a hapten-conjugated protein antigen, control mice showed increased titers of NP-specific IgM and IgG antibodies. In contrast, AID-deficient mice did not exhibit increased NP-specific IgG titers, despite comparable production of the NP-specific IgM class. As with NP-CGG, the SRBC-specific IgG response was abolished completely, despite a normal response of SRBC-specific IgM. The general function of B cells *in vivo* appeared normal because AID-deficient mice could mount an antigen-specific IgM response. Furthermore, B cells in AID-deficient mice were activated as efficiently as B cells from control mice by SRBC administration.

No production of both total and antigen-specific IgGs with normal response of the IgM class is reminiscent of CD40 ligand (CD154) deficiency that causes X-linked hyper-IgM syndrome in humans (Allen *et al.*, 1993; Aruffo *et al.*, 1993; DiSanto *et al.*, 1993; Fuleihan *et al.*, 1993; Korthauer *et al.*, 1993). Defective IgG production in this genetic disorder is not due to a defect in the CSR molecular machinery but in T-cell help. Under conditions of CD40 ligand deficiency, the germinal center, an anatomical niche for B cells to receive T-cell help *in vivo*, does not develop properly (Facchetti *et al.*, 1995). Notably, B cells from CD40 ligand-deficient mice undergo normal CSR *in vitro* (Allen *et al.*, 1993; Aruffo *et al.*, 1993; Durandy *et al.*, 1993; Korthauer *et al.*, 1993). The importance of germinal center formation for IgG production was also reported in other genetically modified mice (Le Hir *et al.*, 1995; Matsumoto *et al.*, 1996; Ryffel *et al.*, 1997). It is now well accepted that the germinal center is essential for efficient production of IgG *in vivo*. Is germinal center formation normal in AID-deficient mice? When histological sections of Peyer's patches and spleens from immunized AID-deficient mice were stained with PNA in combination with other markers, germinal center formation was obvious (even more prominent than in control mice), indicating an intact anatomical microenvironment for CSR (Muramatsu et al., 2000). A specific defect in CSR that does not affect germinal center formation was a very unique phenotype of AID deficiency that had not been described previously.

Because AID is a B-cell-specific gene and the anatomical niche for CSR is intact in AID-deficient mice, the next question was whether AID-deficient B cells have an intrinsic defect in CSR. B cells were cultured with various CSR stimulants *in vitro*, and secretion of each Ig isotype was examined. Proliferation of AID-deficient B cells was not substantially different from that of control B cells (Muramatsu et al., 2000). AID-deficient B cells secrete IgM as efficiently as control B cells; however, no CSR-dependent isotypes were detected from AID-deficient B cells. Moreover, digestion-circularization PCR to detect switched IgH loci and RT-PCR to detect switched Ig transcripts demonstrated a complete lack of detectable CSR in AID-deficient B cells. This result indicated that the CSR defect observed *in vivo* can be attributed to defective CSR at the B-cell level and that the general protein secretion machinery is intact in AID-deficient B cells.

SHM is another genetic alteration that occurs in germinal center B cells. Since AID is specifically expressed in germinal center B cells, SHM was also investigated. After immunization with NP-CGG, the mutation load of the Vh186.2 gene was assessed. Surprisingly, SHM was not detected in AID-deficient mice, whereas control mice showed the expected mutation rate in the Vh186.2 gene (Muramatsu et al., 2000). This was the first example of a single gene disruption that results in complete loss of SHM without affecting B-cell development or activation. Thus, the study of AID-deficient mice revealed that AID is essential for two genetic diversification systems that occur in germinal center B cells after antigen stimulation.

At the same time AID-deficient mice were being analyzed in Japan, the group led by Durandy and Fischer in France were searching for genes responsible for an autosomal recessive form of class switch deficiency, hyper-IgM syndrome type 2 (HIGM2). The French group mapped the HIGM2 locus on chromosome 12p13, to which we mapped the AID gene (*AICDA*) (Muto et al., 2000). The collaboration of the two groups revealed that the coding regions of AID genes of all 18 HIGM2 patients from 12 families had mutations in both AID alleles. On the other hand, AID loci from healthy controls did not have any mutations (Revy et al., 2000). HIGM2 patients and AID-deficient mice share common phenotypes: loss of CSR and SHM, higher IgM levels in sera, and enlarged secondary lymphoid organs. Collectively, these observations clearly indicate that mutation of the AID locus causes HIGM2.

2.3. Enlarged Secondary Lymphoid Organs in AID-Deficient Mice

When secondary lymphoid organs, such as lymph nodes and Peyer's patches, were carefully examined in AID-deficient mice, most of them appeared hypertrophic (Fagarasan et al., 2002; Muramatsu et al., 2000). Histological and FACS analyses with surface markers of various cell types revealed that enlarged secondary lymphoid organs accumulated two to three times more germinal center B cells than those of controls (Fagarasan et al., 2002). All secondary lymphoid organs investigated accumulated germinal center B cells. Among such lymphoid structures, enlargement of the isolated lymphoid follicle (ILF) was most prominent. This secondary lymphoid tissue is thought to control or survey immune status in the gut, and the usual size of this tissue is microscopic (Hamada et al., 2002; Rosner and Keren, 1984). In AID-deficient mice, ILFs are visible by the naked eye from 5 weeks of age, and the number of enlarged ILFs increases with age (Fagarasan et al., 2002).

To elucidate the mechanism of lymphoid organ hypertrophy in AID-deficient mice, intestinal bacterial flora were examined. It was found that the balance of intestinal flora was heavily biased toward nonpathogenic anaerobes in AID-deficient mice, although control mice maintained in the same specific pathogen-free environment did not show expansion of anaerobic intestinal flora (Fagarasan et al., 2002). To reduce the load of anaerobic flora in the guts of AID-deficient mice, anaerobe-specific antibiotics were administered through drinking water. Strikingly, accumulated germinal center B cells in most secondary lymphoid organs were normalized in parallel with the disappearance of the abnormal balance of anaerobic flora. Thus, the accumulated germinal center B cells observed in AID-deficient mice are not due to malignant transformation but are the consequence of continuous antigen stimulation by abnormal gut flora. Without CSR and SHM, mice may not be able to control gut flora properly, and secreted IgM in the gut cannot compensate. In the human AID deficiency HIGM2, lymphoid hyperplasia with germinal center B-cell accumulation was also reported (Revy et al., 2000), raising the possibility that a similar mechanism is also operating in HIGM2 patients.

3. AID Is the Only B-Cell-Specific Factor Required for Both CSR and SHM

The study of AID-deficient mice clearly demonstrated that AID is indispensable to both CSR and SHM. To elucidate whether AID is sufficient for CSR and SHM, artificial substrates for CSR and SHM were established and introduced to nonlymphoid cells.

3.1. Ectopic Expression of AID Induces CSR of an Artificial Switch Construct in Fibroblasts

CSR requires three steps: (1) transcription of a target S region (germ line transcription), (2) DNA cleavage in both Sμ and the downstream S region (in which AID is involved), and (3) repair and joining of DNA double-stranded breaks (DSBs) by the nonhomologous end-joining (NHEJ) machinery. AID is expressed specifically in activated B cells and, like the transcription of S regions, is indispensable to CSR. On the other hand, the NHEJ repair system is constitutively expressed in almost all cell types. Can AID induce CSR in a non-B-cell lineage if an artificial target is offered?

To test the hypothesis that AID is the only B-cell-specific factor required for CSR, Okazaki *et al.* (2002) established a fibroblast cell line with an artificial switch substrate that is stably integrated in the genome. Since the IgH locus including S regions is transcribed only in B cells, an artificial switch construct requires elements that reproduce the fundamental characteristics unique to CSR in B cells: an inducible transcription system that mimics germ line transcription in B cells, S regions that provide nonhomologous but region-specific recombination without consensus sequences, and a broad but defined distribution of recombination sites. Kinoshita *et al.* (1998) established an artificial switch construct fulfilling these requirements in the murine B-cell lymphoma line CH12F3-2 (Kinoshita *et al.*, 1998). In this system, CSR of the artificial switch substrate was detectable by genomic Southern blot analysis. Furthermore, they modified the construct so that recombination between the two S regions was detectable by fluorescence-activated cell sorting (FACS) (Okazaki *et al.*, 2002). In the artificial CSR substrate [termed SCI (μ,α)], transcription of the Sμ and Sα regions was directed by the elongation factor 1α promoter (pEF1α) and the tetracycline-responsive promoter (pTET), respectively. The coding sequences for the extracellular domain of CD8α and for the transmembrane (TM) domain of CD8α fused to green fluorescent protein (GFP) are separated into two transcription units. The extracellular domain of CD8α is detectable on the cell surface only after its fusion with the TM domain by recombination between the two S regions.

To examine whether ectopic expression of AID can induce CSR in non-B cells, Okazaki *et al.* introduced SCI(μ,α) with the tetracycline transactivator into murine fibroblast cell line NIH3T3 in which the CD8α(TM)-GFP unit was transcribed by removal of tetracycline from the culture medium. In the absence of tetracycline, surface CD8α-GFP$^+$ cells were detected in AID-expressing NIH3T3-SCI(μ,α) cells at a level comparable to that in AID-transfected CH12F3–2-SCI(μ,α) cells. In contrast, NIH3T3-SCI(μ,α) cells expressing an

AID loss-of-function mutant (AIDm-1) lacking most of the cytidine deaminase motif did not show detectable CD8α-GFP surface expression. Furthermore, the features of recombination junction points in AID-expressing NIH3T3-SCI (μ,α) cells were similar to those observed in physiological CSR: no consensus sequences around break points and no substantial homology between the two S sequences at the junctions. Recombination junctions were widely distributed in the Sμ and Sα regions. These results indicate that AID-induced CSR in fibroblasts is dependent on transcription of the target S region, and the recombination machinery in fibroblasts works in a manner similar to that in B cells with endogenous immunoglobulin loci. AID is thus the only B-cell-specific factor required for the initiation of CSR, whereas other components required for CSR are expressed constitutively and probably ubiquitously.

3.2. Ectopic Expression of AID Induces SHM of an Artificial Construct in Fibroblasts

The transcriptional requirement for hypermutation in target genes has been demonstrated by several experiments (Bachl et al., 2001; Fukita et al., 1998; Peters and Storb, 1996). The most direct quantitative correlation between transcription level and SHM frequency was demonstrated using the hypermutating pre-B-cell line 18–81 that was transfected with a mutated GFP transgene containing a premature stop codon in the middle of the coding region (Bachl et al., 2001). The tetracycline-inducible promoter controlled transcription of the GFP transgene, and the level of GFP gene transcripts was almost directly correlated with the frequency of SHM measured by expression of functional GFP.

Yoshikawa et al. (2002) took advantage of this system as an artificial SHM substrate for AID in the murine fibroblast cell line NIH3T3. Ectopic expression of AID induced hypermutation of the artificial GFP substrate in NIH3T3 cells, whereas a loss-of-function mutant of AID (AIDm-1) did not. The mutation frequency was closely correlated with the level of transcription of the GFP gene, and the distribution of mutations in NIH3T3 cells was similar to that reported previously in a pre-B-cell line (Bachl et al., 2001; Martin et al., 2002). AID-induced hypermutation in NIH3T3 cells shared common properties with physiological SHM of Ig genes: predominantly point mutations with occasional deletions or duplications, strict dependency on AID, correlation with transcription level of the target gene, weak target specificity to motifs such as RGYW/WRCY, and a preference for transition over transversion (Neuberger and Milstein, 1995). AID also induced occasional deletions and insertions in the mutant GFP substrate in NIH3T3 cells, which are also observed in the Sμ region in B cells stimulated with LPS and IL-4 (Nagaoka et al., 2002;

Petersen *et al.*, 2001). In addition, ectopic expression of AID also introduced mutations in actively transcribed genes in hybridoma, Chinese hamster ovary cells, and T cells (Kotani *et al.*, 2005; Martin and Scharff, 2002; Martin *et al.*, 2002; Okazaki *et al.*, 2003).

In summary, AID is sufficient for SHM of an actively transcribed gene in fibroblasts, as well as in B cells. Thus, all of the required factors other than AID must be expressed in these fibroblasts.

4. Functional Domains of AID

4.1. The C-Terminal Domain of AID Is Required for CSR but Not for SHM

How can a single molecule, AID, differentially regulate CSR and SHM? In other words, how are the V and S regions specifically targeted for each event? Functional analyses of AID mutants has partially answered this question. AID mutants with truncation or replacement of the C-terminus (P20, human AID with a 34-amino acid insertion at residue 182; JP41, human AID190X; JP8B, human AID with a frameshift mutation at residue 183; and mouse AID188X) are almost completely devoid of CSR activity but retain SHM activity *in vitro* as well as *in vivo* (Barreto *et al.*, 2003; Revy *et al.*, 2000; Ta *et al.*, 2003; Zhu *et al.*, 2003). C-terminal mutants retain deaminase activity. In addition, C-terminal deletion mutant (mouse AID188X) was shown to catalyze gene conversion as well but not CSR (Barreto *et al.*, 2003). These results suggest that the C-terminal domain is crucial specifically for CSR, probably due to a mechanism distinct from AID's cytidine deaminase activity (Fig. 2). The C-terminal domain may be important for recruiting putative CSR-specific cofactor(s) that aid in recognition of mRNA target for CSR or for connecting AID to the CSR-specific NHEJ repair machinery (Casellas *et al.*, 1998; Manis *et al.*, 1998; Wu *et al.*, 2005).

4.2. The N-Terminal Domain of AID Is Required for SHM but Not for CSR

Studies of C-terminal AID mutants led to speculation that SHM might require SHM-specific cofactor(s) that interact with a different domain of AID than putative CSR-specific cofactors, so that AID can differentially regulate SHM and CSR. Indeed, five mouse AID mutants (Y13H, V18R, V18SR19V, W20K, and G23S) made by random mutagenesis show almost normal CSR activity but absent SHM activity (Shinkura *et al.*, 2004). All of these point mutations are located in the N-terminal region of AID (amino acids 13–23). Because N-terminal mutants retain deaminase activity, the N-terminal domain

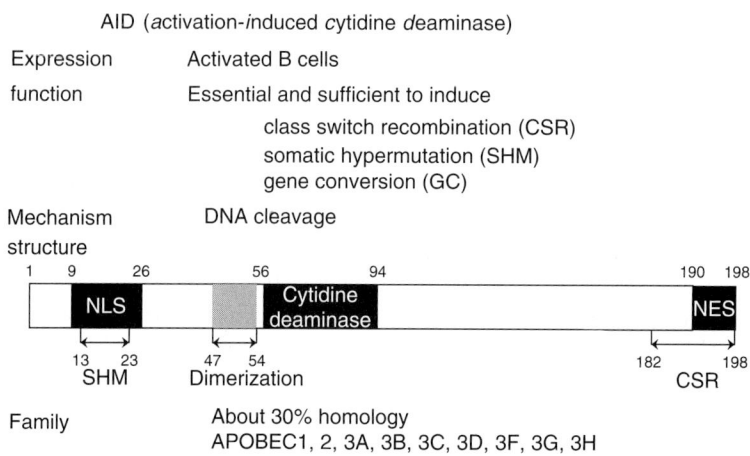

Figure 2 Structural and functional properties of AID. A schematic representation of the primary structure shows the motifs of AID. NLS, nuclear localization signal; NES, nuclear export signal.

must have some other function such as interacting with SHM-specific cofactor(s) that regulate target specificity (Fig. 2).

At present, no definitive AID-specific cofactor has been reported. Although the C-terminus of AID interacts with MDM2 (MacDuff *et al.*, 2006), a ubiquitin ligase that targets cytoplasmic p53 for degradation, the functional relevance of this interaction in CSR is unclear. Replication protein A (RPA), protein kinase A (PKA), DNA-PKcs, and RNA polymerase II have been implicated as AID-interacting molecules (Basu *et al.*, 2005; Chaudhuri *et al.*, 2004; Nambu *et al.*, 2003; Wu *et al.*, 2005). However, it is unclear whether they function in a CSR- or SHM-specific manner or which domain of AID interacts with them.

4.3. AID Shuttles Between the Nucleus and Cytoplasm

APOBEC1 shares the strong homology with AID. APOBEC1 shuttles between the nucleus and the cytoplasm by association with importin α at its N-terminal nuclear localization signal (NLS) and with the nuclear export machinery at its C-terminal nuclear export signal (NES) (Chester *et al.*, 2003). Likewise, AID was shown to shuttle between the nucleus and the cytoplasm (Ito *et al.*, 2004; McBride *et al.*, 2004). An NES (residues 183–198) and potential NLS (residues 8–25) exist at the N- and C-termini of AID, respectively (Brar *et al.*, 2004; Ito *et al.*, 2004; McBride *et al.*, 2004). This biological similarity between AID and APOBEC1 supports functional homology, that is, RNA editing but obviously does not prove it.

Since the NLS and the NES partially overlap the SHM-specific and CSR-specific domains, respectively, correlation between AID cellular localization and activity was expected. AID mutants lacking the 16 C-terminal amino acid residues (including the NES) lose the shuttling ability and accumulate in the nucleus (Ito et al., 2004). These mutants are inactive or severely impaired for CSR but active for SHM, suggesting that efficient export of AID from the nucleus is important for CSR but not for SHM induction. On the other hand, N-terminal AID mutants are able to mediate CSR, although they show defective nuclear accumulation (except for G23S) in the presence of leptomycin B (LMB), an inhibitor of exportin-1-dependent nuclear export (Shinkura et al., 2004). Although a minimal amount of AID in the nucleus might be sufficient for activity, these results suggest that the amount of AID in the nucleus is not directly correlated with the efficiency of CSR. However, nuclear localization of AID is not sufficient for SHM activity, as the SHM-deficient mutant G23S accumulates in the nucleus in the presence of LMB as efficiently as wild-type AID. It is likely that SHM requires not only nuclear localization of AID but also SHM-specific cofactor binding to the N-terminus of AID.

4.4. AID Dimerization Is Necessary for CSR

APOBEC1 has been shown to function as a dimer (Navaratnam et al., 1998; Teng et al., 1999). Dimerization of APOBEC1 creates an active structure capable of RNA-binding and deaminase activity toward apoB mRNA (Teng et al., 1999). Mutations abolishing APOBEC1 dimerization also destroy its RNA-binding and editing activities (Navaratnam et al., 1998), although the dimerization motif, the RNA-binding region, and the catalytic site do not completely overlap in APOBEC1. AID is 31 residues shorter than APOBEC1 with 9 and 24 residues missing in the N- and C-termini, respectively, the residues reported to be critical for APOBEC1 dimerization. Besides, the C-terminal region of APOBEC1 that is important for dimerization is not conserved in AID (Chester et al., 2003). In fact, wild-type AID and even C-terminally deleted mutants are able to form a homomultimeric complex (Ta et al., 2003), indicating AID and APOBEC1 have different dimerization motifs.

Coimmunoprecipitation of differently tagged AID serial deletion mutants in 293T cells showed that a minimal region between Thr27 and His56 is responsible for dimerization (Wang et al., 2006) (Fig. 2). Analyses of point mutations within this region revealed that the residues between Gly47 and Gly 54 are most important for dimer formation. Furthermore, all mutations impairing dimerization are inefficient for CSR, suggesting that dimer formation is necessary for CSR activity.

Because size exclusion chromatography and glycerol gradient sedimentation revealed the presence of AID in a complex larger than 500 kDa (Chaudhuri et al., 2003), AID may require cofactors (including nucleic acids) to stabilize dimer or multimer formation. However, the multimeric AID complex formed *in vivo* is resistant to treatment with DNase, RNase, or EDTA before immunoprecipitation, indicating that AID multimer formation does not require binding to nucleic acids. To examine whether specific posttranslational modifications are required for AID dimerization, recombinant AID purified from *Escherichia coli* was mixed with 293T-produced AID, and the resulting complex was successfully immunoprecipitated (Wang et al., 2006). Because *E. coli* is unlikely to produce posttranslational modifications similar to those in eukaryotic cells, AID dimer formation appears to be independent of posttranslational modification.

In summary, dimer formation is autonomous and independent of modifications and cofactors, including nucleic acids. Once synthesized, AID monomers associate with each other to form a dimer, and then the dimer interacts with putative substrate-specific cofactors for either CSR or SHM at the respective domains described above. Therefore, dimerization of AID is necessary but not sufficient for its activity.

5. AID Is Involved in a DNA Cleavage Step

At the molecular level, CSR can be separated into three successive phases. The first phase is activation of B cells by CSR stimulants such as IL-4, CD40 ligand, and LPS. This stimulation leads to two events: induction of AID expression and transcriptional activation of the I exon promoter located at the 5′ flank of each S region. Transcription of I exon is required for CSR to proceed on B-cell stimulation (Honjo et al., 2002). This transcript is called a "germ line" or "sterile" transcript because it does not encode any meaningful open reading frames (Stavnezer, 1996). It is generally believed that this transcription is required to increase the accessibility of recombinase to specific S regions. In the second phase of CSR, the putative switch recombinase cleaves two S regions. Finally, in the third phase the cleaved ends of two S regions are repaired to form blunt ends and then ligated to complete recombination.

When it was discovered that AID-deficient B cells lack CSR, experiments were performed to determine which phase of CSR is affected in this mutant. To determine whether germ line transcription is affected by AID deficiency, semiquantitative RT-PCR for all isotypes was performed. The results indicated that AID-deficient B cells induced all isotypes of germ line transcripts, responding to CSR stimulants as efficiently as control B cells. Thus, germ line transcription is independent of AID. Therefore, the affected CSR phase should be either DNA cleavage or repair. The role of the NHEJ pathway in CSR is supported by the finding that CSR is defective in Ku70- or Ku80-deficient mice in which B cells have been rescued by the expression of functional Ig transgenes (Casellas et al., 1998; Manis et al., 1998). Because AID-deficient mice appear to undergo normal V(D)J recombination in which the NHEJ pathway plays a major role, AID deficiency should not affect the third phase of CSR (Muramatsu et al., 2000; Revy et al., 2000). As a consequence of these initial studies on AID-deficient B cells, it was postulated that AID controls CSR (and perhaps SHM), most likely at the DNA cleavage step. Series of experiments to elucidate whether AID is indeed involved in DNA cleavage were performed.

Supporting evidence for a role for AID in DNA cleavage was obtained by examining the nucleotide sequence of the Sμ region. B lymphocytes accumulate SHM-like point mutations in their Sμ regions on CSR stimulation, even in the absence of actual switch recombination. These mutations are thought to be markers of past DNA cleavage generated in the Sμ region on CSR stimuli. Such Sμ hypermutation is dependent on AID, suggesting that AID is required for DNA cleavage (Nagaoka et al., 2002; Petersen et al., 2001). Another line of evidence for involvement of AID in the DNA cleavage step of CSR was obtained by microscopically monitoring γH2AX (a phosphorylated form of histone H2A family member X) focus formation, which occurs at sites of DSBs. Petersen et al. (2001) showed that γH2AX foci colocalize with IgH loci in cells undergoing CSR, and this colocalization is dependent on AID. This observation was confirmed by chromatin immunoprecipitation (ChIP) using an anti-γH2AX antibody (Begum et al., 2004a). Begum et al. stimulated $AID^{-/-}$ B cells by LPS and IL-4 and retrovirally infected cells with an AID-expressing construct or mock vector. The cells were fixed and solubilized by sonication. Chromatin associated with γH2AX was enriched by immunoprecipitation, and extracted DNA was subjected to semiquantitative PCR. Sμ region DNA was efficiently enriched by anti-γH2AX from AID-expressing switching cells but was undetectable from the negative control.

Ligation-mediated PCR (LM-PCR) is also used for detecting DSBs associated with CSR. In this procedure, a blunt end linker is ligated onto purified genomic DNA, and subsequent PCR amplification using locus-specific and linker-specific primers directly detects DSBs. This method is sensitive, although it sometimes produces nonspecific background signals (Faili et al., 2002). It was demonstrated that DSBs detected by LM-PCR in the Sμ region of switching cells were nearly absent in $AID^{-/-}$ B cells (Catalan et al., 2003; Rush et al., 2004). This result was further confirmed by a hybridoma study in which the frequency of microdeletions at the Sμ region (which represent past DSBs) was examined (Dudley et al., 2002). In AID deficiency, the frequency of microdeletion was drastically reduced, suggesting that the DNA cleavage phase of CSR is affected. Taken together, these results indicate that AID is crucial for DSB induction of CSR.

AID is also thought to be involved in the DNA cleavage step of SHM. AID overexpression in human lymphoma BL2 cells induced γH2AX accumulation at the IgH locus. Since in that system CSR does not occur efficiently, if at all, γH2AX accumulation is likely associated with SHM (Woo et al., 2003). Furthermore, CSR-inactive but SHM-active AID mutant with C-terminal truncation also induced γH2AX accumulation at IgH, suggesting that AID induces DSBs associated with SHM (Nagaoka et al., 2005). Notably, despite γH2AX foci formation, SHM seems to be more strongly associated with single-stranded breaks than DSBs (Kong and Maizels, 2001). Likely, enhanced single-stranded nicking by AID overexpression causes detectable levels of DSBs with staggered ends. Indeed, γH2AX focus formation at the IgL locus, which is the target of SHM but not CSR, was undetectable in purified germinal center B cells (Odegard et al., 2005).

However, detection of DSBs associated with SHM in the V region by LM-PCR has been inconclusive. Many laboratories reported LM-PCR detection of AID-independent DSBs in the V region (Bross et al., 2002; Catalan et al., 2003; Faili et al., 2002; Papavasiliou and Schatz, 2002). Because such DSBs were also detected in the un-rearranged upstream V segment that is not an efficient target of SHM, many of the DSBs detected by these experiments may not be associated with SHM (Bross et al., 2002; Catalan et al., 2003). The physiological relevance of such DSBs is currently unknown.

Further evidence that AID is involved in DNA cleavage is provided by the fact that ectopic AID overexpression can induce SHM and CSR in other cell lineages (fibroblasts, hybridomas, T cells, and so on) as described in Section 3 in this chapter (Martin and Scharff, 2002; Martin et al., 2002; Okazaki et al., 2002; Yoshikawa et al., 2002). Taking all of the data together, it is concluded that AID is involved in the DNA cleavage steps of CSR and SHM. The major hypotheses for CSR and SHM described below are based on this conclusion.

6. Major Hypotheses for the Action of AID

When Muramatsu et al. (2000) demonstrated the crucial role of AID in CSR and SHM, both RNA and DNA editing hypotheses were considered to explain the function of AID in these processes. Currently, popular models are based on these original ideas. Data supporting both models have been published; therefore, the exact function of AID is still a matter of considerable debate.

6.1. RNA Editing Model

The RNA editing model was proposed based on the observation that AID shares strong homology with the RNA editing enzyme APOBEC1. APOBEC1 deaminates a specific cytidine (C) in the mRNA encoding a component of low-density lipoprotein (ApoB100), generating a stop codon. The edited mRNA with a shorter reading frame encodes a component of chylomicron, ApoB48. This is a well-documented RNA editing reaction in mammalian cells by which two functionally different proteins are generated from a single transcript. According to the RNA editing model, analogous to APOBEC1, AID and an associated cofactor recognize a putative mRNA precursor and convert it to an mRNA encoding an endonuclease (a recombinase and mutator), or a molecule that guides a preexisting nuclease to target sites. The endonuclease cleaves DNA in the V region gene for SHM or in the S region for CSR (Fig. 3).

6.2. Evidence for the RNA Editing Model

AID and APOBEC1 have strong evolutionary conservation. Genes encoding these proteins are located in proximity to each other on chromosomes 6 and 12 in mouse and human, respectively, indicating that they were generated by gene duplication (Conticello *et al.*, 2005; Muto *et al.*, 2000). The similarity is not

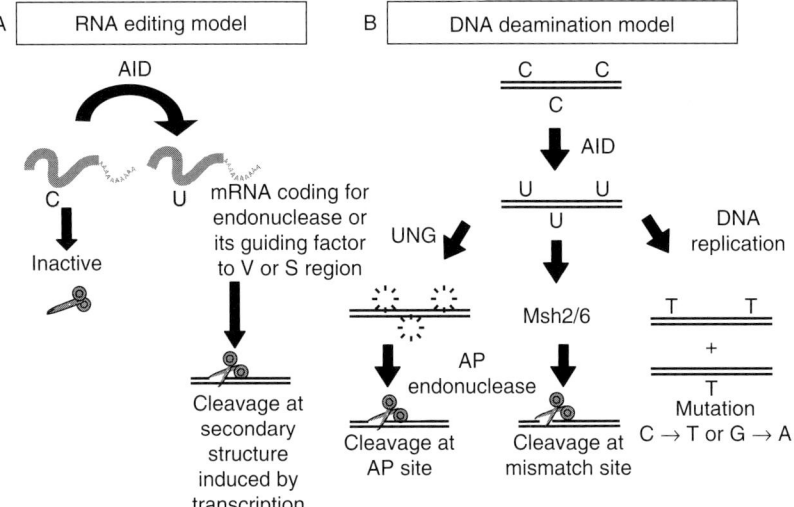

Figure 3 RNA editing and DNA deamination models. Mechanisms that induce DNA cleavage or point mutation are shown. See text for detailed explanation.

limited to overall homology but is also evident in mechanistic features. Both AID and APOBEC1 require cofactors for their function. For specific recognition of the editing site on ApoB mRNA, APOBEC1 requires the cofactor ACF (Mehta et al., 2000). Studies of AID mutants suggested that AID also requires CSR- and SHM-specific cofactors for its function (Shinkura et al., 2004; Ta et al., 2003).

Another similarity between AID and APOBEC1 is in the regulation of their subcellular localization. APOBEC1 is a nuclear-cytoplasmic shuttling protein with a weak NLS and an NES (Chester et al., 2003). Interestingly, APOBEC1 shuttling seems to be involved in the nuclear export of the edited ApoB mRNA. The APOBEC1-ACF complex remains associated with the edited RNA during its export, thereby protecting the RNA from nonsense-mediated decay (Chester et al., 2003). As discussed previously, there are also NES- and NLS-like sequences in the N- and C- termini of AID, respectively. From the study of an AID–GFP fusion protein, it was demonstrated that these signals indeed facilitate nuclear-cytoplasmic shuttling of AID, although the NLS seems to be very weak, as observed for APOBEC1 (Chester et al., 2003; Ito et al., 2004; McBride et al., 2004).

APOBEC1 forms a homodimer, and dimerization is important for its function (Chester et al., 2003; Teng et al., 1993). Homodimerization of AID and the relevance to its function were demonstrated by coimmunoprecipitation of differently tagged AID proteins that were simultaneously expressed by cotransfection (Ta et al., 2003; Wang et al., 2006). Therefore, it has been suggested that dimer formation is a common functional requirement of AID and APOBEC1.

The RNA editing hypothesis predicts that a recombinase and mutator (or their guiding factors) are synthesized from the mRNA after editing by AID. Therefore, experiments to assess the requirement for de novo protein synthesis after AID activation were considered important. Because AID is also newly synthesized on B-cell activation, simple addition of a protein synthesis inhibitor cannot be applied. A new trick for inducible activation of AID independent of protein synthesis was developed by fusing AID and the human estrogen receptor (ER) hormone-binding domain (Doi et al., 2003). This AID-ER protein can be overexpressed in an inactive form and then activated by adding 4-hydroxytamoxifen (OHT), an estrogen analogue. Doi et al. introduced AID-ER protein into AID-deficient B cells that were stimulated by LPS and IL-4, and cycloheximide or puromycin was added before or after the addition of OHT. Inhibition of de novo protein synthesis by addition of these chemicals severely impaired CSR when added 1 h before but not after OHT treatment (Doi et al., 2003).

However, the possibility cannot be excluded that the synthesis of factors required for DNA repair was inhibited. Therefore, Begum et al. examined whether CSR inhibition occurs before or after the DNA cleavage step.

To monitor the formation of DNA DSBs at the S region of the IgH gene, γH2AX foci formation (a specific marker for DSBs) was detected by ChIP analysis. By addition of cycloheximide before OHT, γH2AX focus formation in the IgH locus was severely impaired, indicating that *de novo* protein synthesis is required for the DNA cleavage step of CSR after AID activation (Begum *et al.*, 2004b). A similar result was obtained from cells specifically undergoing SHM (Nagaoka *et al.*, 2005). Collectively, these data strongly suggest that *de novo* protein synthesis is required after AID activation and before DNA cleavage for both CSR and SHM, consistent with the RNA editing hypothesis.

The RNA editing model could easily explain why different AID cofactors are required for CSR and SHM and why CSR and SHM, both of which are induced by AID, can be differentially regulated in activated B cells. Assuming that target RNA specificity of AID is determined by associated cofactors, synthesis of the CSR recombinase and the mutator could be uncoupled. The identification of such cofactors, as well as mRNA targets, is indispensable to proving the model.

6.3. DNA Deamination Model

Petersen-Mahrt *et al.* (2002) published a report showing that overexpression of AID in *E. coli* results in a mutator phenotype. Because it is very unlikely that *E. coli* has specific RNA targets and cofactors for AID, the mutations are considered to be a direct effect of AID on DNA. Mutations preferentially convert C/G to T/A, concordant with the idea that AID directly deaminates C in DNA to generate U. The mutation rate is enhanced under conditions of uracil DNA glycosylase (UNG) deficiency. These observations led to proposal of the DNA deamination model, in which AID directly deaminates C in target DNA to generate U:G mismatch sites (Fig. 4). Mismatch sites are recognized either by base excision repair (BER) enzymes, including UNG and apyrimidinic endonuclease, or by mismatch repair proteins Msh2/Msh6 that induce the patch repair system, resulting in DNA strand cleavage. Alternatively, the U or apyrimidinic site can be repaired by DNA replication in the absence of DNA strand cleavages (Petersen-Mahrt *et al.*, 2002).

7. Critical Examination of the DNA Deamination Model

7.1. *In Vitro* DNA Deamination

Although the *E. coli* system strongly implicates AID in the direct deamination of *E. coli* genomic DNA, the specificity of the effect should have been carefully evaluated. A publication from the same group drew attention to a potential

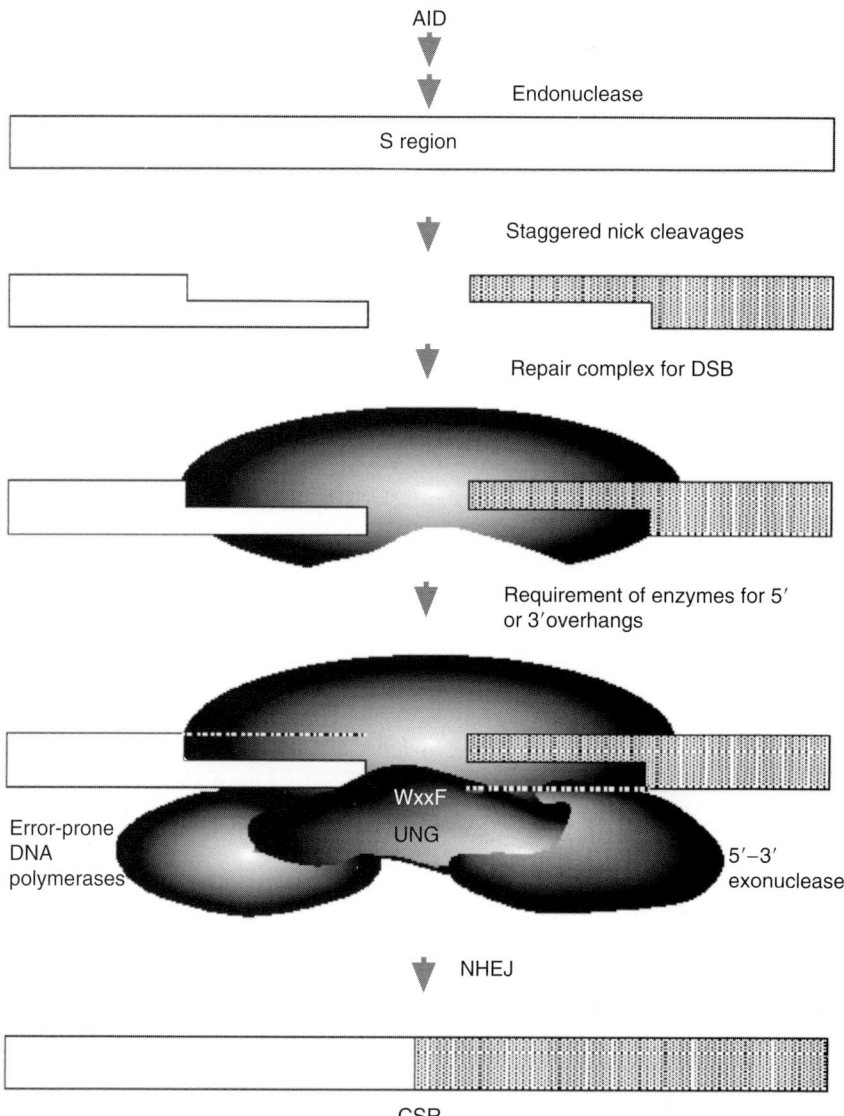

Figure 4 A model of UNG complex during CSR. U removal activity of UNG is dispensable to CSR. UNG does not require interaction with PCNA or RPA for CSR activity, but the Vpr interaction domain of UNG (WXXF) is critical. During repair of AID-induced S region cleavage, UNG might be recruited into the complex via its WXXF motif. A Vpr-like UNG-interacting host protein may exist and contribute to CSR being associated with UNG, which may also interact with error-prone DNA polymerases, 5′–3′ exonucleases, and so on.

problem with the system. When APOBEC1, a *bona fide* RNA editing enzyme, is overexpressed in *E. coli*, a mutator phenotype is observed that is 50 times stronger than that for AID (Harris *et al.*, 2002). Because APOBEC1 cannot rescue CSR or SHM in mammalian cells (Eto *et al.*, 2003; Fugmann *et al.*, 2004), the ability to make valid comparisons between the *E. coli* system and actual CSR and SHM in B cells is severely limited. Direct DNA deamination by AID has been further examined biochemically. In these experiments, it was demonstrated that recombinant AID or AID purified from activated B cells can deaminate C in single-stranded DNA *in vitro* (Bransteitter *et al.*, 2003, 2004; Chaudhuri *et al.*, 2003, 2004; Dickerson *et al.*, 2003; Morgan *et al.*, 2004; Pham *et al.*, 2003; Yu, *et al.*, 2004). Similarly, purified APOBEC1 was shown to deaminate C in single-stranded DNA (Morgan *et al.*, 2004). Thus, both AID and APOBEC1 clearly can deaminate C in single-stranded DNA, but the physiological relevance of these observations should be carefully considered.

Di Noia and Neuberger (2002) demonstrated that inhibition of UNG in eukaryotic cells changes the ratio of transition versus transversion mutations but does not reduce the frequency in SHM. Chicken DT40 B cells spontaneously accumulate mutations in their Ig genes in an AID-dependent manner, and less than 40% of these mutations at G/C bases are transition mutations. When a protein inhibitor for UNG was introduced, the rate of transition mutation drastically increased to as much as 86% (Di Noia and Neuberger, 2002). A similar result was obtained in $ung^{-/-}$ mouse B cells (Rada *et al.*, 2002). Moreover, CSR efficiency in $ung^{-/-}$ mouse B cells decreases to ~10% of the normal level. According to the DNA deamination model, loss of UNG activity should decrease DNA cleavage and increase the amount of U residues remaining in target DNA. Therefore, the observed reduction in CSR and increase in transition mutations at G/C sites in $ung^{-/-}$ cells are thought to provide a support for the DNA deamination model.

SHM with strong bias toward G/C transition mutations, which is frequently seen in AID-overexpressing cells, is often interpreted as an indication of the DNA deamination reaction. However, it appears that the tendency toward G/C transition mutations depends on experimental conditions, including cell type and target genes. In T-cell lymphoma caused by AID overexpression, A/T point mutations preferentially accumulate in CD4 and CD5 genes (Kotani *et al.*, 2005). In addition, AID overexpression in mouse B cells did not cause G/C-biased mutations in Ig genes (Muto *et al.*, 2004).

A direct interaction between AID and the target DNA at the catalytic step would be inevitable for the DNA deamination model. The *in vivo* association of AID with S region DNA in CSR-stimulated cells was demonstrated by ChIP analysis (Chaudhuri *et al.*, 2004; Nambu *et al.*, 2003). AID binding seems to be specific for the S region that is actually undergoing CSR, that is, AID associates with Sγ1 when IgG1 switching is induced by LPS and IL-4, and with Sγ3 when induced by LPS alone (Chaudhuri et al., 2004; Nambu et al., 2003). Formaldehyde, which is used in the ChIP assay, forms protein–protein as well as protein–DNA cross-links; therefore, it is critical to determine whether the association of AID with DNA is direct or indirect. RNA polymerase II was coimmunoprecipitated with AID, suggesting that the interaction with DNA might be through RNA polymerase II (Nambu et al., 2003). Specific targets of CSR and SHM must be transcribed by RNA polymerase II; however, not all transcribed DNA regions undergo SHM or CSR. The guiding mechanism of AID to specific DNA regions should be resolved for the DNA deamination model to be proven.

7.2. UNG Is Dispensable for DSBs

UNG is important for CSR, yet ~10% of normal CSR remains in UNG-deficient mice (Rada et al., 2002). In the DNA deamination model, it is predicted that the Msh2/Msh6 pathway compensates for UNG function to induce DSBs at S regions (Fig. 3). In fact, virtually no CSR is detected in UNG and Msh2 double-deficient B cells. Strikingly, SHMs in the double-knockout B cells are almost exclusively transition mutations at G or C, which has been explained as the result of DNA replication of the initiating dU:dG lesion. Overall, these observations can be explained by the DNA deamination model, but an alternative explanation exists (Honjo et al., 2005). Since the phenotype of the double-knockout B cells is far stronger than the additive effects of two single-knockout B cells, each UNG and Msh2 proteins may have major roles at different steps in the CSR pathway possibly after DNA-DSB formation (Honjo et al., 2005). In fact, U removal activity of Msh2/6 is not proven convincingly. Another puzzling observation is that SMUG1 cannot replace UNG, although SMUG1 is shown to remove U efficiently (Di Noia et al., 2006).

To determine if DSB formation is dependent on UNG activity, DSB assays that utilize γH2AX-ChIP or LM-PCR were performed, but sometimes suffer from various technical drawbacks (Begum et al., 2004a; Imai et al., 2003; Schrader et al., 2005). A CH12F3-2 lymphoma cell line that switches efficiently to IgA (Nakamura et al., 1996) after stimulation with CD40L, IL-4, and TGF β (CIT) was engineered to express AID and Ugi in a regulated fashion. Ugi is a peptide inhibitor of UNG (Wang and Mosbaugh, 1989) and it forms a tight enzyme:inhibitor complex with UNG. Previously Ugi was expressed in chicken B cells to demonstrate the requirement of UNG during gene conversion (Di Noia and Neuberger, 2002, 2004). Ugi expression drastically decreased class switching induced by CIT, AID overexpression, or both. CSR inhibition by Ugi was also documented by the absence of circular transcripts derived from looped-out circular DNA after CSR. In contrast, Ugi expression did not inhibit γH2AX accumulation (DSB marker) at the IgH locus, which was induced under all activation conditions mentioned above for switching to IgA (Begum et al., 2004a). Consistent with earlier observations, these results indicate that γH2AX focus formation at the IgH locus absolutely depends on AID, but not on UNG, although CSR is markedly reduced by UNG inhibition.

In the same cell line, immunohistochemistry combined with a fluorescence *in situ* hybridization (FISH) assay of γH2AX focus formation further demonstrated that the number of IgH loci that overlapped with γH2AX foci increased to a similar level on CIT stimulation and AID induction, regardless of the absence or presence of Ugi. These results indicate that AID-induced DSBs detectable by the nascent DNA-DSB marker like γH2AX are independent of UNG activity. However, other groups reported the opposite observations using UNG-deficient human and mouse B cells with LM-PCR assays (Imai et al., 2003; Schrader et al., 2005).

Detection of intra-Sμ deletion in IgM^+ B cells is another approach to assess the postbreak signature of S region DNA in activated B cells. Therefore, involvement of UNG in DNA cleavage step of CSR was reexamined by analyzing its direct footprints: deletions in the germ line Sμ region and mutations generated during error-prone repair of broken ends (Begum et al., 2006). In addition to UNG-deficient mice, UNG and Msh2 double-deficient mice were included in this study to rule out possible involvement of the Msh2-dependent uracil repair pathway (Rada et al., 2004) that may cause DSBs in the absence of UNG. IgM^+ hybridomas were analyzed from stimulated wild-type, $ung^{-/-}$, $ung^{-/-}msh2^{-/-}$, and $AID^{-/-}$ B cells to compare the occurrence of deletions in the Sμ region. Analysis of the hybridomas revealed that deletion frequencies per locus were 12.8, 20.7, and 9.6% for wild-type, $ung^{-/-}$, and $ung^{-/-}msh2^{-/-}$ cells, respectively (Begum et al., 2006). It is striking that the frequencies of deletion in the S region in the single- and double-knockout B cells were statistically indistinguishable from the wild type. In contrast, AID-deficient B cells barely showed deletion above the background, clearly indicating that Sμ deletions are cleavage dependent. These observations further suggest that neither UNG nor Msh2 is playing critical roles in the DNA cleavage step of CSR.

Recombination break points and switch junctions were more precisely analyzed in germ line and in switched allele in stimulated IgM^+ and IgG^+ B cells, respectively, from $ung^{-/-}$ mice. The distribution of break points in germ line (5′ of Sμ core) in activated $ung^{-/-}$ IgM^+ B cells did not differ compared to that of wild type. Recombination break point analysis in $IgG1^+$ and $IgG3^+$ cells also did not show any biased distribution of break points in $ung^{-/-}$ compared to wild type. As expected, in the absence of UNG both germ line and recombined S regions showed enhanced mutation rates around the break point as a signature of postbreak error-prone repair. Biased mutation to G/C transition, as observed for SHMs in IgV genes due to UNG deficiency (Rada *et al.*, 2004), was also evident in the S region of $ung^{-/-}$ cells. Locations of mutations in germ line S region were not found to be skewed compared with those of junctional break points identified in switched B cells, which favors the notion that germ line Sμ mutations are generated through abortive DNA cleavage during CSR.

However, the increased mutations in the S region in the absence of UNG can be also explained by the DNA deamination model because U generated by DNA deamination by AID remains without repair, resulting in the increase of G/C A/T transition mutation. Nonetheless, there are three observations that are difficult to be explained by the DNA deamination model: (1) SHM frequency is not augmented in spite of increase in CSR-associated mutations in the S region in UNG-deficient B cells, (2) S region mutations always cluster immediately adjacent to the recombination junction and diminish sharply as it goes away from the junction, and (3) the mutation frequencies are higher in the recombined S region than the germ line S region. On the other hand, all these observations can be easily explained by the assumption that S region mutations are introduced during the repair phase of recombination.

DSBs in the S region are resolved with various outcomes, such as generation of mutations by low-fidelity repair, intra-S deletions, CSR, or chromosomal translocation caused by *trans*-recombination. UNG deficiency does not inhibit mutation or deletion events in a single S region, but CSR and *trans*-recombinations are severely affected. Therefore, it is likely that UNG plays a role in the process of union of recombining ends by NHEJ repair during CSR (Casellas *et al.*, 1998; Manis *et al.*, 1998, 2002; Pan-Hammarstrom *et al.*, 2005).

8. Evidence for a Novel Function of UNG in CSR

8.1. Catalytic Site Mutants of UNG Do Not Affect CSR

From a catalytic standpoint, UNG is highly conserved among the species and a well-studied enzyme from hyperthermophilic archae to higher eukaryotes (Aravind and Koonin, 2000; Pearl, 2000). A great deal of data from structural–functional analyses is available for *E. coli* and human UNG enzymes, and all the active site residues responsible for glycosidic bond cleavage and uracil recognition were found to be well conserved (Mol *et al.*, 1995; Parikh *et al.*, 1998; Savva and Pearl, 1995; Xiao *et al.*, 1999). Mol *et al.* conducted an extensive mutagenesis and crystal structure analysis of human UNG and identified the most critical residues for uracil DNA glycosylace (UDG) activity; mutations at the sites severely crippled the enzyme's ability to repair U in DNA. As mouse UNG shows 96% homology with human UNG and the active site residues are identical, loss-of-catalytic function mutants of UNG were easily generated to validate the importance of the catalytic activity of UNG in CSR. Three mutants of human UNG (D145N, N204V, and H268L) had less than 0.6% UNG activity but retained the ability to bind DNA (Mol *et al.*, 1995). Identical mouse mutants also showed loss of UDG activity and retention of DNA-binding activity. The UNG mutants were expressed in UNG-deficient spleen B cells using a retrovirus vector, and class switching to IgG1 was assessed. Surprisingly, all the mutants that lost catalytic activity rescued wild-type levels of CSR in UNG-deficient B cells. However, the double mutants D145N + N204V and H268L + D145N were incapable of rescuing CSR, which may imply to a structural requirement for an unknown function of UNG.

UNG has a second catalytic activity that shares some of its catalytic residues with the uracil glycosylase activity. Evidence of a second UNG activity is arising by the fact that, simply by introducing N204D or Y147A mutation, UNG gains function of cytosine or thymine DNA glycosylase activity, respectively (Kavli *et al.*, 1996). It is important to note that N204D and Y147A mutants cannot rescue CSR (Table 1), although they have residual uracil removing activity (Kavli *et al.*, 1996, 2005). This observation further emphasizes that the trace amount of glycosylase activity or glycosylase activity alone is not sufficient for CSR, which is consistent with the result obtained by the catalytic mutants. Mutations at N204 and F242 positions also showed variable levels of expression, although none of these mutants are unstable *in vitro* expression analyses (Kavli *et al.*, 2005), suggesting that the *in vivo* action of UNG may differ from what we know about structure–function of UNG as purified molecule. Most importantly, the complete rescue of CSR by loss-of-catalytic-function mutants certainly indicates that the CSR reduction in UNG-deficient mice is not due to loss of U removal activity, but to loss of an as-yet-unknown activity of UNG.

8.2. Replication-Coupling Motifs of UNG Are Dispensable for CSR

Structurally, both human and mouse full-length UNG show similar architecture: a short, nonstructural N-terminal domain comprising ~1/3 of the total amino acid length, and a core catalytic domain comprising 1/2 of the length of the protein. Intracellular localization studies using the nuclear form of human UNG suggested that UNG colocalizes with replication foci (Ko and Bennett, 2005; Otterlei *et al.*, 1999). Indeed, both human and mouse UNG N-termini possess consensus binding sites for proliferating cell nuclear antigen (PCNA; QXXLXXFF) and for RPA (as detected in the case of repair factor XPA)

Table 1 CSR Activity of Mouse UNG2 Mutants and Their Human Counterparts in UNG$^{-/-}$ B Cell

Mutation/deletion	Feature/property	CSR	References
D145N	Catalytic inactivation	$(+)^a$	Mol et al., 1995
H268L	Catalytic inactivation	$(+)^a$	Mol et al., 1995
N204V	Catalytic inactivation	$(+)^a$	Mol et al., 1995
F242S	Unknown/instability	$(+)^a$	Imai et al., 2003; Kavli et al., 2005; Mol et al., 1995
D145N + H268L	Catalytic inactivation	$(-)^a$	Mol et al., 1995
D145N + N204V	Catalytic inactivation	$(-)^a$	Mol et al., 1995
N204D	CDG and residual UDG	$(-)^b$	Kavli et al., 1996, 2005
Y147A	TDG and residual UDG	$(-)^b$	Kavli et al., 1996, 2005
L272A	Unable to flip uracil	$(+)^b$	Parikh et al., 1998
L272R	Increased binding to DNA	$(+)^b$	Slupphaug et al., 1996
R276E	SS-specific catalysis	$(+)^b$	Chen et al., 2004, 2005
N-terminal deletion mutants			
Δ28	Lacks PCNA interaction site	$(+)^c$	Otterlei et al., 1999
Δ77	Lacks NLS	$(+)^c$	Otterlei et al., 1998
Δ86	Lacks RPA2 interaction site	$(+)^c$	Mer et al., 2000; Nagelhus et al., 1997
Mutation at Vpr-interacting motif			
W231A + W231G	Double	$(-)^c$	BouHamdan et al., 1998
W231A	Single	$(-)^c$	BouHamdan et al., 1998
W231K	Single	$(-)^c$	BouHamdan et al., 1998
F234G	Single	$(-)^c$	BouHamdan et al., 1998
F234Q	Single	$(-)^c$	BouHamdan et al., 1998

[a] Begum et al. (2004a). CSR rescuing ability of individual mutant was assessed by IgG1 switching efficiency.
[b] Included in this chapter.
[c] Begum et al. (2006).
CDG, cytosine DNA glycosylase; TDG, thymine DNA glycosylase; UDG, uracil deglycosylase; SS, single strand; RPA, replication protein A.

(Nagelhus et al., 1997). Studies using N-terminal-specific immunoprecipitation indicate that nuclear UNG possibly forms a BER complex composed of multiple proteins, including PCNA, APE, Ligase-4, Pol-β, and Fen-1 endonuclease (Akbari et al., 2004). Although association with RPA was not detected in this study, yeast two-hybrid analysis and protein–peptide direct interaction analyses suggested that two RPA interaction sites at the N-terminus of UNG are functional (Mer et al., 2000; Nagelhus et al., 1997). Currently, it is unknown how and when UNG is recruited into the CSR complex, but it has been proposed that UNG might function at the replication fork in conjunction with PCNA and RPA. In addition, AID also has been reported to form a complex with RPA (Chaudhuri et al., 2004). Therefore, it is important to determine how UNG contributes to CSR in the presence or absence of these interactions.

Series of N-terminal truncations and PCNA-binding defective mutants were generated, and their CSR rescue activities were examined in $ung^{-/-}$ B cells. N-terminal truncation of the first 86 residues of UNG showed efficient CSR rescue activity comparable to full-length UNG (Table 1), whereas N-terminal deletions of more than 96 residues did not rescue CSR activity in $ung^{-/-}$ B cells. Consistent with this observation, CSR rescue was also detected using *E. coli* UNG, which lacks the mammalian-type N-terminus and is solely composed of the catalytic domain. Thus, the N-terminal 86 residues of UNG appeared to be dispensable for CSR activity, suggesting that the roles of UNG in CSR and in replication could be distinct. Interestingly, the N-terminally truncated form of UNG showed improved switching efficiency compared to wild-type UNG despite incomplete cellular localization due to truncation of the NLS. It remains to be explored whether UNG can utilize N-terminal-dependent and -independent pathways for CSR. Complete rescue of CSR activity by the N-terminally truncated form also raises the question of how the core domain is targeted to the CSR complex.

8.3. UNG Requires the WXXF Motif for CSR Function

To date, no cellular proteins have been identified that are known to interact with the core structure of UNG. However, it can be easily envisaged that if such proteins exist they may potentially modulate UNG's function and would affect CSR either positively or negatively. UNG has long been known to be associated with HIV propagation in mammalian cells, although its precise function is unclear. Viral accessory protein Vpr, which is essential for HIV replication in nondividing cells (Chen et al., 2004; Priet et al., 2005), was involved in recruiting nuclear UNG to HIV particles. This function of Vpr was dependent on an interaction with the WXXF motif located in the core structure of UNG (BouHamdan et al., 1998; Mansky et al., 2000; Studebaker et al., 2005). Another notable point is that unlike the Ugi–UNG interaction, the Vpr–UNG interaction does not destroy the catalytic activity of UNG. Various mutants in the WXXF site, especially those that fail to interact with Vpr, were analyzed for CSR-rescuing activity (Begum et al., 2006). Mutations in either tryptophan 231 (W231A, W231K) or phenylalanine 234 (F234G, F234Q, and W231A/F234G) caused complete loss of the CSR function of UNG (Table 1). As expected, all of the WXXF motif mutants of UNG retained U removal activity, although some of them showed reduced activity and that could be attributed to differing stabilities of individual mutants. Complete loss of CSR function by WXXF site mutation clearly indicates that this site is a critical protein–protein interaction region of UNG that is essential to CSR.

To elucidate further, the importance of this site, the dominant negative effect of Vpr was evaluated in CH12F3-2 cells (Begum et al., 2006). Overexpression of Vpr drastically decreased IgA class switching in stimulated CH12F3-2 cells. However, Vpr mutants (W54R and H33R) known to be defective (Selig et al., 1997) in interacting with UNG (1.7 and 7% of wild-type binding, respectively) showed much weaker dominant negative effects on CSR. Another Vpr mutant (R90K) that can interact with UNG but does not affect the cell cycle regulation showed a dominant negative effect similar to that of wild-type Vpr. Importantly, infectants expressing less Vpr showed weaker effects, indicating that Vpr is probably competing with an unknown host factor for binding to UNG. Analogous to Vpr-mediated transport of the preintegration complex during the viral life cycle, a Vpr-like host protein might exist that recruits UNG to the CSR machinery. Hence, the WXXF motif is critical for preserving the CSR function of UNG (Fig. 4).

In summary, initial studies demonstrated that S region breaks can be detected in the absence of UNG, and the catalytic activity of UNG is dispensable for CSR. Subsequent studies using N-terminal UNG truncations revealed that the role of UNG in the replication-coupled repair pathway is not mandatory for CSR. The requirement of the WXXF motif further strengthens the previous assumption that UNG might have an alternate function, other than its conventional U-glycosylase activity, that is essential to the postbreak repair-recombination phase of CSR. It is well known that mechanically distinct repair pathways are involved in CSR, SHM, and gene conversion; it remains to be seen how these pathways are controlled, given UNG plays a noncanonical role.

9. Conclusion

The essential function of AID is DNA cleavage at the specific target in SHM and CSR. The target specificity appears to be determined by interaction with specific cofactors at the N-terminal domain for SHM and at the C-terminal domain for CSR. Although strong debate has been continued concerning the mode of AID action in DNA cleavage, RNA editing hypothesis has gained strong support by the evidence showing the requirement of *de novo* protein synthesis for DNA cleavage in SHM and CSR. On the other hand, the strongest evidence for DNA deamination is being reevaluated. UNG is required for CSR, but its U removal activity is dispensable. UNG is not required for DNA cleavage but for DNA repair step. Most recently, a noncanonical function of UNG was shown to be involved in CSR. The final conclusion for the mode of

AID activity has to wait until RNA target is identified and the noncanonical function of UNG is specified.

References

Akbari, M., Otterlei, M., Pena-Diaz, J., Aas, P. A., Kavli, B., Liabakk, N. B., Hagen, L., Imai, K., Durandy, A., Slupphaug, G., and Krokan, H. E. (2004). Repair of U/G and U/A in DNA by UNG2-associated repair complexes takes place predominantly by short-patch repair both in proliferating and growth-arrested cells. *Nucleic Acids Res.* **32**, 5486–5498.

Allen, R. C., Armitage, R. J., Conley, M. E., Rosenblatt, H., Jenkins, N. A., Copeland, N. G., Bedell, M. A., Edelhoff, S., Disteche, C. M., Simoneaux, D. K., Fanslow, W. C., Belmont, J., *et al.* (1993). CD40 ligand gene defects responsible for X-linked hyper-IgM syndrome. *Science* **259**, 990–993.

Aravind, L., and Koonin, E. V. (2000). The α/β fold uracil DNA glycosylases: A common origin with diverse fates. *Genome Biol.* **1**, RESEARCH0007.

Aruffo, A., Farrington, M., Hollenbaugh, D., Li, X., Milatovich, A., Nonoyama, S., Bajorath, J., Grosmaire, L. S., Stenkamp, R., Neubauer, M., Roberts, R. L., Noelle, R. J., *et al.* (1993). The CD40 ligand, gp39, is defective in activated T cells from patients with X-linked hyper-IgM syndrome. *Cell* **72**, 291–300.

Bachl, J., Carlson, C., Gray-Schopfer, V., Dessing, M., and Olsson, C. (2001). Increased transcription levels induce higher mutation rates in a hypermutating cell line. *J. Immunol.* **166**, 5051–5057.

Barreto, V., Reina-San-Martin, B., Ramiro, A. R., McBride, K. M., and Nussenzweig, M. C. (2003). C-terminal deletion of AID uncouples class switch recombination from somatic hypermutation and gene conversion. *Mol. Cell* **12**, 501–508.

Basu, U., Chaudhuri, J., Alpert, C., Dutt, S., Ranganath, S., Li, G., Schrum, J. P., Manis, J. P., and Alt, F. W. (2005). The AID antibody diversification enzyme is regulated by protein kinase A phosphorylation. *Nature* **438**, 508–511.

Begum, N. A., Kinoshita, K., Kakazu, N., Muramatsu, M., Nagaoka, H., Shinkura, R., Biniszkiewicz, D., Boyer, L. A., Jaenisch, R., and Honjo, T. (2004a). Uracil DNA glycosylase activity is dispensable for immunoglobulin class switch. *Science* **305**, 1160–1163.

Begum, N. A., Kinoshita, K., Muramatsu, M., Nagaoka, H., Shinkura, R., and Honjo, T. (2004b). De novo protein synthesis is required for activation-induced cytidine deaminase-dependent DNA cleavage in immunoglobulin class switch recombination. *Proc. Natl. Acad. Sci. USA* **101**, 13003–13007.

Begum, N. A., Izumi, N., Nishikori, M., Nagaoka, H., Shinkura, R., and Honjo, T. (2006). Requirement of non-canonical activity of uracil DNA glycosylase for class switch reccombination. *J. Biol. Chem.* **283**, 732–742.

BouHamdan, M., Xue, Y., Baudat, Y., Hu, B., Sire, J., Pomerantz, R. J., and Duan, L. X. (1998). Diversity of HIV-1 Vpr interactions involves usage of the WXXF motif of host cell proteins. *J. Biol. Chem.* **273**, 8009–8016.

Bransteitter, R., Pham, P., Scharff, M. D., and Goodman, M. F. (2003). Activation-induced cytidine deaminase deaminates deoxycytidine on single-stranded DNA but requires the action of RNase. *Proc. Natl. Acad. Sci. USA* **100**, 4102–4107.

Bransteitter, R., Pham, P., Calabrese, P., and Goodman, M. F. (2004). Biochemical analysis of hypermutational targeting by wild type and mutant activation-induced cytidine deaminase. *J. Biol. Chem.* **279**, 51612–51621.

Brar, S. S., Watson, M., and Diaz, M. (2004). Activation-induced cytosine deaminase (AID) is actively exported out of the nucleus but retained by the induction of DNA breaks. *J. Biol. Chem.* **279,** 26395–26401.

Bross, L., Muramatsu, M., Kinoshita, K., Honjo, T., and Jacobs, H. (2002). DNA double-strand breaks: Prior to but not sufficient in targeting hypermutation. *J. Exp. Med.* **195,** 1187–1192.

Casellas, R., Nussenzweig, A., Wuerffel, R., Pelanda, R., Reichlin, A., Suh, H., Qin, X. F., Besmer, E., Kenter, A., Rajewsky, K., and Nussenzweig, M. C. (1998). Ku80 is required for immunoglobulin isotype switching. *EMBO J.* **17,** 2404–2411.

Catalan, N., Selz, F., Imai, K., Revy, P., Fischer, A., and Durandy, A. (2003). The block in immunoglobulin class switch recombination caused by activation-induced cytidine deaminase deficiency occurs prior to the generation of DNA double strand breaks in switch μ region. *J. Immunol.* **171,** 2504–2509.

Chaudhuri, J., Tian, M., Khuong, C., Chua, K., Pinaud, E., and Alt, F. W. (2003). Transcription-targeted DNA deamination by the AID antibody diversification enzyme. *Nature* **422,** 726–730.

Chaudhuri, J., Khuong, C., and Alt, F. W. (2004). Replication protein A interacts with AID to promote deamination of somatic hypermutation targets. *Nature* **430,** 992–998.

Chen, C. Y., Mosbaugh, D. W., and Bennett, S. E. (2005). Mutations at arginine 276 transform human uracil-DNA glycosylase into a single-stranded DNA-specific uracil-DNA glycosylase. *DNA Repair (Amst.)* **4,** 793–805.

Chen, R., Le Rouzic, E., Kearney, J. A., Mansky, L. M., and Benichou, S. (2004). Vpr-mediated incorporation of UNG2 into HIV-1 particles is required to modulate the virus mutation rate and for replication in macrophages. *J. Biol. Chem.* **279,** 28419–28425.

Chester, A., Somasekaram, A., Tzimina, M., Jarmuz, A., Gisbourne, J., O'Keefe, R., Scott, J., and Navaratnam, N. (2003). The apolipoprotein B mRNA editing complex performs a multifunctional cycle and suppresses nonsense-mediated decay. *EMBO J.* **22,** 3971–3982.

Conticello, S. G., Thomas, C. J., Petersen-Mahrt, S. K., and Neuberger, M. S. (2005). Evolution of the AID/APOBEC family of polynucleotide (deoxy)cytidine deaminases. *Mol. Biol. Evol.* **22,** 367–377.

Di Noia, J., and Neuberger, M. S. (2002). Altering the pathway of immunoglobulin hypermutation by inhibiting uracil-DNA glycosylase. *Nature* **419,** 43–48.

Di Noia, J. M., and Neuberger, M. S. (2004). Immunoglobulin gene conversion in chicken DT40 cells largely proceeds through an abasic site intermediate generated by excision of the uracil produced by AID-mediated deoxycytidine deamination. *Eur. J. Immunol.* **34,** 504–508.

Di Noia, J. M., Rada, C., and Neuberger, M. S. (2006). SMUG1 is able to excise uracil from immunoglobulin genes: Insight into mutation versus repair. *EMBO J.* **25,** 585–595.

Dickerson, S. K., Market, E., Besmer, E., and Papavasiliou, F. N. (2003). AID mediates hypermutation by deaminating single stranded DNA. *J. Exp. Med.* **197,** 1291–1296.

DiSanto, J. P., Bonnefoy, J. Y., Gauchat, J. F., Fischer, A., and de Saint Basile, G. (1993). CD40 ligand mutations in x-linked immunodeficiency with hyper-IgM. *Nature* **361,** 541–543.

Doi, T., Kinoshita, K., Ikegawa, M., Muramatsu, M., and Honjo, T. (2003). De novo protein synthesis is required for the activation-induced cytidine deaminase function in class-switch recombination. *Proc. Natl. Acad. Sci. USA* **100,** 2634–2638.

Dudley, D. D., Manis, J. P., Zarrin, A. A., Kaylor, L., Tian, M., and Alt, F. W. (2002). Internal IgH class switch region deletions are position-independent and enhanced by AID expression. *Proc. Natl. Acad. Sci. USA* **99,** 9984–9989.

Durandy, A., Schiff, C., Bonnefoy, J. Y., Forveille, M., Rousset, F., Mazzei, G., Milili, M., and Fischer, A. (1993). Induction by anti-CD40 antibody or soluble CD40 ligand and cytokines of IgG, IgA and IgE production by B cells from patients with X-linked hyper IgM syndrome. *Eur. J. Immunol.* **23,** 2294–2299.

Eto, T., Kinoshita, K., Yoshikawa, K., Muramatsu, M., and Honjo, T. (2003). RNA-editing cytidine deaminase Apobec-1 is unable to induce somatic hypermutation in mammalian cells. *Proc. Natl. Acad. Sci. USA* **100,** 12895–12898.

Facchetti, F., Appiani, C., Salvi, L., Levy, J., and Notarangelo, L. D. (1995). Immunohistologic analysis of ineffective CD40-CD40 ligand interaction in lymphoid tissues from patients with X-linked immunodeficiency with hyper-IgM. Abortive germinal center cell reaction and severe depletion of follicular dendritic cells. *J. Immunol.* **154,** 6624–6633.

Fagarasan, S., Muramatsu, M., Suzuki, K., Nagaoka, H., Hiai, H., and Honjo, T. (2002). Critical roles of activation-induced cytidine deaminase in the homeostasis of gut flora. *Science* **298,** 1424–1427.

Faili, A., Aoufouchi, S., Gueranger, Q., Zober, C., Leon, A., Bertocci, B., Weill, J. C., and Reynaud, C. A. (2002). AID-dependent somatic hypermutation occurs as a DNA single-strand event in the BL2 cell line. *Nat. Immunol.* **3,** 815–821.

Fu, Y. X., Huang, G., Wang, Y., and Chaplin, D. D. (1998). B lymphocytes induce the formation of follicular dendritic cell clusters in a lymphotoxin α-dependent fashion. *J. Exp. Med.* **187,** 1009–1018.

Fugmann, S. D., Rush, J. S., and Schatz, D. G. (2004). Non-redundancy of cytidine deaminases in class switch recombination. *Eur. J. Immunol.* **34,** 844–849.

Fukita, Y., Jacobs, H., and Rajewsky, K. (1998). Somatic hypermutation in the heavy chain locus correlates with transcription. *Immunity* **9,** 105–114.

Fuleihan, R., Ramesh, N., and Geha, R. S. (1993). Role of CD40-CD40-ligand interaction in Ig-isotype switching. *Curr. Opin. Immunol.* **5,** 963–967.

Hamada, H., Hiroi, T., Nishiyama, Y., Takahashi, H., Masunaga, Y., Hachimura, S., Kaminogawa, S., Takahashi-Iwanaga, H., Iwanaga, T., Kiyono, H., Yamamoto, H., and Ishikawa, H. (2002). Identification of multiple isolated lymphoid follicles on the antimesenteric wall of the mouse small intestine. *J. Immunol.* **168,** 57–64.

Harris, R. S., Petersen-Mahrt, S. K., and Neuberger, M. S. (2002). RNA editing enzyme APOBEC1 and some of its homologs can act as DNA mutators. *Mol. Cell* **10,** 1247–1253.

Honjo, T., Kinoshita, K., and Muramatsu, M. (2002). Molecular mechanism of class switch recombination: Linkage with somatic hypermutation. *Annu. Rev. Immunol.* **20,** 165–196.

Honjo, T., Nagaoka, H., Shinkura, R., and Muramatsu, M. (2005). AID to overcome the limitations of genomic information. *Nat. Immunol.* **6,** 655–661.

Imai, K., Catalan, N., Plebani, A., Marodi, L., Sanal, O., Kumaki, S., Nagendran, V., Wood, P., Glastre, C., Sarrot-Reynauld, F., Hermine, O., Forveille, M., *et al.* (2003). Hyper-IgM syndrome type 4 with a B lymphocyte-intrinsic selective deficiency in Ig class-switch recombination. *J. Clin. Invest.* **112,** 136–142.

Ito, S., Nagaoka, H., Shinkura, R., Begum, N., Muramatsu, M., Nakata, M., and Honjo, T. (2004). Activation-induced cytidine deaminase shuttles between nucleus and cytoplasm like apolipoprotein B mRNA editing catalytic polypeptide 1. *Proc. Natl. Acad. Sci. USA* **101,** 1975–1980.

Kavli, B., Slupphaug, G., Mol, C. D., Arvai, A. S., Peterson, S. B., Tainer, J. A., and Krokan, H. E. (1996). Excision of cytosine and thymine from DNA by mutants of human uracil-DNA glycosylase. *EMBO J.* **15,** 3442–3447.

Kavli, B., Andersen, S., Otterlei, M., Liabakk, N. B., Imai, K., Fischer, A., Durandy, A., Krokan, H. E., and Slupphaug, G. (2005). B cells from hyper-IgM patients carrying UNG mutations lack ability to remove uracil from ssDNA and have elevated genomic uracil. *J. Exp. Med.* **201,** 2011–2021.

Kinoshita, K., Tashiro, J., Tomita, S., Lee, C. G., and Honjo, T. (1998). Target specificity of immunoglobulin class switch recombination is not determined by nucleotide sequences of S regions. *Immunity* **9,** 849–858.

Ko, R., and Bennett, S. E. (2005). Physical and functional interaction of human nuclear uracil-DNA glycosylase with proliferating cell nuclear antigen. *DNA Repair (Amst.)* **4,** 1421–1431.

Kong, Q., and Maizels, N. (2001). DNA breaks in hypermutating immunoglobulin genes: Evidence for a break-and-repair pathway of somatic hypermutation. *Genetics* **158,** 369–378.

Korthauer, U., Graf, D., Mages, H. W., Briere, F., Padayachee, M., Malcolm, S., Ugazio, A. G., Notarangelo, L. D., Levinsky, R. J., and Kroczek, R. A. (1993). Defective expression of T-cell CD40 ligand causes X-linked immunodeficiency with hyper-IgM. *Nature* **361,** 539–541.

Kotani, A., Okazaki, I. M., Muramatsu, M., Kinoshita, K., Begum, N. A., Nakajima, T., Saito, H., and Honjo, T. (2005). A target selection of somatic hypermutations is regulated similarly between T and B cells upon activation-induced cytidine deaminase expression. *Proc. Natl. Acad. Sci. USA* **102,** 4506–4511.

Le Hir, M., Bluethmann, H., Kosco-Vilbois, M. H., Muller, M., di Padova, F., Moore, M., Ryffel, B., and Eugster, H. P. (1995). Tumor necrosis factor receptor-1 signaling is required for differentiation of follicular dendritic cells, germinal center formation, and full antibody responses. *J. Inflamm.* **47,** 76–80.

MacDuff, D. A., Neuberger, M. S., and Harris, R. S. (2006). MDM2 can interact with the C-terminus of AID but it is inessential for antibody diversification in DT40 B cells. *Mol. Immunol.* **43,** 1099–1108.

Mackay, F., Majeau, G. R., Lawton, P., Hochman, P. S., and Browning, J. L. (1997). Lymphotoxin but not tumor necrosis factor functions to maintain splenic architecture and humoral responsiveness in adult mice. *Eur. J. Immunol.* **27,** 2033–2042.

Manis, J. P., Gu, Y., Lansford, R., Sonoda, E., Ferrini, R., Davidson, L., Rajewsky, K., and Alt, F. W. (1998). Ku70 is required for late B cell development and immunoglobulin heavy chain class switching. *J. Exp. Med.* **187,** 2081–2089.

Manis, J. P., Dudley, D., Kaylor, L., and Alt, F. W. (2002). IgH class switch recombination to IgG1 in DNA-PKcs-deficient B cells. *Immunity* **16,** 607–617.

Mansky, L. M., Preveral, S., Selig, L., Benarous, R., and Benichou, S. (2000). The interaction of vpr with uracil DNA glycosylase modulates the human immunodeficiency virus type 1 *in vivo* mutation rate. *J. Virol.* **74,** 7039–7047.

Martin, A., and Scharff, M. D. (2002). Somatic hypermutation of the AID transgene in B and non-B cells. *Proc. Natl. Acad. Sci. USA* **99,** 12304–12308.

Martin, A., Bardwell, P. D., Woo, C. J., Fan, M., Shulman, M. J., and Scharff, M. D. (2002). Activation-induced cytidine deaminase turns on somatic hypermutation in hybridomas. *Nature* **415,** 802–806.

Matsumoto, M., Lo, S. F., Carruthers, C. J., Min, J., Mariathasan, S., Huang, G., Plas, D. R., Martin, S. M., Geha, R. S., Nahm, M. H., and Chaplin, D. D. (1996). Affinity maturation without germinal centres in lymphotoxin-α-deficient mice. *Nature* **382,** 426–462.

McBride, K. M., Barreto, V., Ramiro, A. R., Stavropoulos, P., and Nussenzweig, M. C. (2004). Somatic hypermutation is limited by CRM1-dependent nuclear export of activation-induced deaminase. *J. Exp. Med.* **199,** 1235–1244.

Mehta, A., Kinter, M. T., Sherman, N. E., and Driscoll, D. M. (2000). Molecular cloning of apobec-1 complementation factor, a novel RNA-binding protein involved in the editing of apolipoprotein B mRNA. *Mol. Cell. Biol.* **20**, 1846–1854.

Mer, G., Edwards, A. M., and Chazin, W. J. (2000). 1H, 15N and 13C resonance assignments for the C-terminal protein interaction region of the 32 kDa subunit of human replication protein A. *J. Biomol. NMR* **17**, 179–180.

Mol, C. D., Arvai, A. S., Slupphaug, G., Kavli, B., Alseth, I., Krokan, H. E., and Tainer, J. A. (1995). Crystal structure and mutational analysis of human uracil-DNA glycosylase: Structural basis for specificity and catalysis. *Cell* **80**, 869–878.

Morgan, H. D., Dean, W., Coker, H. A., Reik, W., and Petersen-Mahrt, S. K. (2004). Activation-induced cytidine deaminase deaminates 5-methylcytosine in DNA and is expressed in pluripotent tissues: Implications for epigenetic reprogramming. *J. Biol. Chem.* **279**, 52353–52360.

Muramatsu, M., Sankaranand, V. S., Anant, S., Sugai, M., Kinoshita, K., Davidson, N. O., and Honjo, T. (1999). Specific expression of activation-induced cytidine deaminase (AID), a novel member of the RNA-editing deaminase family in germinal center B cells. *J. Biol. Chem.* **274**, 18470–18476.

Muramatsu, M., Kinoshita, K., Fagarasan, S., Yamada, S., Shinkai, Y., and Honjo, T. (2000). Class switch recombination and hypermutation require activation-induced cytidine deaminase (AID), a potential RNA editing enzyme. *Cell* **102**, 553–563.

Muto, A., Tashiro, S., Nakajima, O., Hoshino, H., Takahashi, S., Sakoda, E., Ikebe, D., Yamamoto, M., and Igarashi, K. (2004). The transcriptional programme of antibody class switching involves the repressor Bach2. *Nature* **429**, 566–571.

Muto, T., Muramatsu, M., Taniwaki, M., Kinoshita, K., and Honjo, T. (2000). Isolation, tissue distribution, and chromosomal localization of the human activation-induced cytidine deaminase (AID) gene. *Genomics* **68**, 85–88.

Nagaoka, H., Muramatsu, M., Yamamura, N., Kinoshita, K., and Honjo, T. (2002). Activation-induced deaminase (AID)-directed hypermutation in the immunoglobulin Sμ region: Implication of AID involvement in a common step of class switch recombination and somatic hypermutation. *J. Exp. Med.* **195**, 529–534.

Nagaoka, H., Ito, S., Muramatsu, M., Nakata, M., and Honjo, T. (2005). DNA cleavage in immunoglobulin somatic hypermutation depends on *de novo* protein synthesis but not on uracil DNA glycosylase. *Proc. Natl. Acad. Sci. USA* **102**, 2022–2027.

Nagelhus, T. A., Haug, T., Singh, K. K., Keshav, K. F., Skorpen, F., Otterlei, M., Bharati, S., Lindmo, T., Benichou, S., Benarous, R., and Krokan, H. E. (1997). A sequence in the N-terminal region of human uracil-DNA glycosylase with homology to XPA interacts with the C-terminal part of the 34-kDa subunit of replication protein A. *J. Biol. Chem.* **272**, 6561–6566.

Nakamura, M., Kondo, S., Sugai, M., Nazarea, M., Imamura, S., and Honjo, T. (1996). High frequency class switching of an IgM$^+$ B lymphoma clone CH12F3 to IgA$^+$ cells. *Int. Immunol.* **8**, 193–201.

Nambu, Y., Sugai, M., Gonda, H., Lee, C. G., Katakai, T., Agata, Y., Yokota, Y., and Shimizu, A. (2003). Transcription-coupled events associating with immunoglobulin switch region chromatin. *Science* **302**, 2137–2140.

Navaratnam, N., Fujino, T., Bayliss, J., Jarmuz, A., How, A., Richardson, N., Somasekaram, A., Bhattacharya, S., Carter, C., and Scott, J. (1998). *Escherichia coli* cytidine deaminase provides a molecular model for ApoB RNA editing and a mechanism for RNA substrate recognition. *J. Mol. Biol.* **275**, 695–714.

Neuberger, M. S., and Milstein, C. (1995). Somatic hypermutation. *Curr. Opin. Immunol.* **7**, 248–254.
Neuberger, M. S., Harris, R. S., Di Noia, J., and Petersen-Mahrt, S. K. (2003). Immunity through DNA deamination. *Trends Biochem. Sci.* **28**, 305–312.
Odegard, V. H., Kim, S. T., Anderson, S. M., Shlomchik, M. J., and Schatz, D. G. (2005). Histone modifications associated with somatic hypermutation. *Immunity* **23**, 101–110.
Okazaki, I. M., Kinoshita, K., Muramatsu, M., Yoshikawa, K., and Honjo, T. (2002). The AID enzyme induces class switch recombination in fibroblasts. *Nature* **416**, 340–345.
Okazaki, I. M., Hiai, H., Kakazu, N., Yamada, S., Muramatsu, M., Kinoshita, K., and Honjo, T. (2003). Constitutive expression of AID leads to tumorigenesis. *J. Exp. Med.* **197**, 1173–1181.
Otterlei, M., Haug, T., Nagelhus, T. A., Slupphaug, G., Lindmo, T., and Krokan, H. E. (1998). Nuclear and mitochondrial splice forms of human uracil-DNA glycosylase contain a complex nuclear localisation signal and a strong classical mitochondrial localisation signal, respectively. *Nucleic Acids Res.* **26**, 4611–4617.
Otterlei, M., Warbrick, E., Nagelhus, T. A., Haug, T., Slupphaug, G., Akbari, M., Aas, P. A., Steinsbekk, K., Bakke, O., and Krokan, H. E. (1999). Post-replicative base excision repair in replication foci. *EMBO J.* **18**, 3834–3844.
Pan-Hammarstrom, Q., Jones, A. M., Lahdesmaki, A., Zhou, W., Gatti, R. A., Hammarstrom, L., Gennery, A. R., and Ehrenstein, M. R. (2005). Impact of DNA ligase IV on nonhomologous end joining pathways during class switch recombination in human cells. *J. Exp. Med.* **201**, 189–194.
Papavasiliou, F. N., and Schatz, D. G. (2002). The activation-induced deaminase functions in a postcleavage step of the somatic hypermutation process. *J. Exp. Med.* **195**, 1193–1198.
Parikh, S. S., Mol, C. D., Slupphaug, G., Bharati, S., Krokan, H. E., and Tainer, J. A. (1998). Base excision repair initiation revealed by crystal structures and binding kinetics of human uracil-DNA glycosylase with DNA. *EMBO J.* **17**, 5214–5226.
Pearl, L. H. (2000). Structure and function in the uracil-DNA glycosylase superfamily. *Mutat. Res.* **460**, 165–181.
Peters, A., and Storb, U. (1996). Somatic hypermutation of immunoglobulin genes is linked to transcription initiation. *Immunity* **4**, 57–65.
Petersen, S., Casellas, R., Reina-San-Martin, B., Chen, H. T., Difilippantonio, M. J., Wilson, P. C., Hanitsch, L., Celeste, A., Muramatsu, M., Pilch, D. R., Redon, C., Ried, T., *et al.* (2001). AID is required to initiate Nbs1/γ-H2AX focus formation and mutations at sites of class switching. *Nature* **414**, 660–665.
Petersen-Mahrt, S. K., Harris, R. S., and Neuberger, M. S. (2002). AID mutates *E. coli* suggesting a DNA deamination mechanism for antibody diversification. *Nature* **418**, 99–103.
Pham, P., Bransteitter, R., Petruska, J., and Goodman, M. F. (2003). Processive AID-catalysed cytosine deamination on single-stranded DNA simulates somatic hypermutation. *Nature* **424**, 103–107.
Priet, S., Gros, N., Navarro, J. M., Boretto, J., Canard, B., Querat, G., and Sire, J. (2005). HIV-1-associated uracil DNA glycosylase activity controls dUTP misincorporation in viral DNA and is essential to the HIV-1 life cycle. *Mol. Cell* **17**, 479–490.
Rada, C., Williams, G. T., Nilsen, H., Barnes, D. E., Lindahl, T., and Neuberger, M. S. (2002). Immunoglobulin isotype switching is inhibited and somatic hypermutation perturbed in UNG-deficient mice. *Curr. Biol.* **12**, 1748–1755.
Rada, C., Di Noia, J. M., and Neuberger, M. S. (2004). Mismatch recognition and uracil excision provide complementary paths to both Ig switching and the A/T-focused phase of somatic mutation. *Mol. Cell* **16**, 163–171.

Ramiro, A. R., Jankovic, M., Eisenreich, T., Difilippantonio, S., Chen-Kiang, S., Muramatsu, M., Honjo, T., Nussenzweig, A., and Nussenzweig, M. C. (2004). AID is required for c-myc/IgH chromosome translocations *in vivo*. *Cell* **118**, 431–438.

Revy, P., Muto, T., Levy, Y., Geissmann, F., Plebani, A., Sanal, O., Catalan, N., Forveille, M., Dufourcq-Labelouse, R., Gennery, A., Tezcan, I., Ersoy, F., *et al.* (2000). Activation-induced cytidine deaminase (AID) deficiency causes the autosomal recessive form of the Hyper-IgM syndrome (HIGM2). *Cell* **102**, 565–575.

Rosner, A. J., and Keren, D. F. (1984). Demonstration of M cells in the specialized follicle-associated epithelium overlying isolated lymphoid follicles in the gut. *J. Leukoc. Biol.* **35**, 397–404.

Rush, J. S., Fugmann, S. D., and Schatz, D. G. (2004). Staggered AID-dependent DNA double strand breaks are the predominant DNA lesions targeted to Sμ in Ig class switch recombination. *Int. Immunol.* **16**, 549–557.

Ryffel, B., Di Padova, F., Schreier, M. H., Le Hir, M., Eugster, H. P., and Quesniaux, V. F. (1997). Lack of type 2 T cell-independent B cell responses and defect in isotype switching in TNF-lymphotoxin α-deficient mice. *J. Immunol.* **158**, 2126–2133.

Savva, R., and Pearl, L. H. (1995). Nucleotide mimicry in the crystal structure of the uracil-DNA glycosylase-uracil glycosylase inhibitor protein complex. *Nat. Struct. Biol.* **2**, 752–757.

Schrader, C. E., Linehan, E. K., Mochegova, S. N., Woodland, R. T., and Stavnezer, J. (2005). Inducible DNA breaks in Ig S regions are dependent on AID and UNG. *J. Exp. Med.* **202**, 561–568.

Selig, L., Benichou, S., Rogel, M. E., Wu, L. I., Vodicka, M. A., Sire, J., Benarous, R., and Emerman, M. (1997). Uracil DNA glycosylase specifically interacts with Vpr of both human immunodeficiency virus type 1 and simian immunodeficiency virus of sooty mangabeys, but binding does not correlate with cell cycle arrest. *J. Virol.* **71**, 4842–4846.

Shinkura, R., Ito, S., Begum, N. A., Nagaoka, H., Muramatsu, M., Kinoshita, K., Sakakibara, Y., Hijikata, H., and Honjo, T. (2004). Separate domains of AID are required for somatic hypermutation and class-switch recombination. *Nat. Immunol.* **5**, 707–712.

Slupphaug, G., Mol, C. D., Kavli, B., Arvai, A. S., Krokan, H. E., and Tainer, J. A. (1996). A nucleotide-flipping mechanism from the structure of human uracil-DNA glycosylase bound to DNA. *Nature* **384**, 82–92.

Stavnezer, J. (1996). Immunoglobulin class switching. *Curr. Opin. Immunol.* **8**, 199–205.

Studebaker, A. W., Ariza, M. E., and Williams, M. V. (2005). Depletion of uracil-DNA glycosylase activity is associated with decreased cell proliferation. *Biochem. Biophys. Res. Commun.* **334**, 509–515.

Ta, V. T., Nagaoka, H., Catalan, N., Durandy, A., Fischer, A., Imai, K., Nonoyama, S., Tashiro, J., Ikegawa, M., Ito, S., Kinoshita, K., Muramatsu, M., *et al.* (2003). AID mutant analyses indicate requirement for class-switch-specific cofactors. *Nat. Immunol.* **4**, 843–848.

Teng, B., Burant, C. F., and Davidson, N. O. (1993). Molecular cloning of an apolipoprotein B messenger RNA editing protein. *Science* **260**, 1816–1819.

Teng, B. B., Ochsner, S., Zhang, Q., Soman, K. V., Lau, P. P., and Chan, L. (1999). Mutational analysis of apolipoprotein B mRNA editing enzyme (APOBEC1). structure-function relationships of RNA editing and dimerization. *J. Lipid Res.* **40**, 623–635.

Tonegawa, S. (1983). Somatic generation of antibody diversity. *Nature* **302**, 575–581.

Wang, J., Shinkura, R., Muramatsu, M., Nagaoka, H., Kinoshita, K., and Honjo, T. (2006). Identification of a specific domain required for dimerization of activation-induced cytidine deaminase. *J. Biol. Chem.* **281**, 19115–19123.

Wang, Z., and Mosbaugh, D. W. (1989). Uracil-DNA glycosylase inhibitor gene of bacteriophage PBS2 encodes a binding protein specific for uracil-DNA glycosylase. *J. Biol. Chem.* **264,** 1163–1171.

Woo, C. J., Martin, A., and Scharff, M. D. (2003). Induction of somatic hypermutation is associated with modifications in immunoglobulin variable region chromatin. *Immunity* **19,** 479–489.

Wu, X., Geraldes, P., Platt, J. L., and Cascalho, M. (2005). The double-edged sword of activation-induced cytidine deaminase. *J. Immunol.* **174,** 934–941.

Xiao, G., Tordova, M., Jagadeesh, J., Drohat, A. C., Stivers, J. T., and Gilliland, G. L. (1999). Crystal structure of Escherichia coli uracil DNA glycosylase and its complexes with uracil and glycerol: Structure and glycosylase mechanism revisited. *Proteins* **35,** 13–24.

Yoshikawa, K., Okazaki, I. M., Eto, T., Kinoshita, K., Muramatsu, M., Nagaoka, H., and Honjo, T. (2002). AID enzyme-induced hypermutation in an actively transcribed gene in fibroblasts. *Science* **296,** 2033–2036.

Yu, K., Huang, F. T., and Lieber, M. R. (2004). DNA substrate length and surrounding sequence affect the activation-induced deaminase activity at cytidine. *J. Biol. Chem.* **279,** 6496–6500.

Zhu, Y., Nonoyama, S., Morio, T., Muramatsu, M., Honjo, T., and Mizutani, S. (2003). Type two hyper-IgM syndrome caused by mutation in activation-induced cytidine deaminase. *J. Med. Dent. Sci.* **50,** 41–46.

DNA Deamination in Immunity: AID in the Context of Its APOBEC Relatives

Silvestro G. Conticello, Marc-Andre Langlois, Zizhen Yang, and Michael S. Neuberger

Medical Research Council Laboratory of Molecular Biology, Cambridge CB2 2QH, United Kingdom

Abstract	37
1. Introduction	38
2. AID: The DNA Deaminase Trigger for Antibody Diversification	38
3. The Zn-Dependent Deaminase Superfamily	39
4. Timeline of AID/APOBEC Evolution	48
5. APOBEC1: An RNA-Editing Enzyme That Can Also Act on DNA	49
6. APOBEC2: A Muscle-Specific Family Member of Unknown Function/Activity	50
7. APOBEC4: A Distant or Ancestral Member of the AID/APOBEC Family	51
8. APOBEC3s: DNA Deaminases Active in Viral Restriction	52
9. Conclusion	63
References	63

Abstract

The activation-induced cytidine deaminase (AID)/apolipoprotein B RNA-editing catalytic component (APOBEC) family is a vertebrate-restricted sub-grouping of a superfamily of zinc (Zn)-dependent deaminases that has members distributed throughout the biological world. AID and APOBEC2 are the oldest family members with APOBEC1 and the APOBEC3s being later arrivals restricted to placental mammals. Many AID/APOBEC family members exhibit cytidine deaminase activity on polynucleotides, although in different physiological contexts. Here, we examine the AID/APOBEC proteins in the context of the entire Zn-dependent deaminase superfamily. On the basis of secondary structure predictions, we propose that the cytosine and tRNA deaminases are likely to provide better structural paradigms for the AID/APOBEC family than do the cytidine deaminases, to which they have conventionally been compared. These comparisons yield predictions concerning likely polynucleotide-interacting residues in AID/APOBEC3s, predictions that are supported by mutagenesis studies. We also focus on a specific comparison between AID and the APOBEC3s. Both are DNA deaminases that function in immunity and are responsible for the hypermutation of their target substrates. AID functions in the adaptive immune system to diversify antibodies with targeted DNA deamination being central to this function. APOBEC3s function as part of an innate pathway of immunity to retroviruses with targeted DNA deamination being central to their activity in retroviral hypermutation. However, the mechanism by which the APOBEC3s fulfill their function of retroviral restriction remains unresolved.

1. Introduction

Aside from the mutations caused by replication errors, incidental DNA damage or the movement of viruses and transposable elements, multicellular organisms reproduce their genomes faithfully during somatic development, without any modifications of the coding sequence. The major (possibly) sole exception to this rule is provided by the adaptive immune system which uses two types of programmed DNA modifications in order to achieve the diversity of antigen receptors: site-specific gene rearrangement and targeted DNA deamination.

In both B and T cells, RAG-mediated gene rearrangement is used to generate a primary repertoire of functional antigen receptor genes, whereas in B (but not T) cells this primary repertoire is then further diversified by somatic hypermutation (SHM) or gene conversion [which diversify the primary repertoire of integrated IgV(D)J genes] and class switch recombination (which underpins the shift from an IgM to IgG/IgA/IgE antibody repertoire). These latter processes of SHM, gene conversion, and switch recombination are all triggered by activation-induced cytidine deaminase (AID)-catalyzed targeted deamination of deoxycytidine residues in the Ig loci.

Unexpectedly, an analogous process of targeted DNA deamination takes place with lentiviruses (e.g., HIV-1) in which a host deaminase belonging to the AID-related APOBEC3 family attacks cytidines in the DNA of lentiviral replication intermediates.

The AID/apolipoprotein B RNA-editing catalytic component (APOBEC) family can be divided into four major groupings (AID, APOBEC1, APOBEC2, and APOBEC3) with AID, APOBEC1, and APOBEC3 members all acting as polynucleotide deaminases. Here we consider the function (and possible structure) of AID as a DNA deaminase in the context of the entire deaminase superfamily and, in particular, compare AID to the APOBEC3s, since they constitute the major grouping of DNA deaminases active in immunity.

2. AID: The DNA Deaminase Trigger for Antibody Diversification

AID was first identified as a cDNA that was induced on activation of a mouse B-cell line (Muramatsu *et al.*, 1999), with disruption of the AID gene being subsequently shown to lead to abolition of immunoglobulin heavy chain class switch recombination as well as IgV SHM in both mouse and man (Arakawa *et al.*, 2002; Harris *et al.*, 2002a; Muramatsu *et al.*, 2000; Revy *et al.*, 2000). Since at that time the only molecular activity that had been ascribed to an

AID/APOBEC family member was that of RNA editing [with APOBEC1 having been discovered as the catalytic component of a complex that edits apolipoprotein B RNA (Navaratnam et al., 1993; Teng et al., 1993)], it was reasonably suggested that AID might also prove to be an RNA-editing enzyme. However, as discussed elsewhere (Neuberger et al., 2003), it subsequently became evident that AID itself acts directly on immunoglobulin gene DNA, diversifying antibodies by active mutation.

Several lines of evidence had come together to give insight into the likely mechanism of AID action. In particular, although it had long been considered that SHM of IgV genes might occur through some form of localized, error-prone DNA synthesis (Brenner and Milstein, 1966), analysis of IgV gene SHM in DNA repair-deficient mice had suggested that SHM might actually occur in two phases, the first targeting C:G pairs and the second (triggered by MSH2-mediated recognition of lesions created in the first phase) targeting A:T pairs (Rada et al., 1998). The fact that AID showed similarity to a family of cytidine deaminases, therefore, made it attractive to consider the possibility that AID acted directly on cytidine in immunoglobulin gene DNA, accounting for the first (C:G-targeted) phase of SHM. Such a DNA deamination model was especially attractive in view of the fact that AID was essential for IgV gene conversion and IgH class switch recombination as well as for SHM (Arakawa et al., 2002; Harris et al., 2002a; Muramatsu et al., 2000; Revy et al., 2000), since there were already pointers that these three distinct processes might show some similarities in their initiating events (Ehrenstein and Neuberger, 1999; Maizels, 1995; Sale et al., 2001; Weill and Reynaud, 1996). The DNA deamination scheme of antibody diversification (Fig. 1A) found support from genetic and biochemical experiments showing that recombinant AID is able to deaminate cytosine in DNA (Beale et al., 2004; Bransteitter et al., 2003; Chaudhuri et al., 2003; Dickerson et al., 2003; Petersen-Mahrt et al., 2002; Pham et al., 2003; Ramiro et al., 2003; Sohail et al., 2003). Furthermore, genetic experiments revealed that antibody diversification pathways are perturbed in cells deficient in uracil-DNA glycosylase, indicating that uracil in DNA is indeed a central intermediate in antibody gene diversification (Di Noia and Neuberger, 2002, 2004; Imai et al., 2003; Rada et al., 2002, 2004; Saribasak et al., 2006).

3. The Zn-Dependent Deaminase Superfamily

3.1. Overview of Family Members

The AID/APOBEC family members (with the exception of APOBEC2; see below) function as polynucleotide deaminases with no activity on free base/nucleotide. Analysis of currently available genomic sequence databases suggests

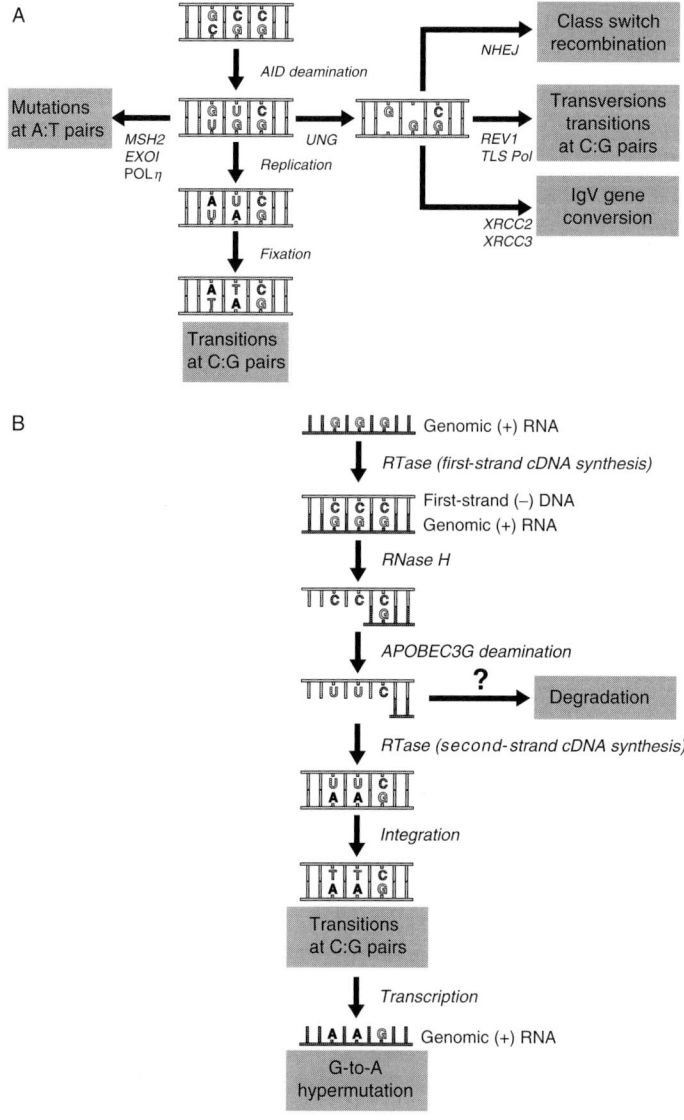

Figure 1 Comparison of AID-triggered antibody hypermutation and APOBEC3-triggered retroviral hypermutation. (A) Antibody hypermutation. AID-mediated deamination of C residues in the immunoglobulin locus DNA generates U:G mispairs. Replication over these mispairs will result in the fixation of C → T and G → A transition mutations. The U:G lesion can also be recognized by components of either the base excision (UNG) or mismatch (MSH2/MSH6) repair pathways leading to alternate pathways of resolution (mutation at A:T pairs; both transition and transversion

that the AID/APOBEC family is restricted to jawed vertebrates. However, the AID/APOBEC proteins are part of a much more widely expressed superfamily of zinc (Zn)-dependent deaminases which act on pyrimidines and purines. While the deaminases involved in guanine and riboflavin metabolism are present only in bacteria and are often composite enzymes which also possess other catalytic activities, the AID/APOBECs are more related to those superfamily members which can act on free cytosine, cytidine, and dCMP as well as other members which act on adenosine in the context of RNA (Table 1).

The vast majority of the characterized cytosine deaminases act on free base/nucleoside/nucleotide, catalyzing the formation of uracil through the hydrolysis of the 4-amino group. These enzymes contribute to the pyrimidine salvage pathway

Table 1 Zinc-Dependent Deaminases[a]

Enzyme	Substrate	Organisms
Cytosine deaminase	Cytosine/methylcytosine	Bacteria, archea, yeast
Cytidine deaminase	Cytidine/deoxycytidine	Bacteria, archea, yeast, plants, metazoa
dCMP deaminase	dCMP	(Archea, bacteria), yeast, plants, metazoa, virus
TadA/Tad2p–3p/ADAT2–3	Adenosine-34 in tRNA	Bacteria, yeast, metazoa
Tad1p/ADAT1	Adenosine-37 in tRNA^{Ala}	Yeast, metazoa
ADAR1–2–3	Adenine in mRNA	Metazoa
AID/APOBECs	Cytosine in DNA/mRNA	Vertebrates
Riboflavin deaminase	Riboflavin synthesis	Bacteria, archea, fungi, plants
Guanine deaminase	Guanine	Some bacteria, (archea)

[a]The group of organisms for which the presence of a given enzyme is uncertain are indicated in parenthesis.

mutations at C:G pairs through replication over the UNG-generated abasic site; IgV gene conversion and class switch recombination). The likely mechanisms of these various pathways of resolution are discussed elsewhere (Di Noia and Neuberger, 2007; Longerich et al., 2006). (B) Retroviral G-to-A hypermutation. Reverse transcription of retroviral RNA generates a single-stranded first-strand cDNA that is available to the action of virally incorporated APOBEC3s. Deamination creates U residues in the first-strand cDNA, which are replicated over during retroviral second-strand cDNA synthesis. This leads to the fixation of C → T and G → A transition mutations in the integrated retroviral cDNA and subsequent G → A hypermutation of the resulting retroviral RNA. It is possible that deamination also triggers a degradation pathway that trashes the entire viral genome before integration, but the existence and nature of such a pathway remains to be defined. Those genomes that escape degradation are integrated and the mutations introduced by APOBEC3 will be fixated. (**See Color Plate 1.**)

and span the entire life tree, though with some variation. Thus, deaminases active on the free cytosine base have been found in prokaryotes and lower eukaryotes but do not have homologues in metazoa (Nishiyama *et al.*, 1985).

With regard to free nucleoside, cytidine deaminases catalyzing the deamination of cytidine/deoxycytidine exist in two varieties: a homotetrameric form which is characteristic of the enzymes from most organisms (Song and Neuhard, 1989) as well as a larger dimeric form, which appears restricted to *Escherichia coli* (Betts *et al.*, 1994) and some other bacteria. Finally, with regard to nucleotide substrates, the enzymes in eukaryotes are specific to dCMP, whereas nucleotide deamination in prokaryotes is carried out by Mg-dependent dCTP/CTP deaminases which are not really part of the superfamily members, only showing homology at the three-dimensional level (Johansson *et al.*, 2005).

Many members of the deaminase superfamily act on adenosine rather than cytosine, removing the amino group from the 6-position yielding inosine. These enzymes work as RNA-editing enzymes active on tRNA or mRNA. Although they deaminate adenosine rather than cytidine, the similarity of these enzymes to the deaminases which work on cytosine, cytidine, or dCMP clearly places them in the deaminase superfamily (Conticello *et al.*, 2005). (Adenosine deaminases that function in purine metabolism and act on free nucleoside belong to an entirely different though structurally related gene family.) There are examples of tRNA deaminases working on the adenosine at the wobble position present in all organisms (Auxilien *et al.*, 1996; Gerber and Keller, 1999; Wolf *et al.*, 2002): inclusion of inosine within the anticodon allows the same tRNA to pair with codons bearing A, C, or U in their third position. In bacteria, only tRNA^{Arg2} is edited by the TadA enzyme. However, in yeast and higher eukaryotes, at least seven or eight tRNAs are edited by the TadA homologues Tad2p/Tad3p (yeast) or ADAT2/ADAT3 (metazoa). The nonviability of yeast deficient in Tad2p/Tad3p indicates that their role is essential (Gerber and Keller, 1999).

In eukaryotes, Tad1p/ADAT1 constitutes another tRNA deaminase, which appears to have evolved from ADAT2/ADAT3 and is responsible for deamination of the adenosine at position 37 of the tRNA^{ala} (Gerber *et al.*, 1998). The importance of tRNA^{ala} editing is not yet clear with Tad1p-deficient mice not showing any apparent phenotype apart from the lack of A$_{37}$ editing of tRNA^{ala}.

Higher eukaryotes also contain a group of adenosine deaminases that act on pre-mRNAs. This group includes three paralogues identified as ADAR1, -2, and -3. They appear to have evolved from ADAT1 but have incorporated additional domains (dsRNA-binding as well as Z-DNA-binding cassettes; Bass, 2002; Keller *et al.*, 1999).

3.2. Correlation of Structure and Function Among Deaminases

3.2.1. The Common Zn-Coordination Motif

Elucidation of the three-dimensional structure of the *E. coli* cytidine deaminase revealed the organization of the domain responsible for the catalytic activity of the deaminases (Betts *et al.*, 1994). This domain is characterized by a pocket where a Zn atom is coordinated by two cysteines and a histidine (or by a third cysteine rather than a histidine in the case of cytidine deaminases) and is located at the N-terminus of two alpha helices that come from opposite directions (Carter, 1995; Ireton *et al.*, 2003; Ko *et al.*, 2003; Xiang *et al.*, 1996, 1997; Fig. 2A). A fourth ligand coordinated to the Zn atom is an activated water molecule that can serve as a donor for the attacking hydroxide in the deamination reaction. The alpha helix that contains the coordinating histidine also provides a glutamate residue that serves as proton donor in the reaction.

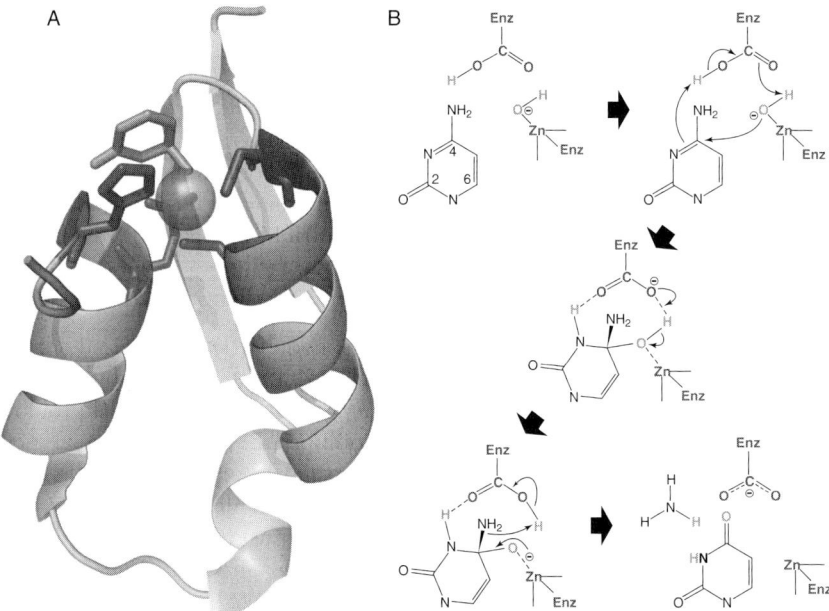

Figure 2 Deamination by Zn-dependent deaminases. (A) Structure of catalytic pocket of the yeast cytosine deaminase (Ko *et al.*, 2003). The zinc atom is coordinated by a histidine and two cysteines (in blue). The glutamate (in red) participates in the nucleophilic attack on C4 of the cytosine (in magenta). (B) Mechanism of reaction. The hydroxide of a Zn-activated water molecule mediates a nucleophilic attack on C4 of the cytosine ring, leading to loss of the amino group. (**See Color Plate 2.**)

The deamination reaction is a hydrolysis initiated by nucleophilic attack from the Zn-coordinated hydroxide onto the C4 position of the cytosine facilitated by a neighboring glutamate residue; the reaction proceeds through two tetravalent intermediates, releasing ammonia and uracil (Fig. 2B). The reaction catalyzed by the *E. coli* cytidine deaminase proceeds at the extremely high rate of 10^{-10} s^{-1}.

3.2.2. Comparison of Known Deaminase Quaternary Structures

Although the structures that have been determined for different cytosine and cytidine deaminases reveal high similarity of their active sites, the two types of deaminase have highly specific and distinct substrate specificities (Carlow and Wolfenden, 1998; Ipata and Cercignani, 1978) with tertiary and quaternary structural differences beyond the catalytic site that probably play an important role in substrate specificity.

Cytidine deaminases from most of the organisms studied form homotetramers with a twofold pseudosymmetry. These tetramers are formed from a pair of dimers with the interface between the monomers in each dimer being mainly provided by alpha helices 3 and 5; the interfaces between the dimers are contributed by various loops (Fig. 3). Each of the four active sites lies at the interface between the subunits in such a way that the cytidine placed in one catalytic pocket makes contact with residues from two other subunits (Johansson *et al.*, 2002; Fig. 3). Similarly, the *E. coli* cytidine deaminase, which contains a C-terminal pseudocatalytic domain, aggregate in a dimeric complex to form a tetramer-like structure containing two Zn-coordinating active sites and two pseudocatalytic sites (Betts *et al.*, 1994).

In contrast to cytidine deaminases, cytosine deaminases form homodimers with the alpha helices 2, 3, and 4 forming the intersubunit boundary. The catalytic sites are located at opposite ends of the two subunits and are completely incorporated within the subunit rather than lying at the subunit interface (Ireton *et al.*, 2002; Ko *et al.*, 2003; Fig. 3). Interestingly, the bacterial tRNA adenosine deaminase TadA (the only deaminase acting on nucleic acids whose structure three-dimensional structure has been determined) exhibits a very similar quaternary structure (Elias and Huang, 2005; Kim *et al.*, 2006; Kuratani *et al.*, 2005; Fig. 3). The relative conformation of the subunits in TadA allows a pair of tRNA molecules to bind at opposite sides of the dimer; the adenosine-34 in the anticodon loop is then flipped out of the tRNA main chain and is accommodated within the catalytic pocket of the enzyme (Losey *et al.*, 2006).

3.2.3. Implications for the Structures of AID/APOBECs

Despite the lack of information on the three-dimensional structure of the AID/APOBEC proteins, analysis of their amino acid sequences suggests that their structure in the catalytic domain will show considerable similarity to those of

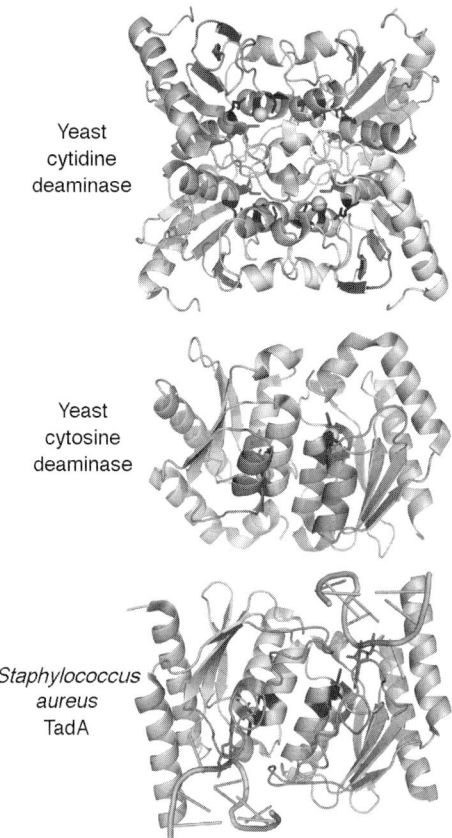

Figure 3 Three-dimensional structures of Zn-dependent deaminases. The yeast cytidine deaminase (Xiang et al., 1997) forms a tetramer. Segments of chains from adjacent subunits come together to form zinc pockets in which the cytidine is deaminated. In contrast, in the yeast cytosine deaminase (Ko et al., 2003) and in the tRNA adenosine deaminase (Losey et al., 2006), each catalytic site is independently and separately formed by each individual subunit. A major structural difference between cytidine deaminases and cytosine/tRNA deaminases is the presence of a stretch of amino acids between the beta sheets 4 and 5 (shown in orange in the cytosine deaminase/TadA structures) forming part of the active site. Part of this region, in TadA, makes contact with the nucleotide that immediately precedes the deaminated adenosine in the tRNA substrate. The Zn atom is shown in yellow. (**See Color Plate 3.**)

the other deaminases. Major interest, however, will focus on the structure of their C-terminal ends, which are notably longer than those of the other deaminases, as well as on the basis of their ability to recognize and bind polynucleotides. In absence of experimental data, it is of some interest to speculate about the likely conformation of the AID/APOBEC proteins on the basis of the available structures of related deaminases.

Given that the cytidine deaminases and cytosine/tRNA deaminases form two distinct classes with respect to quaternary structure and with the two groups binding their substrates in distinct manners, it is appropriate first to ask whether the structures of the AID/APOBEC proteins are likely to resemble those of the cytidine deaminases or of the cytosine/tRNA deaminases.

Being the first deaminases whose structure was analyzed, *E. coli* cytidine deaminase has long been considered the archetypal structure to which the AID/APOBECs will conform. This idea was somehow strengthened by the presence of the long C-terminal tail in APOBEC1 (the first APOBEC family member to be identified) which resembles the pseudocatalytic domain of the *E. coli* cytidine deaminase in length. However, analysis of the primary sequence of the AID/APOBECs shows that their predicted secondary structure more closely resembles that of the cytosine/dCMP/tRNA deaminases than that of the cytidine deaminases, especially regarding the presence of a segment between beta sheets 4 and 5, including a predicted alpha helix 4 (Fig. 4A). Mutational studies reveal that amino acid substitutions in residues located immediately downstream of predicted beta sheet 4 change the DNA target specificity of APOBEC3F (Langlois *et al.*, 2005; Table 2). The equivalent region in TadA is known from crystallographic studies to make contact with the adenosine-34 (as well as the preceding nucleotide) in the tRNA substrate (Fig. 4B).

The similarity of predicted secondary structures (supported by the mutagenesis studies) is the major reason for suggesting that the AID/APOBECs will exhibit a three-dimensional structure closer to that of the cytosine/dCMP/tRNA (as opposed to cytidine) deaminase group. However, the more accessible catalytic site in TadA (as opposed to that in cytidine deaminases) is certainly more appealing from the perspective of activity on a polynucleotide substrate than is the buried catalytic site in the cytidine deaminases (Fig. 3).

It is notable that TadA acts on a base that has been flipped out of a seven-nucleotide single-stranded segment in the stem-loop of tRNA$^{\text{Arg2}}$ (Losey *et al.*, 2006). This base (adenine at position 34) appears to be located in a conformation that is similar to one adopted by the APOBEC1-target, cytosine 6666 in apolipoprotein B RNA (Anant and Davidson, 2000; Maris *et al.*, 2005; Richardson *et al.*, 1998). It may be significant that AID appears to be able to act on single-stranded DNA loops of a similar size (Yu *et al.*, 2004a); it will be interesting to discover whether the cytidine base is also flipped out during AID action.

COMPARISON OF AID WITH APOBEC DNA DEAMINASES

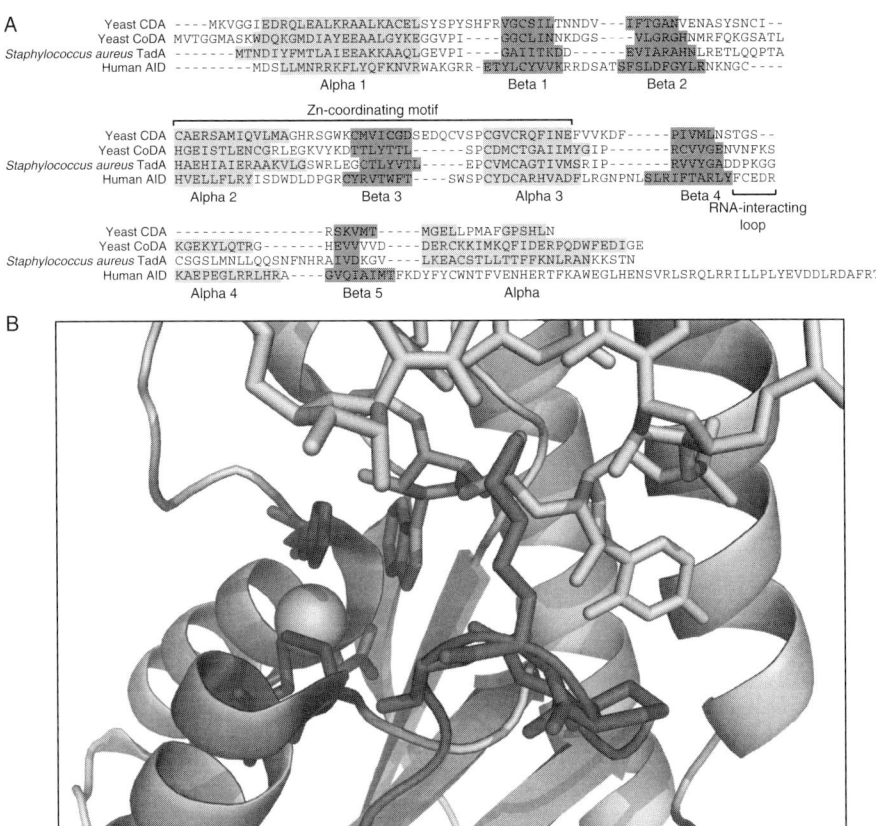

Figure 4 Sequence alignment of Zn-dependent deaminases and suggestion of polynucleotide-interacting residues. (A) Yeast cytidine deaminase, cytosine deaminase, *Staphylococcus aureus* TadA, and human AID are aligned according to their (predicted) secondary structures. Alpha helices and beta sheets are highlighted in light and dark gray, respectively. The Zn-coordinating motif is indicated above the line. The segment of TadA that has been shown to interact with the RNA substrate is indicated. (B) Three-dimensional representation of the RNA-interacting loop in TadA. The tRNA substrate is indicated in magenta (the deaminated adenosine is highlighted in pink); the DPKG residues taking contact with the RNA are indicated in orange. The Zn-coordinating site lies beneath (zinc in yellow, coordinating residues in blue, and glutamate in red). As described in the text, we predict that the aligned region in AID (FCEDR in the human sequence) will be close to the site of interaction with the single-stranded DNA substrate, a suggestion supported by the effects of mutations in this region on substrate specificity (Langlois *et al.*, 2005). (**See Color Plate 4.**)

Table 2 Mutational Analysis of the APOBEC3F Residues Immediately Downstream the Beta Sheet 4

	Interacting loop	Target specificity (position)		
		−2	−1	0
AID	FCEDR	A/T	A	C
APOBEC3F	FWDTD	T	T	C
APOBEC3C	FQYPC	T	C/T	C
APOBEC3F D309Y	FWYTD	T	G/C/T	C
APOBEC3F D311C	FWDTC	G	T	C

Analogously to what has been observed for APOBEC3s (Wiegand et al., 2004), the Tad2p/ADAT2 and Tad3p/ADAT3 (the eukaryotic homologues of bacterial TadA) deaminases form heterodimers (Gerber and Keller, 1999). Indeed, in the tRNA deaminase heterodimers, the Tad3p/ADAT3 subunit contains a catalytically inactive Zn-coordinating domain in which valine replaces the proton-donating glutamate: this is reminiscent of some of the double-domained APOBEC3 proteins (human APOBEC3G and the murine APOBEC3) in which one of the putative active sites seems to be nonfunctional (Shindo et al., 2003; Beale and Neuberger, unpublished data).

Thus, it seems likely that the structures of the AID/APOBEC deaminases will more closely resemble those of the tRNA and cytosine deaminases than that of cytidine deaminase.

4. Timeline of AID/APOBEC Evolution

The AID/APOBECs have evolved as DNA/RNA deaminases relatively late: the analysis of the sequenced genomes of organisms that diverged before the jawed fish do not present any deaminase that might resemble an AID/APOBEC, and despite the efforts to identify AID/APOBECs homologues, AID has been identified only in cartilaginous and bony fish (Conticello et al., 2005; Saunders and Magor, 2004; Zhao et al., 2005). Thus, the bona fide origin of the AID/APOBEC family can be placed at around 500 million years ago, at the time of the divergence of the cartilaginous fish from the teleost/tetrapod lineage.

APOBEC2, for which there is evidence in teleosts, might have originated at a similar time. Given the distinct nature of the APOBEC2 gene structure (which differs significantly from that of other AID/APOBEC family members) with a single exon encompassing the entire AID/APOBEC homology domain and an upstream exon with no similarity to any other known protein, it is possible that APOBEC2 might have arisen as a result of a retrotranspositional event.

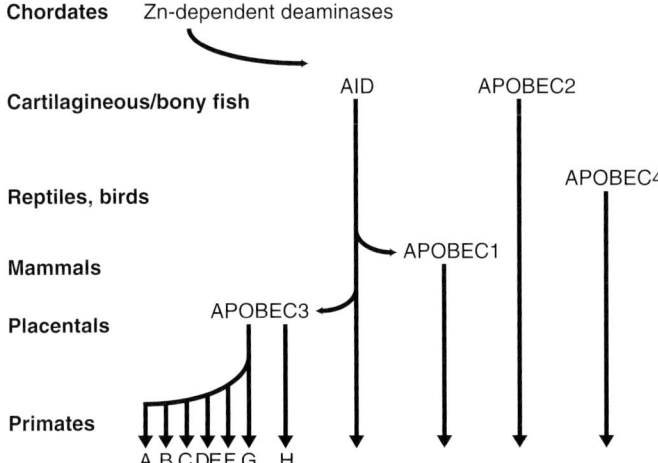

Figure 5 Timeline of AID/APOBEC evolution. AID and APOBEC2 are the ancestral members of the gene family. It seems likely that APOBEC2 evolved from AID since, while APOBEC2 exhibits most of the sequence motifs characteristic of the AID/APOBEC family, it has a quite distinct exon structure (consistent with the central exons having been fused during a cDNA synthesis), whereas AID and the other APOBEC family members share an exon structure similar to that exhibited by the other Zn-dependent deaminases. APOBEC1 and the APOBEC3s appear to have evolved from AID, whereas the origins of APOBEC4 remain obscure.

Thus, until APOBEC1 evolved by duplication of the AID locus in mammals around 300–400 million years ago (Conticello *et al.*, 2005; Fujino *et al.*, 1999), there were probably just two members of the AID/APOBEC gene family, AID and APOBEC2 (Fig. 5). The APOBEC3s then arose as a placental-specific innovation arising again from duplication of AID after the divergence of the placentals from the marsupials (~170 million years ago) (Conticello *et al.*, 2005) and underwent a rapid expansion in primates, where seven APOBEC3s are present (Conticello *et al.*, 2005; Jarmuz *et al.*, 2002; Wedekind *et al.*, 2003).

Yet another member of the AID/APOBECs family, APOBEC4, has been identified, which might have originated before the amphibia/reptile divergence (Rogozin *et al.*, 2005). While we have briefly discussed AID above, we consider each of the other APOBEC groupings below.

5. APOBEC1: An RNA-Editing Enzyme That Can Also Act on DNA

APOBEC1 is the founder member of the AID/APOBEC gene family. It was identified as the catalytic component of the complex that edits apolipoprotein B (ApoB) RNA in the small intestine in man (liver in rodents) (Navaratnam *et al.*, 1993; Teng *et al.*, 1993). The cytidine at position 6666 in ApoB RNA is deaminated to uridine, transforming a glutamine codon into a stop codon and thereby leading to the production of a truncated form of the ApoB polypeptide (ApoB48). APOBEC1 is restricted to mammals and likely arose through gene duplication of AID (Conticello *et al.*, 2005; Fujino *et al.*, 1999). Its function in the production of ApoB48 facilitates efficient transport of dietary lipids from the intestine to the tissues, allowing the synthesis of triglyceride-rich chylomicrons (Chester *et al.*, 2000).

It appears that the APOBEC1-mediated editing of ApoB RNA occurs in the nucleus (Lau *et al.*, 1991) and, similarly to AID, APOBEC1 shuttles between cytoplasm and nucleus using an N-terminal nuclear localization signal and a C-terminal export signal (Chester *et al.*, 2003; Yang and Smith, 1997; Yang *et al.*, 2001).

Although posttranscriptional base modification occurs widely in the biological world, APOBEC1-catalyzed editing of ApoB RNA is the only example identified to date of cytidine deamination being used physiologically in mammals to modify a protein-coding sequence. It is therefore something of a curiosity. APOBEC1 is necessary for ApoB RNA editing with APOBEC1-deficient mice exhibiting no obvious phenotype apart from a lack of ApoB mRNA editing (Hirano *et al.*, 1996; Morrison *et al.*, 1996; Nakamuta *et al.*, 1996). Nevertheless, the possibility cannot be excluded that APOBEC1 may also fulfill some other physiological role. In transfection assays, APOBEC1 has been shown to be able to act on retroviral substrates (Bishop *et al.*, 2004): biochemical assays reveal that recombinant APOBEC1 is able to deaminate cytidine in the context of a single-stranded DNA (as well as RNA) substrate (Harris *et al.*, 2002b; Morgan *et al.*, 2004; Petersen-Mahrt and Neuberger, 2003). Thus, it is conceivable, for example, that APOBEC1 may also function (or may have functioned in the past) as a viral restriction factor analogous to APOBEC3 family members. Such suggestions are, however, entirely speculative.

6. APOBEC2: A Muscle-Specific Family Member of Unknown Function/Activity

APOBEC2 was first identified on the basis of its sequence similarity to APOBEC1 (Anant *et al.*, 2001; Liao *et al.*, 1999). Apart from AID, it is the only AID/APOBEC family member for which evidence can readily be traced back to bony fish (Conticello *et al.*, 2005). Like AID, the sequence of APOBEC2 is well conserved through vertebrate lineages (Liao *et al.*, 1999; Sawyer *et al.*, 2004). Even in bony fish, where two paralogues of APOBEC2 are present, thus theoretically relieving the purifying selection in action on at least one of them, the two paralogues are still maintained with little sequence divergence.

This suggests that, like AID, the evolution of its amino acid sequence is constrained by the need to preserve its function—as opposed, for example, to the APOBEC3s whose rate of sequence evolution appears to be boosted by the arm race with their targets (Sawyer *et al.*, 2004; Zhang and Webb, 2004).

Despite this conservation of sequence, the physiological function of APOBEC2 remains unknown. The APOBEC2 gene is predominantly expressed in skeletal and cardiac muscle [although it has been shown that pro-inflammatory cytokines can induce its expression (Matsumoto *et al.*, 2006)]. APOBEC2-deficient mice do not present any major obvious phenotype (Mikl *et al.*, 2005), indicating that APOBEC2 is not essential for mouse development, health, and fertility. Attempts to ascribe any biochemical activity to APOBEC2 have also been unsuccessful: it does not appear able to edit ApoB RNA (Anant *et al.*, 2001; Liao *et al.*, 1999), it failed to exhibit any DNA deaminase activity in biochemical and genetic assays (Harris *et al.*, 2002b) and, despite early reports, failed to show any activity in deaminating free cytidine (Mikl *et al.*, 2005).

7. APOBEC4: A Distant or Ancestral Member of the AID/APOBEC Family

APOBEC4 was identified by bioinformatic analysis using the AID/APOBECs as queries in psi-BLAST searches: EST as well as array data show that it is probably expressed in testis (Rogozin *et al.*, 2005). Despite having apparently evolved more recently than AID and APOBEC2, it presents the most divergent architecture of all AID/APOBECs, harboring a very long extension C-terminal to the Zn-coordinating domain.

The APOBEC4 catalytic motif bears the Zn-coordinating residues and the glutamic acid characteristic of all the deaminases (H[PA]E–PC–C), but the spacing between the cysteines is different from that of the other AID/APOBECs. There are other important features around the Zn-coordination motif where APOBEC4 differs from all the other members of the AID/APOBEC family. Even though the amino acids within the Zn-coordinating domain are quite variable among the members of the AID/APOBEC family, they all share some specific residues in this region. In particular, a phenylalanine located shortly downstream of the HAE sequence as well as an SWS (or SSS in the case of APOBEC2) motif located just upstream of the PC–C are common. Indeed, mutations in the F or the SWS motif render the deaminases unable to work on polynucleotide substrates (Teng *et al.*, 1999; Langlois and Neuberger, unpublished data). However, both the conserved phenylalanine and the SWS motif are completely absent from APOBEC4. One could speculate whether APOBEC4, with all these differences from the other AID/APOBECs, might represent a distinct class of deaminases, or whether it might resemble an ancestral deaminase form from which the other AID/APOBECs evolved.

8. APOBEC3s: DNA Deaminases Active in Viral Restriction

The latest arrivals in the AID/APOBEC family are the APOBEC3s. These are the only other AID/APOBECs family members that are known to act *in vivo* to deaminate cytidine in DNA. Like AID, they appear to have an important role in the immune system. While AID targets endogenous DNA (the immunoglobulin genes) to generate antibody diversity in the adaptive immune system, APOBEC3s function in the innate immune system where they attack retroviral replication intermediates. The APOBEC3s provide an interesting comparison to AID in the context of targeted DNA deamination in immunity and therefore merit more detailed discussion.

8.1. APOBEC3G

8.1.1. Vif and the Identification of a Host Restriction Factor for HIV-1

In the years following the identification of HIV as the causative agent of acquired immune deficiency syndrome (AIDS) (Barré-Sinoussi *et al.*, 1983; Gallo *et al.*, 1983), the function of most of HIV's nine genes was rapidly identified. The function of HIV-1 *vif* gene product (virion infectivity factor), however, long remained elusive. Vif encodes a 23-kDa protein that is essential under physiological conditions for the production of infectious virions from the integrated HIV provirus. It was soon discovered, however, that Vif was not required for the production of infectious particles in various laboratory T-cell lines (Gabuzda *et al.*, 1992). T-cell lines could then be segregated in two categories depending if they were permissive or nonpermissive for the production of infectious HIV particles in the absence of a functional *vif* gene. Since the expression of Vif is essential only in the virus producer cell, it was then speculated that nonpermissive T cells either lacked an essential component for the production of infectious viral particles or expressed a factor that needed to be neutralized by Vif (Gabuzda *et al.*, 1992; Simon and Malim, 1996; von Schwedler *et al.*, 1993). The answer to this enigma came much later by the identification in nonpermissive cells of an innate antiretroviral factor initially named CEM15 (Sheehy *et al.*, 2002) and subsequently recognized as identical to the APOBEC3G (Jarmuz *et al.*, 2002). The ultimate demonstration that APOBEC3G was indeed responsible for restricting HIV infection came with an experiment showing that enforced expression of APOBEC3G in permissive CEM-SS cells reverted these to a nonpermissive phenotype (Sheehy *et al.*, 2002).

8.1.2. Deamination of Retroviral Replication Intermediates and Restriction of Infection

In contrast to the single-domained AID, APOBEC1, and APOBEC2 proteins, the architecture of APOBEC3G comprises two tandem Zn-coordination domains (Jarmuz et al., 2002). APOBEC3G shows DNA deaminase activity (with a distinct local sequence specificity from that of AID and APOBEC1) (Harris et al., 2002b) and can act in infected target cells when packaged into viral particles to heavily deaminate cytosines into uracils in nascent minus-strand viral DNA following retroviral reverse transcription (Harris et al., 2003; Lecossier et al., 2003; Mangeat et al., 2003; Mariani et al., 2003; Zhang et al., 2003). The uracils that are introduced in the viral DNA can then act as a template for the incorporation of adenines on the opposite plus-strand (Fig. 1B). Thus, the deaminase activity on the minus-strand can be deduced by the accumulation of G-to-A hypermutations mainly on the plus-strand viral DNA following second-strand synthesis. Not only can such hypermutation be detected *in vitro* using experimental systems: the frequent detection of G-to-A hypermutation in viral samples from HIV patients constitutes clear evidence that APOBEC3G does indeed act to deaminate the DNA of HIV-1 replication intermediates during natural infection (discussed in Beale et al., 2004).

A gradient has been noted of APOBEC3G-induced mutation along the proviral HIV cDNA (Chelico et al., 2006; Yu et al., 2004c). The highest level of hypermutation can be observed immediately 5′ of the polypurine tract (as read on the plus-strand DNA) and gradually fades toward the 5′-LTR region (Yu et al., 2004c). An apparent 3′ → 5′ directional processivity of APOBEC3G action can be explained by the slide and jump model of deamination proposed by the Goodman group who used various single-stranded DNA substrates flanking double-stranded DNA spacers to establish the kinetics of the deamination process (Chelico et al., 2006; Yu et al., 2004c).

Apart from binding and mutating single-stranded DNA, APOBEC3G has been shown to also bind RNA although there is no evidence for APOBEC3G-induced deamination of the viral genomic RNA of HIV-1: such deamination would lead to C-to-T hypermutation (as opposed to the G-to-A hypermutation characteristic of action on the first-strand cDNA replication intermediate) (Iwatani et al., 2006; Kozak et al., 2006; Lecossier et al., 2003; Yu et al., 2004c). Binding to RNA may, however, play a critical role in designating active or inactive forms of the protein. Chiu et al. (2005) have shown that APOBEC3G is ineffective in restricting HIV-1 infection in activated CD4+ cells because it apparently binds cellular RNAs to form high molecular mass complexes. However, in resting T cells or when extracts from activated T cells are treated with RNAse, APOBEC3G shifts to low molecular mass complexes where it appears to be active (Chelico et al., 2006; Chiu et al., 2005; Kreisberg et al., 2006).

APOBEC3G-mediated retroviral restriction is dependent on the presence of APOBEC3G in the viral producer cells (Harris et al., 2003; Lecossier et al., 2003; Mangeat et al., 2003; Mariani et al., 2003; von Schwedler et al., 1993; Zhang et al., 2003). Thus, to act as a retroviral restriction agent during reverse transcription in the target cell, APOBEC3G must first get encapsidated into the viral particle in the producer cells. Western blots performed on Vif-negative HIV virions clearly show the presence of APOBEC3G (Mariani et al., 2003). It has been reported that APOBEC3G is lured into assembling HIV particles essentially through interaction of its amino acids 104–156 located between the two Zn-coordination motifs and the nucleocapsid region of the retroviral Gag polyprotein precursor that is responsible for recruiting the viral genomic RNA (Alce and Popik, 2004; Cen et al., 2004; Svarovskaia et al., 2004). It has been strongly argued whether the genomic viral RNA is involved in this interaction, but now it is becoming increasingly likely that APOBEC3G incorporation can be achieved using RNA of either cellular or viral origin (Khan et al., 2005; Luo et al., 2004; Schäfer et al., 2004; Svarovskaia et al., 2004).

8.1.3. The Arms Race Between HIV and APOBEC3G

Primate lentiviruses appear to have evolved a mechanism to circumvent this innate APOBEC3G-mediated defense pathway by acquiring the *vif* gene. A clue as to how Vif neutralized APOBEC3G-mediated restriction came with the observations that APOBEC3G was absent from Vif-positive HIV particles and that APOBEC3G was rapidly degraded in Vif-expressing producer cells (Conticello et al., 2003; Marin et al., 2003; Mehle et al., 2004a; Sheehy et al., 2003; Stopak et al., 2003; Yu et al., 2003). Therefore, the role of Vif in nonpermissive cells is to prevent APOBEC3G encapsidation into viral particles. Vif then recruits an elongin B–elongin C–cullin 5 (E3 ubiquitin ligase) complex through the interaction of Vif BC box motif and elongin C (Kobayashi et al., 2005; Mehle et al., 2004b, 2006; Shirakawa et al., 2005; Yu et al., 2003). Vif acts as a bridge to target APOBEC3G, through its N-terminal domain, for ubiquitination and subsequent proteasomal degradation (Conticello et al., 2003; Marin et al., 2003; Mehle et al., 2004a; Sheehy et al., 2003; Stopak et al., 2003; Wichroski et al., 2006; Yu et al., 2003).

Their role in directly acting on HIV (and probably other pathogens) places the APOBEC3s under different evolutionary selective constraints from those operating on the ancestral AID/APOBECs. Thus, AID and APOBEC2 exhibit a high degree of conservation among the species with values as high as >50% identity between fish and mammalian AID (>70% similarity), suggesting a difficulty in tolerating mutations while retaining function. In contrast, the APOBEC3s show the hallmarks of positive selection (Sawyer et al., 2004; Zhang and Webb, 2004), presumably reflecting the distinctive selective pressures on these molecules as part of the arms race between host and pathogen. In support of this argument, it appears that the N-terminal domain of APOBEC3G, which undergoes the strongest positive selection, is the domain which is recognized in a species-specific way by the Vif proteins of different primate lentiviruses to trigger APOBEC3G degradation and overcome the host restriction (Bogerd et al., 2004; Conticello et al., 2003; Mangeat et al., 2004; Sawyer et al., 2004; Schröfelbauer et al., 2004; Xu et al., 2004; Zhang and Webb, 2004).

8.2. Other APOBEC3 Family Members

The APOBEC3 family has undergone a complex pattern of evolution. The ancestral APOBEC3 gene is presumed to have derived from a duplication of AID after the divergence of the marsupial and placental lineages: all of the APOBEC3s lack the 40-amino acid C-terminal domain characteristic of APOBEC1 and their primary sequence is overall closer to that of AID. This putative ancestral single-domained APOBEC3 gene appears soon to have been duplicated. Placentals then inherited these ancestral forms of the APOBEC3 gene that either fused together to form a single gene or remained independent. In primates, the evolution has been even more tortuous with the APOBEC3 locus now comprising eight genes: seven of which originate from one of the ancestral genes and the single-domained APOBEC3H being a direct descendant of the second ancestral gene only (Conticello et al., 2005).

Three members of the human APOBEC3 family have been shown to have significant antiretroviral activity on HIV-1 *in vitro* (Table 3). Interestingly, these are all double-domained deaminases (APOBEC3B, -F, and -G), although APOBEC3B is poorly expressed and is unlikely to play a significant role *in vivo* (Doehle et al., 2005; Yu et al., 2004b). A major hallmark of their retroviral activity is the presence of hypermutation in the targeted viral genome. APOBEC3F and APOBEC3G each has a particular sequence preference for deamination: APOBEC3G will preferentially deaminate a deoxycytidine if it is preceded by CC dinucleotide, whereas APOBEC3F prefers a deoxycytidine preceded by TT (Harris et al., 2003; Langlois et al., 2005; Mariani et al., 2003; Wiegand et al., 2004; Zheng et al., 2004). Modification of the protein sequence in a region downstream of the Zn-coordinating causes the deamination target-site consensus sequence to be altered, suggesting that this region is likely to be involved in substrate recognition (Langlois et al., 2005). APOBEC3B and APOBEC3C may possibly have a role in preventing zoonotic transmission of

Table 3 Characterized APOBEC3s

Human APOBEC3	Inhibition of retroviruses	Inhibition of other viruses	G → A hypermutation	Deamination context		
				−2	−1	0
A	−	+	N	−		
B	+	N.D.	Y	C/G	T	C
C	+	−	Y	T	C/T	C
D/E	+	N.D.	Y	T/A	T/A	C
F	+	+	Y	T	T	C
G	+	+	Y	C	C	C
H	−	N.D.	N	−		
Mouse A3	+	N.D.	Y	T	C	C

retroviruses. These APOBEC3s have been shown to have a potent antiretroviral activity on SIV *in vitro* (Yu *et al.*, 2004b).

The expansion of the APOBEC3 locus and the apparent positive selection might also have a broader significance. As discussed below, although first characterized as inhibitors of primate lentiviruses, the human APOBEC3 proteins can, in transfection assays, exhibit activity beyond lentiviral substrates and act on other types of retroviruses such as murine leukemia viruses, foamy viruses, as well as on retrotransposons (Delebecque *et al.*, 2006; Esnault *et al.*, 2005; Harris *et al.*, 2003; Löchelt *et al.*, 2005; Mariani *et al.*, 2003). It has also been proposed that AID itself, in addition to its major role in antibody gene diversification, may also function in an innate defense pathway against transforming retroviruses (Gourzi *et al.*, 2006). It will be interesting to learn whether these various observations in different experimental systems actually reflect physiologically significant *in vivo* restriction pathways.

8.3. Action of APOBEC3 Family Members on Viruses Other Than Retroviruses

Hepatitis B virus (HBV) is not a retrovirus; it contains a DNA genome that employs a reverse transcription step as part of its replication process. Studies performed on HBV have shown APOBEC3G (as well as APOBEC3B, -3C, and -3F; Table 3) to be capable of restricting viral replication in cotransfection experiments. Although G-to-A hypermutation of HBV has been seen occasionally in patients, the restriction seen *in vitro* is not accompanied by massive hypermutation loads in the viral genome. In fact, mutations are scarce at best *in vitro* (Noguchi *et al.*, 2005; Rösler *et al.*, 2005; Suspène *et al.*, 2005; Turelli *et al.*, 2004a). Human T-cell leukemia virus-1 (HTLV-1) is also found to be sensitive to restriction by APOBEC3G *in vitro* but with this restriction only rarely being accompanied by hypermutation: no mutated sequences so far have been found from HTLV-1 patients (Mahieux *et al.*, 2005; Sasada *et al.*, 2005). Finally, the case of APOBEC3G restricting the infectivity of the DNA virus adeno-associated virus (AAV) is another example of the APOBEC3 proteins exhibiting an antiviral effect *in vitro* without obvious signs of viral hypermutation (Chen *et al.*, 2006).

8.4. Action of APOBEC3 Family Members on LTR-Containing Endogenous Retroelements

There is a striking evolutionary coincidence, when comparing primates and rodents, between the abrupt drop in retrotransposon activity (Waterston *et al.*, 2002) and the expansion of the APOBEC3 gene cluster. Indeed, many APOBEC3s have been shown to be able to control the retrotransposition of mobile elements, at least as observed using assays in transfected, cultured cell lines (Table 4).

Retrotransposons are classified into two groups—those that bear long terminal repeats (LTRs), also known as endogenous retroviruses, and those that do not (non-LTRs). LTR retrotransposons are analogous to exogenous retroviruses in their replication cycle, and might therefore be expected to be vulnerable to similar host control measures. When tested in tissue culture transfection systems, retrotransposition of the active murine LTR retroelements intracisternal A-particle (IAP) and MusD could be downregulated by human APOBEC3A, -3B, -3C, -3F, -3G, human AID, African green monkey APOBEC3G, and mouse APOBEC3 (Bogerd *et al.*, 2006a; Chen *et al.*, 2006; Esnault *et al.*, 2005, 2006). There is no obvious correlation between the potencies of an APOBEC3 protein as an antiretroviral and as an antiretrotransposon. For example, APOBEC3A, which is not presently known to inhibit any retroviruses, was found to have the highest inhibitory activity against IAP (Bogerd *et al.*, 2006a). Whereas restriction of retrotransposition by most APOBEC3s in these assays is accompanied by an accumulation of G-to-A mutations in the integrated retrotransposon DNA (Bogerd *et al.*, 2006a; Esnault *et al.*, 2005, 2006), this was not the case for APOBEC3A (Bogerd *et al.*, 2006a; Chen *et al.*, 2006). Furthermore, mutations of the APOBEC3A Zn-binding and active sites reportedly had no effect on its ability to restrict IAP transposition (Bogerd *et al.*, 2006a). This suggested the possibility of an alternative, deaminase-independent pathway of retrotransposon restriction. In mediating the restriction, the APOBEC3s could access transposition intermediates via the retrotransposon Gag protein, since (similar to what has been observed with

Table 4 Effects of the APOBEC3s on Mobile Elements[a]

APOBEC3	Cellular localization	Inhibits LTR retrotransposons			Inhibits non-LTR retrotransposons		G → A hypermutation					Reduced proviral integration			Intact CDA activity required for inhibition			
		MusD	IAP	Ty1	L1	Alu	MusD	IAP	Ty1	L1	Alu	MusD	IAP	Ty1	MusD	IAP	Ty1	L1
A	N	+	+		+	+	−	−	−	−	−				+	−		+
B	N/C	+/−	+		+	+				−						−		+/−
C	N	+/−	+	+	+	+		+	−	−	−							
D/E	C				−			+		−	−							
F	C	+/−	+	+	−		+	+	+	−		+						
G	C	+	+/−	+	−		+	+	+			+	+	+				
H	N+C				−												+	
Mouse		+/−	+		+/−		+	+				+						

[a]Bogerd et al. (2006a,b), Chen et al. (2006), Dutko et al. (2005), Esnault et al. (2005, 2006), Muckenfuss et al. (2006), Schumacher et al. (2005), Stenglein and Harris (2006), and Turelli et al. (2004b).

retroviruses) APOBEC3G, -3B, and -3A have been shown to be able to interact with the IAP Gag (Bogerd et al., 2006a).

It has been proposed that the endogenous IAP and MusD sequences naturally present in the mouse genome bear evidence of GXA-to-AXA substitutions (Esnault et al., 2005), which shows some similarity to but is clearly distinct from the mAPOBEC3 sequence preference previously reported (Yu et al., 2004c). No such mutation patterns were observed in L1Md (murine LINE-1, a non-LTR retroelement) sequences analyzed. These observations, therefore, provide a measured degree of support to the idea that APOBEC3 proteins may indeed have played a role in the hypermutation of LTR (but not non-LTR) retroelements during their evolution in mouse, possibly also functioning to control such retrotransposition. However, APOBEC3-deficient mice breed well with little obvious phenotype indicating that maintaining an endogenous retrotransposition that is low enough to ensure viability, health, and fertility does not require APOBEC3 (Mikl et al., 2005).

In addition to an effect on mammalian retrotransposons, expression of human APOBEC3C, -3F, -3G, or of mouse APOBEC3 in yeast can lead to an inhibition of transposition of yeast Ty element constructs with accompanying G-to-A mutations on the Ty1 plus-strand (Dutko et al., 2005; Schumacher et al., 2005). These observations made using a Ty1 element transposition assay suggest that yeast might provide an attractive system in which to dissect aspects of APOBEC3 activity. However, since the APOBEC3s are clearly a vertebrate-specific gene family, the observations in yeast also caution that even if effects can be observed by enforced expression of APOBEC3 proteins in a contrived *in vitro* retrotransposition assay, care must be taken in extrapolating to conclusions regarding a natural physiological role in regulating transposition *in vivo*. The APOBEC3 proteins bind nucleic acid and artifactual effects of ectopic expression can readily be envisaged.

8.5. Action of APOBEC3 Family Members on Non-LTR-Containing Endogenous Retroelements

In the human genome, the L1 element is the only autonomous non-LTR retrotransposon with, on average, only 80–100 of the ~520,000 L1 copies being retrotransposition competent (Brouha et al., 2003; Lander et al., 2001). A functional full-length L1 element is ~6-kb long and includes two open-reading frames (ORFs) (Dombroski et al., 1991). Functional L1 ORF2 protein (ORF2p) can also mobilize nonautonomous non-LTR retrotransposons such as Alu in trans (Dewannieux et al., 2003).

Using cell line assays to monitor *in vitro* retrotransposition of L1 element constructs, it has been found that L1 transposition activity was reduced significantly by APOBEC3A, -3B, and -3C, but not by APOBEC3D, -3G, and -3H (Bogerd et al., 2006b; Chen et al., 2006; Esnault et al., 2005; Muckenfuss et al., 2006; Stenglein and Harris, 2006; Turelli et al., 2004b; Table 4). Contradicting results were obtained for APOBEC3F and mAPOBEC3. There appears to be no correlation between L1 restriction by an APOBEC3 protein and its intracellular localization, or the potency of its antiretroviral or anti-LTR retrotransposon activity (Bogerd et al., 2006b; Chen et al., 2006; Esnault et al., 2005; Muckenfuss et al., 2006; Stenglein and Harris, 2006; Turelli et al., 2004b). Transfected human APOBEC3A and -3B are also able to reduce Alu element mobility in cell line assays which utilize either a cotransfected full-length L1 or just its ORF2p-coding region. The restriction therefore appears to be independent of the retroviral Gag equivalent ORF1p (Bogerd et al., 2006b). APOBEC3B and -3F have similar inhibitory potentials, and are 96% identical between residues 66–190 and 65–189, respectively, whereas the remainders of the proteins share <57% identity. The corresponding region of APOBEC3G is <50% identical, and is required for association with HIV-1 Gag during encapsidation. Thus, it is possible that this region in APOBEC3B and -3F may mediate L1 and Alu inhibition by associating with ORF2p (Stenglein and Harris, 2006).

It appears that at least one intact Zn-coordination domain in both APOBEC3A and -3B is required in order to inhibit L1 retrotransposition (Bogerd et al., 2006b; Chen et al., 2006; Muckenfuss et al., 2006; Stenglein and Harris, 2006). Indeed, it is notable that the transposition-restricting activity of the APOBEC3B N-terminal domain (which displays no deaminase activity on its own) is destroyed by disruption of its Zn-binding consensus sequence. This is reminiscent of the requirement for a Zn-binding domain in the enzymatically inactive APOBEC3G N-terminus for efficient packaging of APOBEC3G into HIV-1 virions (Navarro et al., 2005; Newman et al., 2005). Furthermore, L1 retrotransposition appears similarly inhibited by wild-type APOBEC3B as by a catalytically dead mutant carrying amino acid substitutions outside the Zn-coordination domain (Stenglein and Harris, 2006). Perhaps the Zn-coordination domain sequence mediates L1 inhibition by APOBEC3A and -3B by allowing a specific interaction with L1 nucleic acid complexes (possibly involving the cytosine base), although enzymatic activity per se may not be important. In support of this, L1 or Alu elements retrotransposed in the presence of APOBEC3A, -3B, or -3C contained no detectable G-to-A hypermutations (Bogerd et al., 2006b; Stenglein and Harris, 2006), and no such footprints of cytidine deamination could be detected in 30 full-length pre-existing endogenous L1 sequences (Muckenfuss et al., 2006; Zingler et al., 2005). L1 cDNA integration was reduced in the presence of APOBEC3B (Stenglein and Harris, 2006) and so it seems that, at least in these assay systems,

APOBEC3 proteins can interfere with L1 retrotransposition at a step prior to integration and by a process that does not require DNA cytosine deamination.

To investigate the physiological relevance of the restriction of artificial L1 substrates by APOBEC3 proteins observed in these assays, Muckenfuss *et al.* (2006) knocked down expression of endogenous APOBEC3C in HeLa cells using a specific siRNA. Retrotransposition frequency of transfected L1 was found to increase by ~78%, compared to cells expressing a control siRNA. In order to propagate, retroelements must transpose in germ cells and/or during the earliest stages in human embryonic development (Moran *et al.*, 1996). RT-PCR analyses showed that both APOBEC3B and L1 mRNA, but not APOBEC3A mRNA, could be detected in three distinct undifferentiated human ES cell lines (Bogerd *et al.*, 2006b). It is possible, therefore, that APOBEC3B might exert an antiretrotransposon function in very early embryonic tissues, where novel L1 and Alu retrotransposition events could lead to new heritable insertions. Furthermore, immunohistochemistry data from Uhlén *et al.* (Uhlén and Ponten, 2005; Uhlén *et al.*, 2005) showed strong APOBEC3F expression in the seminiferous epithelium region of human testes, consistent with APOBEC3F possibly constituting a male germ cell-specific barrier to L1 retrotransposition.

Taken together, the data suggest that the inhibition of L1 transposition by APOBEC3s observed in these *in vitro* assays occurs by a mechanism distinct from cytidine deamination of the L1 genome. It is possible that the APOBEC3 proteins might interfere with RNP assembly in the cytoplasm, through sequestering RNA or protein, or by competitive binding. Alternatively, APOBEC3s could directly inhibit L1-encoded protein activity, or repress other steps of the L1 replication cycle, such as transcription, RNA export, or L1 protein translation. It remains to be established, however, whether the observations made using these *in vitro* culture systems reflect any natural role of APOBEC3 family members in the restriction of L1 element transposition *in vivo*.

8.6. Mechanism of APOBEC3-Mediated Restriction

All human APOBEC3 proteins except APOBEC3A and APOBEC3H have been shown to exhibit DNA deaminase activity coupled to antiretroviral activity *in vitro*. Their enzymatic activity targets retroviral replication intermediates to induce G-to-A hypermutations. Such hypermutations occur during natural HIV-1 infection in man, as witnessed by the existence of hypermutated HIV-1 sequences with the mutation patterns bearing the hallmarks of DNA deamination by APOBEC3 family members. Therefore, that some APOBEC3 family members can and do act on retroviral replication intermediates *in vivo* is not in doubt.

However, it is also clear that, at least in *in vitro* experimental assay systems, some APOBEC3 family members are capable of restricting the infectivity of retroviral and nonretroviral particles, as well as retroelement transposition by pathways that appear not to depend on DNA deamination. Major questions therefore arise associated with the issues of (1) Does DNA deamination underpin the major pathway of APOBEC3-mediated retroviral restriction and, if so, what is the restriction pathway downstream of the deamination event? (2) Does the DNA deamination-independent restriction observed using *in vitro* assays reflect a physiologically important pathway of retroelement restriction and, if so, how does it work?

With regard to deamination-dependent pathways of APOBEC3-mediated retrovirus restriction, it has been speculated that aside from causing deleterious mutations in the viral genome, the presence of uracils in the minus-strand DNA might lead to the recruitment of uracil-excision enzymes which would lead to the generation of abasic sites. Such abasic sites might compromise the processivity of the reverse-transcriptase or could provide a target for apurinic-apyrimidic endonucleases leading to the destruction of the viral cDNA before its genomic integration. If such mechanisms apply, then it is clear that the UNG2 enzyme cannot be the sole glycosylase responsible for uracil excision since experiments performed using a UNG-deficient human cell line revealed that UNG2 activity is dispensable for APOBEC3G-mediated restriction of HIV-1 infectivity (Kaiser and Emerman, 2006). Alternatively, it could be imagined that the deamination of the retroviral replication intermediates could restrict retroviral infectivity simply by virtue of its mutagenic effect on the viral genome or through some process involving recognition of the uracilation of the DNA replication intermediates that does not directly involve uracil excision.

With regard to possible deamination-independent pathways, these have been observed in cotransfection experiments using cultured cell lines and mutated APOBEC3G proteins that exhibit little or no deaminase activity but can nevertheless retain some ability to restrict retroviral infectivity (Bishop *et al.*, 2006; Iwatani *et al.*, 2006; Navarro *et al.*, 2005; Newman *et al.*, 2005; Opi *et al.*, 2006; Zhang *et al.*, 2003). This has been proposed to suggest that APOBEC3G (possibly by virtue of its RNA-binding capacity) may act as a retroviral restriction factor independently of its own deaminase activity, although these observations need to be extended to more physiological assays (Alce and Popik, 2004; Cen *et al.*, 2004; Iwatani *et al.*, 2006; Schäfer *et al.*, 2004; Svarovskaia *et al.*, 2004). Thus, mutants in the first, second, or both Zn-binding domains of APOBEC3G have mapped the RNA-binding region to the first domain of APOBEC3G and the main contributor to the cytidine deaminase activity on DNA to the second domain (Bishop *et al.*, 2006; Iwatani *et al.*, 2006; Navarro *et al.*,

2005; Newman *et al.*, 2005; Opi *et al.*, 2006; Zhang *et al.*, 2003). The viral restriction activity of APOBEC3G is severely compromised by mutation of the Zn-binding motif in the second domain but much less so by mutation of the first domain. It is only when both domains of the protein are mutated that deaminase activity and the viral restriction can both completely be abolished. It is also becoming clear that the potency of retroviral inhibition does not correlate with the hypermutation load, although it is possible that just a few deamination events in the viral genome could suffice to induce restriction (Bishop *et al.*, 2006; Iwatani *et al.*, 2006; Navarro *et al.*, 2005; Opi *et al.*, 2006).

Taken together with analogous studies on APOBEC3-mediated restriction of retroelement transposition discussed above, it seems probable that—at least following enforced expression in cell culture systems—the APOBEC3s are able to act on retroviruses/retroelements by pathways that do not require cytidine deamination. While one could readily imagine numerous other ways by which APOBEC3 proteins could act (presumably involving protein–protein or DNA–RNA interaction) such pathways remain to be delineated and their importance in physiological situations (especially in the absence of enforced overexpression) remains to be assessed.

9. Conclusion

The AID/APOBEC family of polynucleotide deaminases constitutes a vertebrate-restricted grouping related to a larger deaminase superfamily. With regard to structure, the AID/APOBEC proteins have conventionally be compared to deaminases active on free cytidine; some of the deaminases active on cytosine or tRNA are likely, however, to provide better paradigms. With regard to function, although AID, APOBEC1 and APOBEC3s are all able to deaminate DNA *in vitro*, only in the case of AID and APOBEC3s is it clear that such deamination also occurs *in vivo*. Whereas DNA deamination is central to the activity of AID in antibody diversification and of APOBEC3s in retroviral hypermutation, the molecular mechanism by which the APOBEC3s restrict retroviral infection remains to be elucidated.

References

Alce, T. M., and Popik, W. (2004). APOBEC3G is incorporated into virus-like particles by a direct interaction with HIV-1 Gag nucleocapsid protein. *J. Biol. Chem.* **279**, 34083–34086.

Anant, S., and Davidson, N. O. (2000). An AU-rich sequence element (UUUN[A/U]U) downstream of the edited C in apolipoprotein B mRNA is a high-affinity binding site for Apobec-1: Binding of Apobec-1 to this motif in the 3′ untranslated region of c-myc increases mRNA stability. *Mol. Cell. Biol.* **20**, 1982–1992.

Anant, S., Mukhopadhyay, D., Sankaranand, V., Kennedy, S., Henderson, J. O., and Davidson, N. O. (2001). ARCD-1, an apobec-1-related cytidine deaminase, exerts a dominant negative effect on C to U RNA editing. *Am. J. Physiol. Cell Physiol.* **281,** C1904–C1916.

Arakawa, H., Hauschild, J., and Buerstedde, J. M. (2002). Requirement of the activation-induced deaminase (AID) gene for immunoglobulin gene conversion. *Science* **295,** 1301–1306.

Auxilien, S., Crain, P. F., Trewyn, R. W., and Grosjean, H. (1996). Mechanism, specificity and general properties of the yeast enzyme catalysing the formation of inosine 34 in the anticodon of transfer RNA. *J. Mol. Biol.* **262,** 437–458.

Barré-Sinoussi, F., Chermann, J. C., Rey, F., Nugeyre, M. T., Chamaret, S., Gruest, J., Dauguet, C., Axler-Blin, C., Vézinet-Brun, F., Rouzioux, C., Rozenbaum, W., and Montagnier, L. (1983). Isolation of a T-lymphotropic retrovirus from a patient at risk for acquired immune deficiency syndrome (AIDS). *Science* **220,** 868–871.

Bass, B. L. (2002). RNA editing by adenosine deaminases that act on RNA. *Annu. Rev. Biochem.* **71,** 817–846.

Beale, R. C., Petersen-Mahrt, S. K., Watt, I. N., Harris, R. S., Rada, C., and Neuberger, M. S. (2004). Comparison of the differential context-dependence of DNA deamination by APOBEC enzymes: Correlation with mutation spectra *in vivo. J. Mol. Biol.* **337,** 585–596.

Betts, L., Xiang, S., Short, S. A., Wolfenden, R., and Carter, C. W. (1994). Cytidine deaminase. The 2.3 Å crystal structure of an enzyme: Transition-state analog complex. *J. Mol. Biol.* **235,** 635–656.

Bishop, K. N., Holmes, R. K., Sheehy, A. M., and Malim, M. H. (2004). APOBEC-mediated editing of viral RNA. *Science* **305,** 645.

Bishop, K. N., Holmes, R. K., and Malim, M. H. (2006). Antiviral potency of APOBEC proteins does not correlate with cytidine deamination. *J. Virol.* **80,** 8450–8458.

Bogerd, H. P., Doehle, B. P., Wiegand, H. L., and Cullen, B. R. (2004). A single amino acid difference in the host APOBEC3G protein controls the primate species specificity of HIV type 1 virion infectivity factor. *Proc. Natl. Acad. Sci. USA* **101,** 3770–3774.

Bogerd, H. P., Wiegand, H. L., Doehle, B. P., Lueders, K. K., and Cullen, B. R. (2006a). APOBEC3A and APOBEC3B are potent inhibitors of LTR-retrotransposon function in human cells. *Nucleic Acids Res.* **34,** 89–95.

Bogerd, H. P., Wiegand, H. L., Hulme, A. E., Garcia-Perez, J. L., O'shea, K. S., Moran, J. V., and Cullen, B. R. (2006b). Cellular inhibitors of long interspersed element 1 and Alu retrotransposition. *Proc. Natl. Acad. Sci. USA* **103,** 8780–8785.

Branstetter, R., Pham, P., Scharff, M. D., and Goodman, M. F. (2003). Activation-induced cytidine deaminase deaminates deoxycytidine on single-stranded DNA but requires the action of RNase. *Proc. Natl. Acad. Sci. USA* **100,** 4102–4107.

Brenner, S., and Milstein, C. (1966). Origin of antibody variation. *Nature* **211,** 242–243.

Brouha, B., Schustak, J., Badge, R. M., Lutz-Prigge, S., Farley, A. H., Moran, J. V., and Kazazian, H. H. (2003). Hot L1s account for the bulk of retrotransposition in the human population. *Proc. Natl. Acad. Sci. USA* **100,** 5280–5285.

Carlow, D., and Wolfenden, R. (1998). Substrate connectivity effects in the transition state for cytidine deaminase. *Biochemistry* **37,** 11873–11878.

Carter, C. W. (1995). The nucleoside deaminases for cytidine and adenosine: Structure, transition state stabilization, mechanism, and evolution. *Biochimie* **77,** 92–98.

Cen, S., Guo, F., Niu, M., Saadatmand, J., Deflassieux, J., and Kleiman, L. (2004). The interaction between HIV-1 Gag and APOBEC3G. *J. Biol. Chem.* **279,** 33177–33184.

Chaudhuri, J., Tian, M., Khuong, C., Chua, K., Pinaud, E., and Alt, F. W. (2003). Transcription-targeted DNA deamination by the AID antibody diversification enzyme. *Nature* **422,** 726–730.

Chelico, L., Pham, P., Calabrese, P., and Goodman, M. F. (2006). APOBEC3G DNA deaminase acts processively 3′–5′ on single-stranded DNA. *Nat. Struct. Mol. Biol.* **13**, 392–399.

Chen, H., Lilley, C. E., Yu, Q., Lee, D. V., Chou, J., Narvaiza, I., Landau, N. R., and Weitzman, M. D. (2006). APOBEC3A is a potent inhibitor of adeno-associated virus and retrotransposons. *Curr. Biol.* **16**, 480–485.

Chester, A., Scott, J., Anant, S., and Navaratnam, N. (2000). RNA editing: Cytidine to uridine conversion in apolipoprotein B mRNA. *Biochim. Biophys. Acta* **1494**, 1–13.

Chester, A., Somasekaram, A., Tzimina, M., Jarmuz, A., Gisbourne, J., O'Keefe, R., Scott, J., and Navaratnam, N. (2003). The apolipoprotein B mRNA editing complex performs a multifunctional cycle and suppresses nonsense-mediated decay. *EMBO J.* **22**, 3971–3982.

Chiu, Y. L., Soros, V. B., Kreisberg, J. F., Stopak, K., Yonemoto, W., and Greene, W. C. (2005). Cellular APOBEC3G restricts HIV-1 infection in resting CD4(+) T cells. *Nature* **435**, 108–114.

Conticello, S. G., Harris, R. S., and Neuberger, M. S. (2003). The Vif protein of HIV triggers degradation of the human antiretroviral DNA deaminase APOBEC3G. *Curr. Biol.* **13**, 2009–2013.

Conticello, S. G., Thomas, C. J., Petersen-Mahrt, S. K., and Neuberger, M. S. (2005). Evolution of the AID/APOBEC family of polynucleotide (deoxy)cytidine deaminases. *Mol. Biol. Evol.* **22**, 367–377.

Delebecque, F., Suspène, R., Calattini, S., Casartelli, N., Saïb, A., Froment, A., Wain-Hobson, S., Gessain, A., Vartanian, J. P., and Schwartz, O. (2006). Restriction of foamy viruses by APOBEC cytidine deaminases. *J. Virol.* **80**, 605–614.

Dewannieux, M., Esnault, C., and Heidmann, T. (2003). LINE-mediated retrotransposition of marked Alu sequences. *Nat. Genet.* **35**, 41–48.

Di Noia, J., and Neuberger, M. S. (2002). Altering the pathway of immunoglobulin hypermutation by inhibiting uracil-DNA glycosylase. *Nature* **419**, 43–48.

Di Noia, J. M., and Neuberger, M. S. (2004). Immunoglobulin gene conversion in chicken DT40 cells largely proceeds through an abasic site intermediate generated by excision of the uracil produced by AID-mediated deoxycytidine deamination. *Eur. J. Immunol.* **34**, 504–508.

Di Noia, J., and Neuberger, M. S. (2007). Molecular mechanisms of antibody somatic hypermutation. *Ann. Rev. Biochem.* **76** (in press).

Dickerson, S. K., Market, E., Besmer, E., and Papavasiliou, F. N. (2003). AID mediates hypermutation by deaminating single stranded DNA. *J. Exp. Med.* **197**, 1291–1296.

Doehle, B. P., Schäfer, A., Wiegand, H. L., Bogerd, H. P., and Cullen, B. R. (2005). Differential sensitivity of murine leukemia virus to APOBEC3-mediated inhibition is governed by virion exclusion. *J. Virol.* **79**, 8201–8207.

Dombroski, B. A., Mathias, S. L., Nanthakumar, E., Scott, A. F., and Kazazian, H. H. (1991). Isolation of an active human transposable element. *Science* **254**, 1805–1808.

Dutko, J. A., Schäfer, A., Kenny, A. E., Cullen, B. R., and Curcio, M. J. (2005). Inhibition of a yeast LTR retrotransposon by human APOBEC3 cytidine deaminases. *Curr. Biol.* **15**, 661–666.

Ehrenstein, M. R., and Neuberger, M. S. (1999). Deficiency in Msh2 affects the efficiency and local sequence specificity of immunoglobulin class-switch recombination: Parallels with somatic hypermutation. *EMBO J.* **18**, 3484–3490.

Elias, Y., and Huang, R. H. (2005). Biochemical and structural studies of A-to-I editing by tRNA: A34 deaminases at the wobble position of transfer RNA(,). *Biochemistry* **44**, 12057–12065.

Esnault, C., Heidmann, O., Delebecque, F., Dewannieux, M., Ribet, D., Hance, A. J., Heidmann, T., and Schwartz, O. (2005). APOBEC3G cytidine deaminase inhibits retrotransposition of endogenous retroviruses. *Nature* **433**, 430–433.

Esnault, C., Millet, J., Schwartz, O., and Heidmann, T. (2006). Dual inhibitory effects of APOBEC family proteins on retrotransposition of mammalian endogenous retroviruses. *Nucleic Acids Res.* **34,** 1522–1531.

Fujino, T., Navaratnam, N., Jarmuz, A., von Haeseler, A., and Scott, J. (1999). C → U editing of apolipoprotein B mRNA in marsupials: Identification and characterisation of APOBEC-1 from the American opossum Monodelphus domestica. *Nucleic Acids Res.* **27,** 2662–2671.

Gabuzda, D. H., Lawrence, K., Langhoff, E., Terwilliger, E., Dorfman, T., Haseltine, W. A., and Sodroski, J. (1992). Role of vif in replication of human immunodeficiency virus type 1 in CD4+ T lymphocytes. *J. Virol.* **66,** 6489–6495.

Gallo, R. C., Sarin, P. S., Gelmann, E. P., Robert-Guroff, M., Richardson, E., Kalyanaraman, V. S., Mann, D., Sidhu, G. D., Stahl, R. E., Zolla-Pazner, S., Leibowitch, J., and Popovic, M. (1983). Isolation of human T-cell leukemia virus in acquired immune deficiency syndrome (AIDS). *Science* **220,** 865–867.

Gerber, A., Grosjean, H., Melcher, T., and Keller, W. (1998). Tad1p, a yeast tRNA-specific adenosine deaminase, is related to the mammalian pre-mRNA editing enzymes ADAR1 and ADAR2. *EMBO J.* **17,** 4780–4789.

Gerber, A. P., and Keller, W. (1999). An adenosine deaminase that generates inosine at the wobble position of tRNAs. *Science* **286,** 1146–1149.

Gourzi, P., Leonova, T., and Papavasiliou, F. N. (2006). A role for activation-induced cytidine deaminase in the host response against a transforming retrovirus. *Immunity* **24,** 779–786.

Harris, R. S., Petersen-Mahrt, S. K., and Neuberger, M. S. (2002a). RNA editing enzyme APOBEC1 and some of its homologs can act as DNA mutators. *Mol. Cell* **10,** 1247–1253.

Harris, R. S., Sale, J. E., Petersen-Mahrt, S. K., and Neuberger, M. S. (2002b). AID is essential for immunoglobulin V gene conversion in a cultured B cell line. *Curr. Biol.* **12,** 435–438.

Harris, R. S., Bishop, K. N., Sheehy, A. M., Craig, H. M., Petersen-Mahrt, S. K., Watt, I. N., Neuberger, M. S., and Malim, M. H. (2003). DNA deamination mediates innate immunity to retroviral infection. *Cell* **113,** 803–809.

Hirano, K., Young, S. G., Farese, R. V., Ng, J., Sande, E., Warburton, C., Powell-Braxton, L. M., and Davidson, N. O. (1996). Targeted disruption of the mouse apobec-1 gene abolishes apolipoprotein B mRNA editing and eliminates apolipoprotein B48. *J. Biol. Chem.* **271,** 9887–9890.

Imai, K., Slupphaug, G., Lee, W. I., Revy, P., Nonoyama, S., Catalan, N., Yel, L., Forveille, M., Kavli, B., Krokan, H. E., Ochs, H. D., Fischer, A., et al. (2003). Human uracil-DNA glycosylase deficiency associated with profoundly impaired immunoglobulin class-switch recombination. *Nat. Immunol.* **4,** 1023–108.

Ipata, P. L., and Cercignani, G. (1978). Cytosine and cytidine deaminase from yeast. *Methods Enzymol.* **51,** 394–400.

Ireton, G. C., McDermott, G., Black, M. E., and Stoddard, B. L. (2002). The structure of *Escherichia coli* cytosine deaminase. *J. Mol. Biol.* **315,** 687–697.

Ireton, G. C., Black, M. E., and Stoddard, B. L. (2003). The 1.14 A crystal structure of yeast cytosine deaminase: Evolution of nucleotide salvage enzymes and implications for genetic chemotherapy. *Structure* **11,** 961–972.

Iwatani, Y., Takeuchi, H., Strebel, K., and Levin, J. G. (2006). Biochemical activities of highly purified, catalytically active human APOBEC3G: Correlation with antiviral effect. *J. Virol.* **80,** 5992–6002.

Jarmuz, A., Chester, A., Bayliss, J., Gisbourne, J., Dunham, I., Scott, J., and Navaratnam, N. (2002). An anthropoid-specific locus of orphan C to U RNA-editing enzymes on chromosome 22. *Genomics* **79,** 285–296.

Johansson, E., Mejlhede, N., Neuhard, J., and Larsen, S. (2002). Crystal structure of the tetrameric cytidine deaminase from *Bacillus subtilis* at 2.0 A resolution. *Biochemistry* **41**, 2563–2570.

Johansson, E., Fanø, M., Bynck, J. H., Neuhard, J., Larsen, S., Sigurskjold, B. W., Christensen, U., and Willemoës, M. (2005). Structures of dCTP deaminase from *Escherichia coli* with bound substrate and product: Reaction mechanism and determinants of mono- and bifunctionality for a family of enzymes. *J. Biol. Chem.* **280**, 3051–3059.

Kaiser, S. M., and Emerman, M. (2006). Uracil DNA glycosylase is dispensable for human immunodeficiency virus type 1 replication and does not contribute to the antiviral effects of the cytidine deaminase Apobec3G. *J. Virol.* **80**, 875–882.

Keller, W., Wolf, J., and Gerber, A. (1999). Editing of messenger RNA precursors and of tRNAs by adenosine to inosine conversion. *FEBS Lett.* **452**, 71–76.

Khan, M. A., Kao, S., Miyagi, E., Takeuchi, H., Goila-Gaur, R., Opi, S., Gipson, C. L., Parslow, T. G., Ly, H., and Strebel, K. (2005). Viral RNA is required for the association of APOBEC3G with human immunodeficiency virus type 1 nucleoprotein complexes. *J. Virol.* **79**, 5870–5874.

Kim, J., Malashkevich, V., Roday, S., Lisbin, M., Schramm, V. L., and Almo, S. C. (2006). Structural and kinetic characterization of *Escherichia coli* TadA, the Wobble-specific tRNA deaminase. *Biochemistry* **45**, 6407–6416.

Ko, T. P., Lin, J. J., Hu, C. Y., Hsu, Y. H., Wang, A. H., and Liaw, S. H. (2003). Crystal structure of yeast cytosine deaminase. Insights into enzyme mechanism and evolution. *J. Biol. Chem.* **278**, 19111–19117.

Kobayashi, M., Takaori-Kondo, A., Miyauchi, Y., Iwai, K., and Uchiyama, T. (2005). Ubiquitination of APOBEC3G by an HIV-1 Vif-cullin5-elonginB-elonginC complex is essential for Vif function. *J. Biol. Chem.* **280**, 18573–18578.

Kozak, S. L., Marin, M., Rose, K. M., Bystrom, C., and Kabat, D. (2006). The anti-HIV-1 editing enzyme APOBEC3G Binds HIV-1 RNA and messenger RNAs that shuttle between polysomes and stress granules. *J. Biol. Chem.* **281**, 29105–29119.

Kreisberg, J. F., Yonemoto, W., and Greene, W. C. (2006). Endogenous factors enhance HIV infection of tissue naive CD4 T cells by stimulating high molecular mass APOBEC3G complex formation. *J. Exp. Med.* **203**, 865–870.

Kuratani, M., Ishii, R., Bessho, Y., Fukunaga, R., Sengoku, T., Sekine, S. I., and Yokoyama, S. (2005). Crystal structure of tRNA adenosine deaminase TadA from aquifex aeolicus. *J. Biol. Chem.* **280**, 16002–16008.

Lander, E. S., Linton, L. M., Birren, B., Nusbaum, C., Zody, M. C., Baldwin, J., Devon, K., Dewar, K., Doyle, M., FitzHugh, W., Funke, R., Gage, D., *et al.* (2001). Initial sequencing and analysis of the human genome. *Nature* **409**, 860–921.

Langlois, M. A., Beale, R. C., Conticello, S. G., and Neuberger, M. S. (2005). Mutational comparison of the single-domained APOBEC3C and double-domained APOBEC3F/G antiretroviral cytidine deaminases provides insight into their DNA target site specificities. *Nucleic Acids Res.* **33**, 1913–1923.

Lau, P. P., Xiong, W. J., Zhu, H. J., Chen, S. H., and Chan, L. (1991). Apolipoprotein B mRNA editing is an intranuclear event that occurs posttranscriptionally coincident with splicing and polyadenylation. *J. Biol. Chem.* **266**, 20550–20554.

Lecossier, D., Bouchonnet, F., Clavel, F., and Hance, A. J. (2003). Hypermutation of HIV-1 DNA in the absence of the Vif protein. *Science* **300**, 1112.

Liao, W., Hong, S. H., Chan, B. H., Rudolph, F. B., Clark, S. C., and Chan, L. (1999). APOBEC-2, a cardiac- and skeletal muscle-specific member of the cytidine deaminase supergene family. *Biochem. Biophys. Res. Commun.* **260**, 398–404.

Losey, H. C., Ruthenburg, A. J., and Verdine, G. L. (2006). Crystal structure of *Staphylococcus aureus* tRNA adenosine deaminase TadA in complex with RNA. *Nat. Struct. Mol. Biol.* **13**, 153–159.

Löchelt, M., Romen, F., Bastone, P., Muckenfuss, H., Kirchner, N., Kim, Y. B., Truyen, U., Rösler, U., Battenberg, M., Saib, A., Flory, E., Cichutek, K., *et al.* (2005). The antiretroviral activity of APOBEC3 is inhibited by the foamy virus accessory Bet protein. *Proc. Natl. Acad. Sci. USA* **102**, 7982–7987.

Longerich, S., Basu, U., Alt, F., and Storb, U. (2006). AID in somatic hypermutation and class switch recombination. *Curr. Opin. Immunol.* **18**, 164–174.

Luo, K., Liu, B., Xiao, Z., Yu, Y., Yu, X., Gorelick, R., and Yu, X. F. (2004). Amino-terminal region of the human immunodeficiency virus type 1 nucleocapsid is required for human APOBEC3G packaging. *J. Virol.* **78**, 11841–11852.

Mahieux, R., Suspène, R., Delebecque, F., Henry, M., Schwartz, O., Wain-Hobson, S., and Vartanian, J. P. (2005). Extensive editing of a small fraction of human T-cell leukemia virus type 1 genomes by four APOBEC3 cytidine deaminases. *J. Gen. Virol.* **86**, 2489–2494.

Maizels, N. (1995). Somatic hypermutation: How many mechanisms diversify V region sequences? *Cell* **83**, 9–12.

Mangeat, B., Turelli, P., Caron, G., Friedli, M., Perrin, L., and Trono, D. (2003). Broad antiretroviral defence by human APOBEC3G through lethal editing of nascent reverse transcripts. *Nature* **424**, 99–103.

Mangeat, B., Turelli, P., Liao, S., and Trono, D. (2004). A single amino acid determinant governs the species-specific sensitivity of APOBEC3G to Vif action. *J. Biol. Chem.* **279**, 14481–14483.

Mariani, R., Chen, D., Schröfelbauer, B., Navarro, F., König, R., Bollman, B., Münk, C., Nymark-McMahon, H., and Landau, N. R. (2003). Species-specific exclusion of APOBEC3G from HIV-1 virions by Vif. *Cell* **114**, 21–31.

Marin, M., Rose, K. M., Kozak, S. L., and Kabat, D. (2003). HIV-1 Vif protein binds the editing enzyme APOBEC3G and induces its degradation. *Nat. Med.* **9**, 1398–1403.

Maris, C., Masse, J., Chester, A., Navaratnam, N., and Allain, F. H. (2005). NMR structure of the apoB mRNA stem-loop and its interaction with the C to U editing APOBEC1 complementary factor. *RNA* **11**, 173–186.

Matsumoto, T., Marusawa, H., Endo, Y., Ueda, Y., Matsumoto, Y., and Chiba, T. (2006). Expression of APOBEC2 is transcriptionally regulated by NF-kappaB in human hepatocytes. *FEBS Lett.* **580**, 731–735.

Mehle, A., Goncalves, J., Santa-Marta, M., McPike, M., and Gabuzda, D. (2004a). Phosphorylation of a novel SOCS-box regulates assembly of the HIV-1 Vif-Cul5 complex that promotes APOBEC3G degradation. *Genes Dev.* **18**, 2861–2866.

Mehle, A., Strack, B., Ancuta, P., Zhang, C., McPike, M., and Gabuzda, D. (2004b). Vif overcomes the innate antiviral activity of APOBEC3G by promoting its degradation in the ubiquitin-proteasome pathway. *J. Biol. Chem.* **279**, 7792–7798.

Mehle, A., Thomas, E. R., Rajendran, K. S., and Gabuzda, D. (2006). A zinc-binding region in Vif binds CUL5 and determines cullin selection. *J. Biol. Chem.* **281**, 17259–17265.

Mikl, M. C., Watt, I. N., Lu, M., Reik, W., Davies, S. L., Neuberger, M. S., and Rada, C. (2005). Mice deficient in APOBEC2 and APOBEC3. *Mol. Cell. Biol.* **25**, 7270–7277.

Moran, J. V., Holmes, S. E., Naas, T. P., DeBerardinis, R. J., Boeke, J. D., and Kazazian, H. H. (1996). High frequency retrotransposition in cultured mammalian cells. *Cell* **87**, 917–927.

Morgan, H. D., Dean, W., Coker, H. A., Reik, W., and Petersen-Mahrt, S. K. (2004). Activation-induced cytidine deaminase deaminates 5-methylcytosine in DNA and is expressed in pluripotent tissues: Implications for epigenetic reprogramming. *J. Biol. Chem.* **279**, 52353–52360.

Morrison, J. R., Pászty, C., Stevens, M. E., Hughes, S. D., Forte, T., Scott, J., and Rubin, E. M. (1996). Apolipoprotein B RNA editing enzyme-deficient mice are viable despite alterations in lipoprotein metabolism. *Proc. Natl. Acad. Sci. USA* **93**, 7154–7159.

Muckenfuss, H., Hamdorf, M., Held, U., Perkovic, M., Löwer, J., Cichutek, K., Flory, E., Schumann, G. G., and Münk, C. (2006). APOBEC3 proteins inhibit human LINE-1 retrotransposition. *J. Biol. Chem.* **281**, 22161–22172.

Muramatsu, M., Sankaranand, V. S., Anant, S., Sugai, M., Kinoshita, K., Davidson, N. O., and Honjo, T. (1999). Specific expression of activation-induced cytidine deaminase (AID), a novel member of the RNA-editing deaminase family in germinal center B cells. *J. Biol. Chem.* **274**, 18470–18476.

Muramatsu, M., Kinoshita, K., Fagarasan, S., Yamada, S., Shinkai, Y., and Honjo, T. (2000). Class switch recombination and hypermutation require activation-induced cytidine deaminase (AID), a potential RNA editing enzyme. *Cell* **102**, 553–563.

Nakamuta, M., Chang, B. H., Zsigmond, E., Kobayashi, K., Lei, H., Ishida, B. Y., Oka, K., Li, E., and Chan, L. (1996). Complete phenotypic characterization of apobec-1 knockout mice with a wild-type genetic background and a human apolipoprotein B transgenic background, and restoration of apolipoprotein B mRNA editing by somatic gene transfer of Apobec-1. *J. Biol. Chem.* **271**, 25981–25988.

Navaratnam, N., Morrison, J. R., Bhattacharya, S., Patel, D., Funahashi, T., Giannoni, F., Teng, B. B., Davidson, N. O., and Scott, J. (1993). The p27 catalytic subunit of the apolipoprotein B mRNA editing enzyme is a cytidine deaminase. *J. Biol. Chem.* **268**, 20709–20712.

Navarro, F., Bollman, B., Chen, H., König, R., Yu, Q., Chiles, K., and Landau, N. R. (2005). Complementary function of the two catalytic domains of APOBEC3G. *Virology* **333**, 374–386.

Neuberger, M. S., Harris, R. S., Di Noia, J., and Petersen-Mahrt, S. K. (2003). Immunity through DNA deamination. *Trends Biochem. Sci.* **28**, 305–312.

Newman, E. N., Holmes, R. K., Craig, H. M., Klein, K. C., Lingappa, J. R., Malim, M. H., and Sheehy, A. M. (2005). Antiviral function of APOBEC3G can be dissociated from cytidine deaminase activity. *Curr. Biol.* **15**, 166–170.

Nishiyama, T., Kawamura, Y., Kawamoto, K., Matsumura, H., Yamamoto, N., Ito, T., Ohyama, A., Katsuragi, T., and Sakai, T. (1985). Antineoplastic effects in rats of 5-fluorocytosine in combination with cytosine deaminase capsules. *Cancer Res.* **45**, 1753–1761.

Noguchi, C., Ishino, H., Tsuge, M., Fujimoto, Y., Imamura, M., Takahashi, S., and Chayama, K. (2005). G to A hypermutation of hepatitis B virus. *Hepatology* **41**, 626–633.

Opi, S., Takeuchi, H., Kao, S., Khan, M. A., Miyagi, E., Goila-Gaur, R., Iwatani, Y., Levin, J. G., and Strebel, K. (2006). Monomeric APOBEC3G is catalytically active and has antiviral activity. *J. Virol.* **80**, 4673–4682.

Petersen-Mahrt, S. K., and Neuberger, M. S. (2003). In vitro deamination of cytosine to uracil in single-stranded DNA by apolipoprotein B editing complex catalytic subunit 1 (APOBEC1). *J. Biol. Chem.* **278**, 19583–19586.

Petersen-Mahrt, S. K., Harris, R. S., and Neuberger, M. S. (2002). AID mutates *E. coli* suggesting a DNA deamination mechanism for antibody diversification. *Nature* **418**, 99–103.

Pham, P., Bransteitter, R., Petruska, J., and Goodman, M. F. (2003). Processive AID-catalysed cytosine deamination on single-stranded DNA simulates somatic hypermutation. *Nature* **424**, 103–107.

Rada, C., Ehrenstein, M. R., Neuberger, M. S., and Milstein, C. (1998). Hot spot focusing of somatic hypermutation in MSH2-deficient mice suggests two stages of mutational targeting. *Immunity* **9**, 135–141.

Rada, C., Williams, G. T., Nilsen, H., Barnes, D. E., Lindahl, T., and Neuberger, M. S. (2002). Immunoglobulin isotype switching is inhibited and somatic hypermutation perturbed in UNG-deficient mice. *Curr. Biol.* **12**, 1748–1755.

Rada, C., Di Noia, J. M., and Neuberger, M. S. (2004). Mismatch recognition and uracil excision provide complementary paths to both Ig switching and the A/T-focused phase of somatic mutation. *Mol. Cell* **16**, 163–171.

Ramiro, A. R., Stavropoulos, P., Jankovic, M., and Nussenzweig, M. C. (2003). Transcription enhances AID-mediated cytidine deamination by exposing single-stranded DNA on the nontemplate strand. *Nat. Immunol.* **4**, 452–456.

Revy, P., Muto, T., Levy, Y., Geissmann, F., Plebani, A., Sanal, O., Catalan, N., Forveille, M., Dufourcq-Labelouse, R., Gennery, A., Tezcan, I., Ersoy, F., et al. (2000). Activation-induced cytidine deaminase (AID) deficiency causes the autosomal recessive form of the Hyper-IgM syndrome (HIGM2). *Cell* **102**, 565–575.

Richardson, N., Navaratnam, N., and Scott, J. (1998). Secondary structure for the apolipoprotein B mRNA editing site. Au-binding proteins interact with a stem loop. *J. Biol. Chem.* **273**, 31707–31717.

Rogozin, I. B., Basu, M. K., Jordan, I. K., Pavlov, Y. I., and Koonin, E. V. (2005). APOBEC4, a new member of the AID/APOBEC family of polynucleotide (Deoxy)cytidine deaminases predicted by computational analysis. *Cell Cycle* **4**, 1281–1285.

Rösler, C., Köck, J., Kann, M., Malim, M. H., Blum, H. E., Baumert, T. F., and von Weizsäcker, F. (2005). APOBEC-mediated interference with hepadnavirus production. *Hepatology* **42**, 301–309.

Sale, J. E., Calandrini, D. M., Takata, M., Takeda, S., and Neuberger, M. S. (2001). Ablation of XRCC2/3 transforms immunoglobulin V gene conversion into somatic hypermutation. *Nature* **412**, 921–926.

Saribasak, H., Saribasak, N. N., Ipek, F. M., Ellwart, J. W., Arakawa, H., and Buerstedde, J. M. (2006). Uracil DNA glycosylase disruption blocks Ig gene conversion and induces transition mutations. *J. Immunol.* **176**, 365–371.

Sasada, A., Takaori-Kondo, A., Shirakawa, K., Kobayashi, M., Abudu, A., Hishizawa, M., Imada, K., Tanaka, Y., and Uchiyama, T. (2005). APOBEC3G targets human T-cell leukemia virus type 1. *Retrovirology* **2**, 32.

Saunders, H. L., and Magor, B. G. (2004). Cloning and expression of the AID gene in the channel catfish. *Dev. Comp. Immunol.* **28**, 657–663.

Sawyer, S. L., Emerman, M., and Malik, H. S. (2004). Ancient adaptive evolution of the primate antiviral DNA-editing enzyme APOBEC3G. *PLoS Biol.* **2**, E275.

Schäfer, A., Bogerd, H. P., and Cullen, B. R. (2004). Specific packaging of APOBEC3G into HIV-1 virions is mediated by the nucleocapsid domain of the gag polyprotein precursor. *Virology* **328**, 163–168.

Schröfelbauer, B., Chen, D., and Landau, N. R. (2004). A single amino acid of APOBEC3G controls its species-specific interaction with virion infectivity factor (Vif). *Proc. Natl. Acad. Sci. USA* **101**, 3927–3932.

Schumacher, A. J., Nissley, D. V., and Harris, R. S. (2005). APOBEC3G hypermutates genomic DNA and inhibits Ty1 retrotransposition in yeast. *Proc. Natl. Acad. Sci. USA* **102**, 9854–9859.

Sheehy, A. M., Gaddis, N. C., Choi, J. D., and Malim, M. H. (2002). Isolation of a human gene that inhibits HIV-1 infection and is suppressed by the viral Vif protein. *Nature* **418**, 646–650.

Sheehy, A. M., Gaddis, N. C., and Malim, M. H. (2003). The antiretroviral enzyme APOBEC3G is degraded by the proteasome in response to HIV-1 Vif. *Nat. Med.* **9**, 1404–1407.

Shindo, K., Takaori-Kondo, A., Kobayashi, M., Abudu, A., Fukunaga, K., and Uchiyama, T. (2003). The enzymatic activity of CEM15/Apobec-3G is essential for the regulation of the infectivity of HIV-1 virion but not a sole determinant of its antiviral activity. *J. Biol. Chem.* **278**, 44412–44416.

Shirakawa, K., Takaori-Kondo, A., Kobayashi, M., Tomonaga, M., Izumi, T., Fukunaga, K., Sasada, A., Abudu, A., Miyauchi, Y., Akari, H., Iwai, K., and Uchiyama, T. (2005). Ubiquitination of APOBEC3 proteins by the Vif-Cullin5-ElonginB-ElonginC complex. *Virology* **344**, 263–266.

Simon, J. H., and Malim, M. H. (1996). The human immunodeficiency virus type 1 Vif protein modulates the postpenetration stability of viral nucleoprotein complexes. *J. Virol.* **70**, 5297–5305.

Sohail, A., Klapacz, J., Samaranayake, M., Ullah, A., and Bhagwat, A. S. (2003). Human activation-induced cytidine deaminase causes transcription-dependent, strand-biased C to U deaminations. *Nucleic Acids Res.* **31**, 2990–2994.

Song, B. H., and Neuhard, J. (1989). Chromosomal location, cloning and nucleotide sequence of the *Bacillus subtilis* cdd gene encoding cytidine/deoxycytidine deaminase. *Mol. Gen. Genet.* **216**, 462–468.

Stenglein, M. D., and Harris, R. S. (2006). APOBEC3B and APOBEC3F inhibit L1 retrotransposition by a DNA deamination-independent mechanism. *J. Biol. Chem.* **281**, 16837–16841.

Stopak, K., de Noronha, C., Yonemoto, W., and Greene, W. C. (2003). HIV-1 Vif blocks the antiviral activity of APOBEC3G by impairing both its translation and intracellular stability. *Mol. Cell* **12**, 591–601.

Suspène, R., Guétard, D., Henry, M., Sommer, P., Wain-Hobson, S., and Vartanian, J. P. (2005). Extensive editing of both hepatitis B virus DNA strands by APOBEC3 cytidine deaminases *in vitro* and *in vivo*. *Proc. Natl. Acad. Sci. USA* **102**, 8321–8326.

Svarovskaia, E. S., Xu, H., Mbisa, J. L., Barr, R., Gorelick, R. J., Ono, A., Freed, E. O., Hu, W. S., and Pathak, V. K. (2004). Human apolipoprotein B mRNA-editing enzyme-catalytic polypeptide-like 3G (APOBEC3G) is incorporated into HIV-1 virions through interactions with viral and nonviral RNAs. *J. Biol. Chem.* **279**, 35822–35828.

Teng, B. B., Burant, C. F., and Davidson, N. O. (1993). Molecular cloning of an apolipoprotein B messenger RNA editing protein. *Science* **260**, 1816–1819.

Teng, B. B., Ochsner, S., Zhang, Q., Soman, K. V., Lau, P. P., and Chan, L. (1999). Mutational analysis of apolipoprotein B mRNA editing enzyme (APOBEC1). Structure-function relationships of RNA editing and dimerization. *J. Lipid Res.* **40**, 623–635.

Turelli, P., Mangeat, B., Jost, S., Vianin, S., and Trono, D. (2004a). Inhibition of hepatitis B virus replication by APOBEC3G. *Science* **303**, 1829.

Turelli, P., Vianin, S., and Trono, D. (2004b). The innate antiviral factor APOBEC3G does not affect human LINE-1 retrotransposition in a cell culture assay. *J. Biol. Chem.* **279**, 43371–43373.

Uhlén, M., and Ponten, F. (2005). Antibody-based proteomics for human tissue profiling. *Mol. Cell Proteomics* **4**, 384–393.

Uhlén, M., Björling, E., Agaton, C., Szigyarto, C. A., Amini, B., Andersen, E., Andersson, A. C., Angelidou, P., Asplund, A., Asplund, C., Berglund, L., Bergström, K., *et al.* (2005). A human protein atlas for normal and cancer tissues based on antibody proteomics. *Mol. Cell Proteomics* **4**, 1920–1932.

von Schwedler, U., Song, J., Aiken, C., and Trono, D. (1993). Vif is crucial for human immunodeficiency virus type 1 proviral DNA synthesis in infected cells. *J. Virol.* **67**, 4945–4955.

Waterston, R. H., Lindblad-Toh, K., Birney, E., Rogers, J., Abril, J. F., Agarwal, P., Agarwala, R., Ainscough, R., Alexandersson, M., An, P., Antonarakis, S. E., Attwood, J., et al. (2002). Initial sequencing and comparative analysis of the mouse genome. *Nature* **420**, 520–562.

Wedekind, J. E., Dance, G. S., Sowden, M. P., and Smith, H. C. (2003). Messenger RNA editing in mammals: New members of the APOBEC family seeking roles in the family business. *Trends Genet.* **19**, 207–216.

Weill, J. C., and Reynaud, C. A. (1996). Rearrangement/hypermutation/gene conversion: When, where and why? *Immunol. Today* **17**, 92–97.

Wichroski, M. J., Robb, G. B., and Rana, T. M. (2006). Human retroviral host restriction factors APOBEC3G and APOBEC3F localize to mRNA processing bodies. *PLoS Pathog.* **2**, e41.

Wiegand, H. L., Doehle, B. P., Bogerd, H. P., and Cullen, B. R. (2004). A second human antiretroviral factor, APOBEC3F, is suppressed by the HIV-1 and HIV-2 Vif proteins. *EMBO J.* **23**, 2451–2458.

Wolf, J., Gerber, A. P., and Keller, W. (2002). tadA, an essential tRNA-specific adenosine deaminase from *Escherichia coli*. *EMBO J.* **21**, 3841–3851.

Xiang, S., Short, S. A., Wolfenden, R., and Carter, C. W. (1996). Cytidine deaminase complexed to 3-deazacytidine: A "valence buffer" in zinc enzyme catalysis. *Biochemistry* **35**, 1335–1341.

Xiang, S., Short, S. A., Wolfenden, R., and Carter, C. W. (1997). The structure of the cytidine deaminase-product complex provides evidence for efficient proton transfer and ground-state destabilization. *Biochemistry* **36**, 4768–4774.

Xu, H., Svarovskaia, E. S., Barr, R., Zhang, Y., Khan, M. A., Strebel, K., and Pathak, V. K. (2004). A single amino acid substitution in human APOBEC3G antiretroviral enzyme confers resistance to HIV-1 virion infectivity factor-induced depletion. *Proc. Natl. Acad. Sci. USA* **101**, 5652–5657.

Yang, Y., and Smith, H. C. (1997). Multiple protein domains determine the cell type-specific nuclear distribution of the catalytic subunit required for apolipoprotein B mRNA editing. *Proc. Natl. Acad. Sci. USA* **94**, 13075–13080.

Yang, Y., Sowden, M. P., and Smith, H. C. (2001). Intracellular trafficking determinants in APOBEC-1, the catalytic subunit for cytidine to uridine editing of apolipoprotein B mRNA. *Exp. Cell Res.* **267**, 153–164.

Yu, K., Huang, F. T., and Lieber, M. R. (2004a). DNA substrate length and surrounding sequence affect the activation-induced deaminase activity at cytidine. *J. Biol. Chem.* **279**, 6496–6500.

Yu, Q., Chen, D., König, R., Mariani, R., Unutmaz, D., and Landau, N. R. (2004b). APOBEC3B and APOBEC3C are potent inhibitors of simian immunodeficiency virus replication. *J. Biol. Chem.* **279**, 53379–53386.

Yu, Q., König, R., Pillai, S., Chiles, K., Kearney, M., Palmer, S., Richman, D., Coffin, J. M., and Landau, N. R. (2004c). Single-strand specificity of APOBEC3G accounts for minus-strand deamination of the HIV genome. *Nat. Struct. Mol. Biol.* **11**, 435–442.

Yu, X., Yu, Y., Liu, B., Luo, K., Kong, W., Mao, P., and Yu, X. F. (2003). Induction of APOBEC3G ubiquitination and degradation by an HIV-1 Vif-Cul5-SCF complex. *Science* **302**, 1056–1060.

Zhang, H., Yang, B., Pomerantz, R. J., Zhang, C., Arunachalam, S. C., and Gao, L. (2003). The cytidine deaminase CEM15 induces hypermutation in newly synthesized HIV-1 DNA. *Nature* **424**, 94–98.

Zhang, J., and Webb, D. M. (2004). Rapid evolution of primate antiviral enzyme APOBEC3G. *Hum. Mol. Genet.* **13**, 1785–1791.

Zhao, Y., Pan-Hammarström, Q., Zhao, Z., and Hammarström, L. (2005). Identification of the activation-induced cytidine deaminase gene from zebrafish: An evolutionary analysis. *Dev. Comp. Immunol.* **29,** 61–71.

Zheng, Y. H., Irwin, D., Kurosu, T., Tokunaga, K., Sata, T., and Peterlin, B. M. (2004). Human APOBEC3F is another host factor that blocks human immunodeficiency virus type 1 replication. *J. Virol.* **78,** 6073–6076.

Zingler, N., Willhoeft, U., Brose, H. P., Schoder, V., Jahns, T., Hanschmann, K. M., Morrish, T. A., Löwer, J., and Schumann, G. G. (2005). Analysis of 5′ junctions of human LINE-1 and Alu retrotransposons suggests an alternative model for 5′-end attachment requiring microhomology-mediated end-joining. *Genome Res.* **15,** 780–789.

The Role of Activation-Induced Deaminase in Antibody Diversification and Chromosome Translocations

Almudena Ramiro,* Bernardo Reina San-Martin,[†] Kevin McBride,[‡] Mila Jankovic,[‡] Vasco Barreto,[‡] André Nussenzweig,[§] and Michel C. Nussenzweig[‡,¶]

*DNA Hypermutation and Cancer Group, Spanish National Cancer Center (CNIO),
Melchor Fernandez Almagro, 3, 28029 Madrid, Spain
[†]Institut de Génétique et de Biologie Moléculaire et Cellulaire, Département de,
Pathologie Moléculaire, 1 rue Laurent Fries, 67404 Illkirch CEDEX, France
[‡]Laboratory of Molecular Immunology, The Rockefeller University, New York, New York
[§]Experimental Immunology Branch, National Cancer Institute,
National Institutes of Health, Bethesda, Maryland
[¶]Howard Hughes Medical Institute, Maryland

Abstract 75
1. Introduction 76
2. Events Preceding the DNA Lesion 77
3. The DNA Lesion 78
4. DNA Damage Detection and Resolution During CSR 85
5. AID and Lymphomagenic Lesions 93
6. Conclusions and Perspectives 96
   References 96

Abstract

Although B and T lymphocytes are similar in many respects including diversification of their antigen receptor genes by V(D)J recombination, 95% of all lymphomas diagnosed in the western world are of B-cell origin. Many of these are derived from mature B cells [Kuppers, R. (2005). Mechanisms of B-cell lymphoma pathogenesis. Nat. Rev. Cancer **5**, 251–262] and display hallmark chromosome translocations involving immunoglobulin genes and a protooncogene partner whose expression becomes deregulated as a result of the translocation reaction [Kuppers, R. (2005). Mechanisms of B-cell lymphoma pathogenesis. Nat. Rev. Cancer **5**, 251–262; Kuppers, R., and Dalla-Favera, R. (2001). Mechanisms of chromosomal translocations in B cell lymphomas. Oncogene **20**, 5580–5594]. These translocations are essential to the etiology of B-cell neoplasms. Here we will review how the B-cell specific molecular events required for immunoglobulin class switch recombination are initiated and how they contribute to chromosome translocations in vivo.

1. Introduction

Antibody molecules recognize diverse pathogens and help to eliminate them by activating a variety of immune effector mechanisms. In humans and mice, three different molecular events help create the diversity necessary to deal with the antigenic universe: V(D)J recombination, somatic hypermutation (SHM), and class switch recombination (CSR). Some species, such as the chicken and sheep, also diversify Ig gene by gene conversion, but we will not discuss this here.

V(D)J recombination assembles antibody variable regions from random germ line gene segments in developing B cells in the bone marrow to produce the initial antibody repertoire. B cells that have successfully rearranged their immunoglobulin genes express a cell surface antigen receptor composed of IgM and associated signal transducers Igα and Igβ. Because V(D)J recombination is random, it produces numerous self-reactive receptors which are eliminated from the repertoire before B cells can leave the bone marrow and enter the peripheral lymphoid organs (Wardemann et al., 2003). Although the antibodies produced by V(D)J recombination are sufficiently diverse to recognize nearly all potential antigens, the antibodies produced by naive B cells are generally of low affinity.

B cells develop high-affinity antibodies after initiation of immune responses by SHM in the germinal center reaction in secondary lymphoid organs (McKean et al., 1984). The germinal center reaction entails two molecular processes that modify rearranged Ig loci namely, the SHM and the CSR reactions. SHM involves the introduction of single nucleotide substitutions and occasional deletions or duplications in the variable genes of the Ig heavy and light chain loci. B cells that acquire antibodies with increased affinity for the immunogen are clonally expanded and induced to differentiate into memory cells or antibody producing plasma cells (Meffre et al., 2000; Rajewsky, 1996). Conversely, when SHM gives rise to an autoantibody or an antibody with decreased antigen-binding affinity, the cell will become anergic. CSR is a region-specific recombination reaction which replaces the IgM constant region by a downstream constant region, thereby allowing the expression of an antibody with specialized functional properties (Stavnezer, 1996). The recombination reaction takes place between two highly repetitive sequences called switch regions that precede each of the constant regions (except δ) in the Ig heavy chain locus and involves the excision of the intervening DNA sequence. It has long been known that transcription is an absolute requirement for both SHM and CSR. In the case of SHM, the region of DNA-mutated spans ~1-kb downstream of the Ig promoter. Similarly, CSR is targeted downstream of a series of promoters which precede the switch regions and that are activated by specific cytokines (Barreto et al., 2005b).

Activation-induced deaminase (AID), a cytidine deaminase that was discovered independently by Honjo *et al.* and Durandy *et al.* (reviewed in Honjo *et al.*, 2002), initiates both SHM and CSR. Although there is still some debate about how AID functions, most investigators believe that AID catalyzes the deamination of cytidine residues in single-stranded DNA (ssDNA), thereby producing U:G mismatches which can be repaired by alternative DNA repair pathways to produce either SHM or CSR (reviewed in Neuberger *et al.*, 2005). These DNA lesions also initiate some of the chromosome translocations that are frequently associated with mature B-cell lymphomas (reviewed in de Yebenes and Ramiro, 2006).

2. Events Preceding the DNA Lesion

2.1. Epigenetic Modifications and Transcription

Eukaryotic DNA is folded and compacted by histone and nonhistone proteins into a higher-order structure called chromatin which plays a crucial role in the regulation of a number of processes, including transcription, DNA replication, recombination, and repair. Euchromatin or active chromatin is generally associated with acetylated histones and hypomethylated DNA. Consistent with this idea, blocking histone deacetylases with trichostatin A (TSA) enhanced both the transcriptional activity and the mutation rate of a green fluorescent protein target gene in a hypermutating cell line (Bachl *et al.*, 2001). In addition, histone H3 acetylation is correlated with hypermutation of the Ig heavy chain variable region *in vitro* (Woo *et al.*, 2003). Similarly, switch region transcription and recombination is associated with histone H3 acetylation in primary mouse B lymphocytes (Li *et al.*, 2004a; Nambu *et al.*, 2003; Wang *et al.*, 2006b). However, there was no association between this histone mark and Ig heavy chain V region mutation in primary B cells (Odegard *et al.*, 2005). Translocations between Ig switch regions and IgH are initiated by the same molecular mechanism as CSR (see below, Ramiro *et al.*, 2006), and therefore histone H3 acetylation of Ig switch regions and c-myc is likely to correlate with translocation, but this has not yet been examined.

2.2. Transcriptional Activation

As mentioned above, transcriptional activation of the variable and the switch regions is essential for SHM and CSR, respectively. In the case of the variable region, transcription is initiated at the Ig promoter immediately preceding the rearranged variable region. Transcription of switch regions initiates upstream of an I exon that precedes each switch region giving rise to noncoding germ line transcripts that span the I exon, the switch region, and the immediately downstream CH exons. Different combinations of LPS, cytokines, and costimulatory molecules drive the transcriptional activation of individual I promoters and determine the switch region—and therefore the CH region—that will be involved in the CSR event (reviewed in Stavnezer, 2000). A number of early studies addressed the role of *cis*-acting sequences in SHM and CSR. Removal of the Ig promoter and of the I exon promoter resulted in a dramatic decrease of SHM (Fukita *et al.*, 1998) and CSR (Jung *et al.*, 1993; Zhang *et al.*, 1993), respectively. However, replacement of the endogenous promoters by heterologous promoters could reconstitute, at least in part, both SHM and CSR (reviewed in Li *et al.*, 2004c) and (Honjo *et al.*, 2002). Furthermore, duplication of the Ig promoter in front of a transgenic Cκ region promoted the accumulation of mutations in this constant region. The frequency of SHM frequency decreases with distance from promoter and roughly correlates with transcription rate (see below). All these results indicated that transcriptional activation is closely linked to the SHM and CSR reactions. Today it is believed that the primary function of transcription during SHM and CSR is to provide AID with the proper DNA substrate (see below).

3. The DNA Lesion

3.1. AID Function

AID was identified by Honjo and his colleagues in 1999 as a cDNA selectively expressed in a murine B-cell line activated to undergo CSR (Muramatsu *et al.*, 1999). Sequence analysis suggested that AID is a deaminase and that it is most closely related to APOBEC1 (34% amino acid identity), which is an mRNA-editing cytidine deaminase (Muramatsu *et al.*, 1999). However, there is no known mRNA substrate for AID and all of the biochemical, cell biological, and genetic evidence suggests that AID initiates SHM, CSR, Ig gene conversion, and chromosome translocations by directly deaminating cytidines in DNA. The DNA deamination model posits that cytidine deamination produces a uracyl leading to a U:G mismatch in DNA that is processed by one of several alternative repair pathways leading to SHM or CSR or chromosome translocations. Below we summarize the data supporting this idea.

3.1.1. Genetic Evidence

Uracils in genomic DNA are normally removed by ubiquitous uracil deglicosylases (UDGs), leaving an abasic site that is repaired by one of several different mechanisms. In the absence of UDGs, uracil-containing DNA is replicated resulting in a daughter cell harboring a C to T transition. The first evidence that DNA is the substrate for AID came from experiments in which AID expressed in *Escherichia coli* induced C to T mutations, whose frequency increased dramatically in the absence of UDG (Petersen-Mahrt *et al.*, 2002; Ramiro *et al.*, 2003; Sohail *et al.*, 2003). These experiments lend strong support to the DNA deamination model since an mRNA intermediate shared by eukaryotes and prokaryotes is highly unlikely and uracil removal from DNA was an important feature of the reaction. Furthermore, mice, chickens, and humans lacking uracil-*N*-glycosylase 1 (UNG) showed the predicted abnormalities in SHM (increased transitions) (Di Noia and Neuberger, 2002; Imai *et al.*, 2003; Rada *et al.*, 2002b) and pronounced deficiencies in CSR and translocation (Imai *et al.*, 2003; Rada *et al.*, 2002b; Ramiro *et al.*, 2006).

U:G mismatches can also be recognized and processed by the mismatch repair (MMR) machinery and mutations in MMR proteins Msh2 and Msh6 in mice, chickens, and humans show alterations in SHM and CSR consistent with the DNA deamination model (Li *et al.*, 2004b; Martomo *et al.*, 2004; Rada *et al.*, 1998; Schrader *et al.*, 1999; Wiesendanger *et al.*, 2000). Moreover, the combined deficiency of UNG and Msh2 results in a complete absence of CSR and SHM which is entirely limited to transitions from C to T suggesting that deaminated cytidines can only be recognized by these two repair pathways (Rada *et al.*, 2004). In summary, the genetic evidence shows that AID promotes the introduction of mutations by a pathway that involves cytidine deamination and that U:G mismatches are obligate intermediates in the SHM, CSR, and chromosome translocation reactions (see below).

3.1.2. Biochemical Evidence

AID can bind ssDNA and RNA *in vitro* (Dickerson *et al.*, 2003) but it only deaminates ssDNA (Bransteitter *et al.*, 2003; Chaudhuri *et al.*, 2003; Dickerson *et al.*, 2003). Strikingly, APOBEC1, whose *bona fide* substrate is ApoB mRNA, is also able to deaminate ssDNA *in vitro*, although with low efficiency (Petersen-Mahrt and Neuberger, 2003). Further support for the DNA deamination model comes from analyzing the sequence specificity of the deamination reaction *in vitro*. SHM is focused on WRC hot spots (W = A or T and R = A or G) and AID shows the same sequence preference *in vitro* suggesting that AID recognizes WRC directly (Pham *et al.*, 2003). Finally, AID has been found to be physically associated with switch region DNA in B cells induced to undergo CSR *in vitro* (Nambu *et al.*, 2003), although others were unable to confirm this result in a murine B-cell line (Begum *et al.*, 2004).

3.2. Substrate ssDNA Is Liberated During Transcription

Transcription is required for both CSR and SHM and the rate of transcription is directly related to the frequency of mutation and CSR (Bachl *et al.*, 2001; Fukita *et al.*, 1998; Okazaki *et al.*, 2002; Ramiro *et al.*, 2003; Yoshikawa *et al.*, 2002). In *vitro* biochemistry and *E. coli* experiments suggest that the role of transcription is to make ssDNA available to AID. Whereas ssDNA is deaminated by AID *in vitro*, double-stranded DNA (dsDNA) substrates can only serve as substrates when transcribed and the substrate strand is the nontemplate strand (Chaudhuri *et al.*, 2003; Dickerson *et al.*, 2003; Pham *et al.*, 2003). Similarly in *E. coli*, it is the nontemplate strand which is preferentially mutated by AID (Ramiro *et al.*, 2003; Sohail *et al.*, 2003). The precise DNA structure that is liberated during transcription is not defined and could include both transcription bubbles and R-loop structures, produced by RNA–DNA hybrids that displace the G-rich nontranscribed strand in single-stranded configuration (Shinkura *et al.*, 2003; Tian and Alt, 2000; Yu *et al.*, 2003, 2005).

Less is known about the mechanism by which transcription facilitates AID function *in vivo*. In contrast to the biochemical and *E. coli* experiments, mutations are observed on both strands of Ig genes *in vivo*. The lack of strand bias *in vivo* is likely due to AID targeting because mutations in Sμ (Nagaoka *et al.*, 2002; Reina-San-Martin *et al.*, 2003) appear on both DNA strands in mice that are deficient in Ung and Msh2 where the mutation spectrum can be attributed to AID targeting alone and not to downstream processing of the initial DNA lesion (Xue *et al.*, 2006). Two groups have proposed that DNA supercoiling during transcription may liberate ssDNA on both strands to produce AID substrates (Besmer *et al.*, 2006; Shen and Storb, 2004; Shen *et al.*, 2005). Consistent with this idea, supercoiled plasmids exposed to AID *in vitro* were mutated on both strands (Besmer *et al.*, 2006; Shen and Storb, 2004; Shen *et al.*, 2005).

3.3. AID Transcriptional Regulation

AID is specifically expressed in germinal center B cells (Muramatsu *et al.*, 1999). A number of activation stimuli promote AID expression in splenic B cells, such as LPS alone or in combination with interleukin-4 (IL-4) or TGFβ (Muramatsu *et al.*, 1999) and CD40 ligation (Dedeoglu *et al.*, 2004). Therefore, under physiological conditions, expression of AID is linked to the B-cell activation program taking place in germinal centers. JAK/STAT and NF-κB pathways have been shown to be involved in IL-4-induced AID expression in B cells (Dedeoglu *et al.*, 2004; Zhou *et al.*, 2003).

E-proteins are helix-loop-helix (HLH) transcription factors that bind E boxes at DNA. E-proteins can also form heterodimers with antagonist HLH proteins that lack the DNA-binding domain preventing transcription, known as inhibitors of differentiation (Id1–4). It has been shown that the E47 E-protein can induce the expression of AID in B cells through the activation of an intronic enhancer in the Aicda gene. This activation seems negatively regulated by Id3. Accordingly, E47 deficiency and Id3 overexpression result in a decrease in CSR (Sayegh et al., 2003). Another Id protein, Id2, has been reported to repress AID expression by antagonizing the activity of the Pax5 transcription factor (Gonda et al., 2003). Further, Blimp1, a master transcription factor involved in plasma cell differentiation, represses the expression of Pax5 (Lin et al., 2002) and AID (Shaffer et al., 2002) and in the absence of the Blimp1 regulator interferon regulatory factor-4 (IRF-4) CSR and AID expression are severely impaired (Klein et al., 2006; Sciammas et al., 2006). These results provide evidence that regulation of AID expression is intertwined in the B-cell activation and developmental programs to ensure a tight restriction.

3.4. The AID Protein

3.4.1. The AID Protein

AID is one of the ancestral members of the AID/APOBEC family of cytidine deaminases and it is highly conserved from cartilaginous fish to humans (Conticello et al., 2005; Zhao et al., 2005). SHM developed before CSR, but AID's ability to catalyze CSR developed before the CSR reaction itself (Barreto et al., 2005a; Ichikawa et al., 2006; Wakae et al., 2006). On the basis of modeling by threading and comparative computational models that rely on the crystal structure of a yeast cytidine deaminase, AID is believed to be organized in an N-terminal catalytic domain spanning roughly the first 150 residues whose fold may resemble that of yeast and *E. coli* cytidine deaminase catalytic domains, and a C-terminal pseudocatalytic domain of more uncertain structure (Xie et al., 2004; Zaim and Kierzek, 2003). Numerous inactivating AID mutations have been found in HIGM2 patients affecting both the catalytic and the pseudocatalytic domains, implying a strong structural constraint in the molecule (Quartier et al., 2004; Revy et al., 2000).

Similarly to other cytidine deaminases AID forms dimers and/or multimers when overexpressed in 293T cells (Ta et al., 2003). A careful analysis of deletion and point mutants showed that AID forms homodimers in the absence of DNA or other cofactors, and mapped the region responsible for dimerization between residues 27 and 56 (Wang et al., 2006a). Functional analysis of mutants in this region showed that dimer formation is required for efficient CSR (Wang *et al.*, 2006a).

3.4.2. Functional Domains

AID-induced DNA lesions are repaired by different pathways to produce SHM or CSR. For example, Ku, H2AX, and 53BP1 are required for CSR but not for SHM. How the choice of repair pathway is made in each case is not known but may involve specific domains of AID. For example, the C-terminal region (residues 189–198) of AID is required for CSR but dispensable for SHM and therefore targeting to Ig loci (Barreto *et al.*, 2003; Durandy *et al.*, 2006; Imai *et al.*, 2005; Ta *et al.*, 2003), and the N-terminal region of AID is more important for SHM than for CSR (Shinkura *et al.*, 2004). Interestingly, the R190X mutation in AICDA has an *in vivo* CSR phenotype inherited as an autosomal dominant trait (Imai *et al.*, 2005). These observations suggest that there could be reaction-specific cofactors that interact with different portions of the AID protein and that AID might also influence lesion resolution.

3.5. AID Nuclear Transport and Posttranslational Modification

AID activity, like that of many proteins with nuclear function, is regulated in part by active nuclear export. Expression of epitope-tagged AID or AID–GFP fusions in cells revealed that AID predominantly resides in the cytoplasm (Rada *et al.*, 2002a). The C-terminus of AID, which is essential for CSR (residues 188–198, see above), is a consensus nuclear export signal (NES) recognized by the exporting chromosome region maintenance-1 (CRM1) (Brar *et al.*, 2004; Ito *et al.*, 2004; McBride *et al.*, 2004). CRM1 is a soluble shuttling factor of the Karyopherin family that binds and exports NES-containing proteins out of the nucleus. Mutation of the AID NES or inhibition of CRM1, with the specific inhibitor leptomycin B, results in an accumulation of nuclear AID. This also leads to a marked increase in mutation frequency in fibroblasts (McBride *et al.*, 2004). However, in B cells the rate of CSR and associated hypermutation of switch regions is not affected, indicating that AID nuclear export may function to limit AID mutations on non-Ig loci.

It is unclear how AID gains access to the nucleus. By itself AID is small enough to passively diffuse into the nucleus; however, most nuclear proteins are actively transported. Ito *et al.* (2004) have reported that the N-terminal domain is critical for nuclear accumulation of AID. A similar role for the N-terminus of APOBEC1, with sequence similarity, has also been described (Yang *et al.*, 2001). Although both proteins contain sequence similar to a bipartite nuclear localization signals (NLS) neither one can act as an autonomous NLS when fused to a large indicator protein (Brar et al., 2004; McBride et al., 2004; Yang et al., 2001). Furthermore, mutation of the arginine and lysine residues, normally critical to NLS function, have negligible effects. Therefore, it remains possible that AID contains a nonclassical NLS or interacts with a chaperone protein to translocate to the nucleus.

AID activity is augmented by cAMP-dependent protein kinase A (PKA) phosphorylation on serine 38 (S38) (Basu et al., 2005). In B cells undergoing CSR, the phosphorylated form is a small fraction, perhaps 5–10% of the overall AID population, but this fraction is preferentially enriched on chromatin and contributes disproportionately to hypermutation and CSR activity (McBride et al., 2006). AID with S38 mutated to alanine mutation (AID^{S38A}) has greatly diminished capacity for CSR and hypermutation (Basu et al., 2005; McBride et al., 2006; Pasqualucci et al., 2006). PKA is a ubiquitous kinase and AID phosphorylation is not B-cell specific since AID expressed in fibroblasts is phosphorylated and mutant AID^{S38A} has greatly diminished hypermutation activity in fibroblasts (McBride et al., 2006). One way S38 phosphorylation augments AID activity is by facilitating interaction with replication protein A (RPA), a ssDNA-binding protein that contributes to AID function (Basu et al., 2005; Chaudhuri et al., 2004). On the basis of *in vitro* studies, RPA targets phospho-AID activity to ssDNA and may also facilitate its interaction with UNG.

AID S38 is within a consensus phosphorylation motif of the PKA and is phosphorylated by PKA *in vitro* (Basu et al., 2005). Cells treated with activators of PKA such as forskolin and IBMX also showed enhanced AID phosphorylation, and an inhibitor, H89, diminished CSR (Basu et al., 2005; Pasqualucci et al., 2006). PKA, normally exists as an inactive tetramer of two catalytic units together with two regulatory units (PKAR). On stimulation with cAMP, PKA is released from PKAR and activated. Coimmunoprecipitation studies revealed that AID is in complex with one of the regulatory units PKA regulatory subunit 1α (PKAR1A) (Pasqualucci et al., 2006). Phosphorylation of substrates is often controlled at the level of localization due to PKA anchoring at subcellular sites and limited substrate interaction within subcellular regions. We speculate that in the case of AID phosphorylation may be regulated by nuclear-anchored forms of PKA.

3.6. AID Targeting

Cytidine deamination takes place spontaneously during normal cell metabolism and is normally repaired faithfully. For reasons not yet understood, AID-induced cytidine deamination is channeled to mutations, and in the case of CSR to dsDNA breaks. Under normal circumstances, AID expression is restricted to activated mature B cells (see above), and is mostly localized in the cell cytoplasm, which may decrease the risk of DNA damage. However, the mechanisms responsible for AID targeting of Ig genes, and for sparing other sequences, remains one of the most intriguing issues in the field.

Variable regions are rich in WRC motifs, which constitute mutational hot spots for AID activity (see above). Targeting to these motifs seems an intrinsic feature of AID deaminase activity, although it might be enhanced or modulated by RPA (Chaudhuri et al., 2004), Msh6 (Li et al., 2006), or both. However, neither the AID requirement for these hot spots is absolute nor is their complexity sufficient to ensure specificity for Ig sequences. In addition, the variable region of Ig transgenes has been replaced by a number of heterologous sequences (Li et al., 2004c) and targeting is still achieved. Likewise, heterologous palindromic sequences can substitute for the switch regions in supporting CSR, at least to some extent (Honjo et al., 2002). Therefore, primary sequence is not a major determinant for AID targeting.

As discussed above, transcriptional activation of target sequences—that is, Ig variable and switch regions—is required for AID activity and therefore can be considered a targeting mechanism. Since not all transcribed genes are mutated the role of specific *cis* elements of Ig genes in supporting SHM has been extensively studied [reviewed in Li et al. (2004c) and see above]. However, since removal or mutation of *cis* sequences results in a decreased transcriptional rate of Ig genes, the decrease in SHM observed in these experiments does not allow one to discriminate a targeting effect from an effect on AID accessibility. Similarly, some epigenetic modifications associated with the Ig locus (see above) could be envisioned as a targeting mechanism. However, there is no evidence so far to assign a role to these modifications—in particular to H3 hyperacetylation—different from the transcriptional activation of these regions.

It is tempting to speculate that the main role of Ig *cis* elements might be to allow AID activity by promoting transcriptional activation rather than to serve a targeting/recruiting mechanism specific to the Ig locus. It is counterintuitive that restriction for AID mutagenic activity would be provided only by the transcriptional activity of the locus, unless transcriptional rates of Ig genes are exceptionally high compared to other genes expressed in activated B cells. More likely, targeting specificity may be achieved by other mechanisms, related or not to transcriptional activation. One way or another AID targeting to Ig genes is not infallible, which may be of great consequence to lymphomagenesis (see below).

4. DNA Damage Detection and Resolution During CSR

CSR is a deletional recombination reaction and the joining of two heterologous S regions results in the loss of up to 200 kbps of intervening DNA, which is released as a circular episome. Because of the deletional nature of CSR, double-strand breaks (DSBs) in donor and acceptor S regions are obligate intermediates. The precise mechanism by which DSBs in S regions are generated is not known, but appears to involve the processing of AID-mediated lesions by MMR and base excision repair enzymes (Honjo et al., 2005; Rada et al., 2004; Schrader et al., 2005). For CSR to succeed, DSBs in donor and acceptor S regions need to be detected, brought to close proximity and ligated.

4.1. Nonhomologous End-Joining and DSB Resolution During CSR

In eukaryotes, DSBs are repaired through two pathways: homologous recombination (HR) and nonhomologous end-joining (NHEJ) (Sancar et al., 2004). HR is used to accurately repair DSBs by copying information from a homologous template during S/G2-phases of the cell cycle, where sister chromatids are available (Sancar et al., 2004). NHEJ, on the other hand, is an error-prone process that operates primarily during the G1-phase of the cell cycle to rejoin DNA ends bearing little or no homology (Sancar et al., 2004). Seven factors specifically required for mammalian NHEJ have been described to date: the DNA-dependent protein kinase (DNA-PK) composed of two DNA-binding subunits (Ku70, Ku80) and a catalytic subunit (DNA-PK$_{CS}$), the Artemis endonuclease, the XRCC4 and DNA-ligase IV complex, and their recently identified partner Cernunnos/XLF, which is believed to potentiate the ligase activity of the complex (Ahnesorg et al., 2006; Buck et al., 2006). Mutation in any of these genes results in a severe combined immunodeficiency (SCID) phenotype due to abnormalities in resolution of DNA ends produced by the RAG1/2 endonuclease during V(D)J recombination (Ahnesorg et al., 2006; Buck et al., 2006; de Villartay et al., 2003).

4.1.1. Ku70 and Ku80

Direct evidence for NHEJ in CSR came from the analysis of mice deficient in the DNA-binding subunits of DNA-PK: Ku70 and Ku80 (Casellas et al., 1998; Manis et al., 1998). Mice deficient in these factors fail to develop B lymphocytes due to abnormal V(D)J recombination, but B-cell development can be rescued by introducing prerearranged variable regions into the immunoglobulin heavy and light chain loci by gene targeting (Casellas et al., 1998; Manis et al., 1998). These mice displayed normal numbers of mature peripheral IgM$^+$ cells but had no detectable levels of serum Ig other than IgM (Casellas et al., 1998; Manis *et al.*, 1998). This phenotype appeared to be B-cell intrinsic and was not due to the absence of T cells since Ku70/80-deficient B cells were unable to produce secondary isotypes when cultured *in vitro* in the presence of LPS, LPS and IL-4, and anti-CD40 and IL-4. The CSR defect in the absence of Ku70/80 was independent of abnormal transcription of S regions as sterile transcripts were readily detected by RT-PCR and was not due to reduced DSB formation as assessed by ligation-mediated PCR (Casellas *et al.*, 1998; Manis *et al.*, 1998). Furthermore, failure to undergo CSR was pinpointed to defective recombination at the DNA level since no mature switch recombination products were found by digestion–circularization PCR (Casellas *et al.*, 1998). Ku70/80 deficiency is associated with growth retardation and it remained possible that abnormalities in proliferation per se may have accounted for the CSR defect observed. This issue was, however, addressed by using the vital dye CFSE to show that Ku80-deficient B cells that respond to stimulation and that undergo several rounds of cell division are still unable to undergo CSR (Reina-San-Martin *et al.*, 2003). Therefore, Ku70 and Ku80 are required for CSR.

4.1.2. DNA-PK_{CS}

The role of the catalytic subunit DNA-PK_{CS} in CSR is less clear. The first indication that it might be involved in CSR was obtained by inducing CSR *in vitro* of immature B cells from mice bearing a homozygous mutation in the DNA-PK_{CS} gene (SCID mice) (Rolink *et al.*, 1996). *In vitro* stimulation of SCID pre-B cells with anti-CD40 and IL-4 resulted in a CSR defect to IgE, suggesting that DNA-PK_{CS} is involved in DSB resolution during CSR (Rolink *et al.*, 1996). In this study, however, CSR to other isotypes was not addressed and CSR normally involves mature B cells and not pre-B cells.

In an attempt to clarify the role of DNA-PK_{CS} in CSR, Manis *et al.* (1998) rescued B-cell development in DNA-$PK_{CS}^{-/-}$ mice using the same approach as for $Ku70^{-/-}$ mice. Intriguingly, they found that CSR was impaired to all isotypes except IgG1 (Manis *et al.*, 2002). The defect was not due to altered switch region transcription or AID expression. Furthermore, they showed that DNA-PK_{CS}-deficient B cells do not display proliferation defects and that CSR can occur in both alleles as in the wild type. Analysis of $S\mu$–$S\gamma1$ switch region junctions obtained from DNA-$PK_{CS}^{-/-}$ B cells showed that S region breakpoint locations were unaltered and that these junctions were not different from wild type in the extent of microhomology or in mutation frequency at the junctions. They concluded that CSR is dependent on DNA-PK_{CS} and that switching to IgG1 may be mechanistically different from other isotypes, perhaps due to intrinsic sequence properties and/or to independence of regulation by the 3' IgH enhancer (Manis *et al.*, 2002).

In another study, Bosma et al. (2002) showed that DNA-PK$_{CS}$ is not required for CSR by examining IgM$^+$ mature B cells from SCID mice with site-directed heavy and light (κ) chain transgenes and where the T-cell compartment was reconstituted with thymocytes from JH$^{-/-}$ mice (Bosma et al., 2002). They found that reconstitution of the B- and T-cell compartments in an SCID background resulted in the accumulation of serum immunoglobulins of all isotypes at levels comparable to wild-type mice. When tested in vitro for CSR with LPS, IL-4, and/or TGFβ, SCID B cells were able to undergo CSR as determined by surface expression of IgG1, IgG2b, and IgG3. The percentage of IgG$^+$ cells in SCID homozygous transgenic B cells was similar to SCID heterozygous transgenic controls but two- to threefold lower than in nontransgenic heterozygous B cells. The formation of post-switch and circle transcripts was assessed by semiquantitative RT-PCR and was found to be produced at similar levels in SCID and control heterozygous mice, thus indicating successful CSR events. After failing to detect any DNA-dependent kinase in nuclear extracts obtained from SCID pre-B and mature B cells, they concluded that CSR is not severely impaired in DNA-PK$_{CS}$$^{-/-}$ B cells (Bosma et al., 2002). Similarly, Cook et al. (2003) reported that when the SCID mutation is introduced into anti-hen egg lysozyme transgenic B cells capable of undergoing CSR, switching to all isotypes (including IgG1) is detectable but at reduced levels when compared to control B cells of the same specificity and lacking the *RAG1* gene (Cook et al., 2003). One potential explanation for the difference between SCID and the engineered mutant is that the latter is a null, while the SCID mutation results in the expression of a truncated protein lacking kinase activity that could potentially serve as a scaffold for other proteins involved in CSR (Bosma et al., 2002; Cook et al., 2003; Manis et al., 2002).

4.1.3. Artemis

Artemis is an endonuclease that processes hairpin ends for ligation and it is required to open coding ends during V(D)J recombination (Moshous et al., 2001) but it is not required for CSR (Moshous et al., 2001; Rooney et al., 2005). Artemis-deficient mice displayed normal levels of circulating switched antibodies and Artemis-deficient B cells were able to undergo CSR to all isotypes at wild-type frequencies in in vitro cultures (Rooney et al., 2005). This result indicates that end processing of DNA ends by Artemis is dispensable for CSR.

4.1.4. Cernunnos/XLF, XRCC4, and DNA Ligase IV

Cernunnos/XLF, XRCC4, and DNA ligase IV have yet to be analyzed for CSR by gene targeting. Human patients bearing mutations in Cernunnos display growth retardation, microcephaly, and immunodeficiency characterized by severe T and B lymphocytopenia (Ahnesorg et al., 2006; Buck et al., 2006). Although these patients display hypoglobulinemia, IgM serum levels were found to be occasionally elevated as is observed in CSR-deficient hyper-IgM syndromes (Buck et al., 2006; Durandy et al., 2006). This suggests that Cernnunos may play a role in CSR but further investigation is required.

Inactivation of XRCC4 or DNA ligase IV results in embryonic lethality and conditional inactivation mouse models have not yet been generated (Barnes et al., 1998; Frank et al., 1998; Gao et al., 1998). In contrast to Ku70/80 or DNA-PK$_{CS}$, the XRCC4 and ligase IV ligase complex has no reported roles outside NHEJ and analysis of CSR in B cells deficient for these genes may provide clues as to which DSB repair pathways operate during CSR. Pan-Hammarstrom et al. (2005) reported the analysis of CSR in peripheral B cells obtained from human patients bearing homozygous mutations in the ligase IV gene. Ligase IV-deficient patients appear to accumulate switched IgA$^+$ cells as determined by a semiquantitative genomic DNA PCR assay amplifying Sµ–Sα productive switch junctions. The frequency of IgA$^+$ cells in the patients appears to be lower than in healthy controls but this was not assessed by flow cytometry. Although functional in vitro assays were not done in this study, sequence analysis of Sµ–Sα, Sµ–Sγ2, and Sµ–Sγ3 switch junctions revealed that DSB resolution in B cells from these patients was altered and was characterized by a significant increase in microhomology and insertions. These results link the NHEJ pathway to DSB resolution during CSR and suggest that the requirement for DNA ligase in CSR may not be absolute and that alternative pathways may operate to resolve DSBs during CSR. This point, however, needs to be further clarified by gene targeting in mouse models, as the mutations in the patients are hypomorphic and one cannot exclude the possibility of some residual DNA ligase IV activity.

4.2. DNA Damage Response During CSR

DNA DSBs represent a severe threat for genome integrity and therefore highly sensitive DNA damage signaling and amplification mechanisms have evolved (Sancar et al., 2004). In response to DSB formation, a complex network of proteins is activated in order to impose cell cycle checkpoints, regulate cell survival, and induce DNA repair (Sancar et al., 2004). These responses are tightly coordinated by a family of serine/threonine kinases, containing a phospatidylinositol-3-kinase domain that includes ataxia–telangiectasia mutated (ATM), DNA-PK$_{CS}$, and ATM- and Rad3-related (ATR) (Shiloh, 2003). These kinases are the prototype transducers of the DNA damage signal (Shiloh, 2003). Among these, the ATM kinase plays a prominent role in the response to DSB and disruption of ATM in mice or in humans results in ataxia–telangiectasia (A–T), a syndrome characterized by radiosensitivity, chromosomal instability, cancer predisposition, and immunodeficiency (Barlow et al., 1996; Borghesani et al., 2000; Elson et al., 1996; Savitsky et al., 1995; Xu et al., 1996). ATM is reported to exist as an inactive homodimer which in response to DSBs dissociate by an unknown mechanism leading to the release of active ATM monomers which are autophosphorylated in the serine residue at position 1981 (Bakkenist and Kastan, 2003; Pellegrini et al., 2006). However, in mice, this serine phosphorylation does not affect the oligomerization status of ATM, its activity, or ability to undergo class switch recombination (Pellegrini et al., 2006). Activated ATM monomers then phosphorylate and activate a plethora of substrates including the histone variant H2AX, the nijmegen syndrome protein 1 (Nbs1), p53-binding protein 1 (53BP1) among others, that control cell cycle checkpoints and promote DNA repair (Anderson et al., 2001; Burma et al., 2001; Paull et al., 2000; Rappold et al., 2001; Rogakou et al., 1998; Shiloh, 2003). Although ATM activation is crucial in the responding to DSB formation, ATM is not a DNA damage sensor and its full activation is dependent on the evolutionarily conserved protein complex composed by Mre11, Rad50, and Nbs1 (MRN). The MRN complex has been implicated in many aspects of DSB detection and processing (D'Amours and Jackson, 2002; Stracker et al., 2004). Patients with hypomorphic mutations in Mre11 or Nbs1 display a syndrome that is similar to A–T patients (Carney et al., 1998; Stewart et al., 1999; Varon et al., 1998), indicating that MRN and ATM function in similar pathways *in vivo*. Indeed, Nbs1 and Mre11 are required for the efficient autophosphorylation of ATM on serine 1981, the recruitment of activated ATM into irradiation-induced foci, and for the phosphorylation of downstream ATM targets (Anderson et al., 2001; Burma et al., 2001; Paull et al., 2000; Rappold et al., 2001; Rogakou et al., 1998; Shiloh, 2003). Similarly, 53BP1 is phosphorylated by ATM in response to DSB formation, and it accumulates at sites of DNA damage in a manner dependent on the phosphorylated form of histone H2AX (Celeste et al., 2003; Fernandez-Capetillo et al., 2002; Mochan et al., 2004; Ward et al., 2003a). Although 53BP1 was originally described as a mediator of DNA damage checkpoints, 53BP1 also senses DNA damage by binding to the methylated lysine 79 of histone H3, a residue which is buried within the nucleosome and only exposed after DSB formation (Huyen et al., 2004).

4.2.1. γ-H2AX

One of the earliest events in response to a DSB is the phosphorylation of the histone variant H2AX (γ-H2AX) (Fernandez-Capetillo et al., 2004). γ-H2AX foci formation is believed to mark the site of a DSB and to facilitate the accumulation, but not the initial recruitment, of cell cycle checkpoint and DNA repair proteins including ATM, Nbs1, and 53BP1 (Fernandez-Capetillo et al., 2004). The first indication that the DNA damage response is involved in the mechanism of CSR came from studies by Petersen et al. (2001) who showed that γ-H2AX and the Nbs1 protein form foci specifically at the heavy chain locus in B cells undergoing CSR. γ-H2AX/Nbs1 focus formation was dependent on AID expression and γ-H2AX/Nbs1 foci formed preferentially during the G1-phase of the cell cycle, a result that is consistent with DSB resolution through NHEJ (Petersen et al., 2001). Inactivation of the H2AX gene revealed that γ-H2AX is not required for V(D)J recombination as mature B and T cells were observed, albeit at lower numbers, but bearing normal V(D)J recombination signal and coding joints (Petersen et al., 2001). H2AX deficiency, however, resulted in genomic instability and defective CSR (Celeste et al., 2002; Petersen et al., 2001). These experiments strengthened the idea that DSB are intermediates in the CSR mechanism, directly linked the DNA damage response to CSR and demonstrated that the function of AID is upstream of the generation of DSBs.

Having linked the DNA damage response to the CSR mechanism, Reina-San-Martin et al. (2003) characterized how H2AX deficiency impacts on SHM and CSR. Interestingly, while H2AX deficiency resulted in defective CSR, SHM was unaffected, suggesting that DNA damage inflicted by AID in immunoglobulin genes is processed through alternative pathways during SHM and CSR (Reina-San-Martin et al., 2003). The defect in CSR in H2AX$^{-/-}$ B cells was cell autonomous and independent of proliferation abnormalities. Switch region transcription and AID accessibility to switch regions were unaffected as determined by real time RT-PCR and by the induction of mutation in switch region DNA, respectively. In addition, switch region junctions appeared to be normal in terms of microhomology, mutation frequency, and distribution. B cells stimulated to undergo CSR frequently undergo intraswitch region recombination, an event that is believed to reflect failed attempts at CSR as it is dependent on AID and Ku80 (Dudley et al., 2002; Reina-San-Martin et al., 2003). Unexpectedly, the frequency of short-range intraswitch region recombination in H2AX$^{-/-}$ B cells appeared to occur at wild-type levels, indicating that only long-range interswitch region recombination is affected by H2AX deficiency (Reina-San-Martin et al., 2003). On the basis of these observations, it was proposed that phosphorylation of the C-terminal tail of histone H2AX alters the structure of nucleosomes in switch regions inducing conformational changes that facilitate the synapsis of heterologous switch regions during CSR (Reina-San-Martin et al., 2003).

4.2.2. ATM

Consistent with H2AX phosphorylation by ATM in response to γ-irradiation and AID-dependent γ-H2AX focus formation during CSR, Reina-San-Martin *et al.* (2004) and Lumsden *et al.* (2004) showed that ATM deficiency resulted in inefficient CSR. As in H2AX-deficient mice, SHM appeared to be unaffected by ATM deficiency (Lumsden *et al.*, 2004; Reina-San-Martin *et al.*, 2004). The defect in CSR was not due to alterations in switch region transcription, accessibility, or DNA damage checkpoint protein recruitment (Lumsden *et al.*, 2004; Reina-San-Martin *et al.*, 2004). These results showed that ATM is indeed involved in responding to AID-triggered DNA damage during CSR. However, given the prominent role of ATM in mediating DNA damage responses, it was surprising to find that CSR was reduced but not abrogated in ATM-deficient B cells. This suggested that DNA damage transduction during CSR in the absence of ATM may be compensated by other serine/threonine kinases, possibly by DNA-PK_{CS} and/or ATR and is in agreement with the observation that H2AX phosphorylation is detectable in $ATM^{-/-}$ $DNA\text{-}PK^{-/-}$ and $ATR^{-/-}$ cells (Brown and Baltimore, 2003; Elson *et al.*, 1996; Fernandez-Capetillo *et al.*, 2002, 2003; Ward and Chen, 2001). Consistent with the phenotype observed in H2AX-deficient B cells, in the absence of ATM intraswitch region recombination appeared to occur at wild-type frequency and only long-range interswitch recombination was affected, indicating that H2AX phosphorylation by ATM is involved in facilitating long-range interswitch region recombination during CSR (Reina-San-Martin *et al.*, 2004).

4.2.3. The MRN Complex

On the basis of the AID-dependent γ-H2AX/Nbs1 foci formation during CSR, it was predicted that the DNA damage sensor Nbs1 and the MRN complex would play a role in sensing AID-triggered DNA damage during CSR (Petersen *et al.*, 2001). In addition, switch region junctions cloned from peripheral B cells isolated from patients with hypomorphic mutations in Nbs1 and Mre11 showed abnormalities and suggested that the MRN complex may be involved in the processing of DNA ends prior to joining (Lahdesmaki *et al.*, 2004; Pan-Hammarstrom *et al.*, 2003). To analyze the role of Nbs1 in CSR (Luo *et al.*, 2004; Xiao and Weaver, 1997; Zhu *et al.*, 2001), Reina-San-Martin *et al.* (2005) and Kracker *et al.* (2005) conditionally inactivated Nbs1 in B cells using the CRE/LoxP recombination system. Disruption of Nbs1 resulted in impaired proliferation, chromosomal endoreduplication, high levels of spontaneous DNA damage, and diminished cell survival (Kracker *et al.*, 2005;

Reina-San-Martin et al., 2005). In addition, Nbs1 deficiency in B cells led to a cell intrinsic defect in CSR which was independent of switch region transcription or proliferation abnormalities and due to inefficient recombination at the DNA level (Kracker et al., 2005; Reina-San-Martin et al., 2005). Interestingly, the efficiency of CSR in the absence of Nbs1 was similar to that observed in $ATM^{-/-}$ B cells and would be consistent with a role of Nbs1 in sensing DNA damage, regulating ATM activation and accumulation at switch regions and thus potentiating the phosphorylation of downstream targets, and the transduction of the DNA damage signal during CSR.

4.2.4. 53BP1

Among the ATM targets activated in response to DSB formation, 53BP1 has been implicated in regulating cell cycle arrest at the G2-M and intra-S-cell cycle checkpoints (DiTullio et al., 2002; Fernandez-Capetillo et al., 2002; Wang et al., 2002). 53BP1 forms γ-H2AX-dependent foci in response to DNA damage and at the immunoglobulin heavy chain locus during CSR (Celeste et al., 2003; Fernandez-Capetillo et al., 2002; Mochan et al., 2004; Reina-San-Martin et al., 2004; Ward et al., 2003a). In addition, as mentioned above, 53BP1 senses DNA damage by directly binding to methylated histone H3 (Huyen et al., 2004). Similar to ATM and H2AX, 53BP1 is not required for V(D)J recombination or SHM and its inactivation is associated with hypersensitivity to irradiation, predisposition to T-cell lymphoma, and genomic instability (Manis et al., 2004; Morales et al., 2003; Ward et al., 2003b, 2004). However, 53BP1 differs from other DNA damage response genes in that its inactivation completely abolishes CSR (Manis et al., 2004; Ward et al., 2004). The CSR defect is again B-cell intrinsic and independent of abnormalities in switch region transcription, AID accessibility, or proliferation (Manis et al., 2004; Ward et al., 2004). A notable difference between 53BP1, ATM, and H2AX is that inactivation of 53BP1 results in a significant increase in the frequency of internal deletions in both donor and acceptor switch regions (Reina-San-Martin et al., 2007). Therefore, absence of 53BP1 favors short-range over long-range recombination events and is consistent with the almost complete absence of CSR.

The precise mechanism by which the DNA damage response genes ATM, H2AX, Nbs1 and 53BP1 facilitate the joining of distal switch regions is not fully understood. It has been proposed that the accumulation of these proteins at the site of lesion might facilitate end-joining of switch regions by directly anchoring DNA ends (Bassing and Alt, 2004; Franco et al., 2006; Manis et al., 2004). Alternatively, it is possible that DNA damage sensors like 53BP1 and MRN recognize AID-induced DSB in switch regions, recruit DNA damage transducers ATM and DNA-PK$_{CS}$ which once activated will phosphorylate numerous substrates including histone H2AX. Phosphorylation of H2AX extends over large regions away from the break site, inducing chromatin alterations that may facilitate the synapsis of distal broken DNA ends.

5. AID and Lymphomagenic Lesions

5.1. Mutations in Non-Ig Genes

AID can target a number of non-Ig genes. This effect has been observed in *E. coli*, yeast, fibroblasts, and B-cell lines (Martin and Scharff, 2002; Okazaki *et al.*, 2002; Parsa *et al.*, 2006; Petersen-Mahrt *et al.*, 2002; Poltoratsky *et al.*, 2004; Ramiro *et al.*, 2003; Sohail *et al.*, 2003; Wang *et al.*, 2004; Yoshikawa *et al.*, 2002). An important requirement in all of these experiments is that the target gene is transcribed and the rate of mutation is directly related to the rate of transcription (Martin and Scharff, 2002; Okazaki *et al.*, 2002; Ramiro *et al.*, 2003; Sohail *et al.*, 2003; Yoshikawa *et al.*, 2002). In B-cell lines, the rate of off target mutation is lower than the rate of somatic mutation in B cells and the mutations occurred preferentially at WRC hot spots but were biased toward mutation at G/C pairs, suggesting that the pathways leading to A/T mutations are compromised in these experimental systems.

How off target mutations in B-cell lines and heterologous cell systems relate to the mechanism of targeting in authentic germinal center B cells is still debated. However, B cells from normal donors have been reported to bear mutations, in a number of non-Ig genes, including Bcl-6 (Pasqualucci *et al.*, 1998; Shen *et al.*, 1998), Fas (Muschen *et al.*, 2000), B29 (Igβ), and mb1 (Igα) (Gordon *et al.*, 2003), but not in other genes expressed in B cells such as c-myc, S14, β-globin (Shen *et al.*, 1998), or in genes mutated in large cell lymphomas PIM1, Pax5, and RhoH (Pasqualucci *et al.*, 2001). AID has not formally been proved to produce these off target mutations, but it is likely that it does because mutations are clustered downstream of active promoters, biased toward G/C transitions and WRC hot spots, and they are found in germinal center and memory but not naive B cells. Therefore, physiological levels of AID expression are likely to produce mutations in genes other than Ig.

5.2. Non-Ig Mutations and Lymphomas

Mature B-cell lymphomas, including diffuse large B-cell lymphoma, chronic lymphocytic lymphoma, and follicular lymphoma, frequently harbor mutations in multiple proto-oncogenic loci (Klein *et al.*, 1998; Migliazza *et al.*, 1995; Pasqualucci *et al.*, 2001). These mutations bear the hallmarks of AID-mediated

SHM in non-Ig genes, namely they are transcription dependent, WRC focused and highly biased to G/C pairs.

Some of these mutations are in genes such as Fas or Bcl-6 that might contribute to malignant transformation but this has yet to be proven directly (Muschen *et al.*, 2000; Pasqualucci *et al.*, 2001, 2003). However, the fact that some of the genes mutated in lymphomas, such as PIM1, Pax5, or RhoH, are not mutated in germinal center B cells from normal donors (Pasqualucci *et al.*, 2003), is very suggestive of a selective growth of cells harboring mutations.

In mouse models, AID-induced mutations can promote lymphoma development. Constitutive and ubiquitous expression of AID in transgenic mice leads to T-cell lymphomas (Okazaki *et al.*, 2003; Rucci *et al.*, 2006) and lung microadenomas (Okazaki *et al.*, 2003) but not B-cell lymphomas. The thymomas harbored mutations in the T-cell receptor β gene and in a number of transcribed genes including c-myc and PIM1 (Kotani *et al.*, 2005; Okazaki *et al.*, 2003). Interestingly, CD19 promoter-driven AID expression did not produce B-cell lymphomas or accumulation of aberrant of mutations (Muto *et al.*, 2006). These results suggest that there may be a negative regulation of AID that might protect B cells against excessive DNA damage by AID.

5.3. AID and Chromosome Translocations

Recurrent, reciprocal chromosomal translocations are a hallmark of malignant lymphomas. Many of these translocations juxtapose Ig loci to proto-oncogenes whose expression comes under the control of Ig transcriptional regulatory elements (Kuppers and Dalla-Favera, 2001). For example, Bcl-1 to Ig translocations are found in mantle-zone lymphoma, Bcl-2 to Ig translocations in follicular lymphoma, and c-myc to Ig translocations in Burkitt lymphoma (Kuppers, 2005) and each of these plays an essential but nonexclusive role in the etiology of the lymphoma. Many of the translocation breakpoints associated with lymphoma occur at Ig variable and switch regions supporting the long standing speculation that these events might be related to DNA damage incurred during the SHM and CSR reactions in germinal centers (Kuppers and Dalla-Favera, 2001).

The idea that AID might catalyze the initiation of chromosome translocations was tested in mouse models of plasmacytoma induced by pristane injection or IL-6 overexpression in transgenic mice (reviewed in Potter, 2003). Pristane is a mineral oil that induces chronic inflammation and granuloma when injected intraperitoneally and this is associated with the development of plasmacytomas bearing c-myc/IgH translocations. These translocations were among the first chromosome translocations to be characterized molecularly and they involve the switch region of the Ig heavy chain gene and the 5′-untranslated region of the c-myc proto-oncogene, closely resembling translocations in sporadic Burkitt lymphomas (Potter, 2003). A similar phenotype is observed in IL-6 transgenic mice, and in fact IL-6 is required for the generation of pristane-induced plasmacytomas (reviewed in Potter, 2003).

In the absence of AID, IL-6 transgenic mice developed hyperplastic lymph nodes and plasmacytosis but c-myc/IgH translocations were absent, indicating that in this model AID is indeed required for translocations (Ramiro et al., 2004). The initial studies did not distinguish between a direct catalytic role for AID or an indirect role in facilitating the outgrowth of cells that acquired c-myc/IgH translocations by an AID independent mechanism (Unniraman et al., 2004). However, later experiments proved that the translocations were dependent on AID cytidine deaminase activity and UNG glycosylase, indicating that CSR and c-myc/IgH translocations are initiated by a common mechanism requiring cytidine deaminase activity (Ramiro et al., 2006). In contrast, Ku80, one of the components of the classical NHEJ pathway was not required for c-myc/IgH translocations, suggesting that the resolution of DSBs intermediates during CSR and chromosome translocations may proceed through different pathways (Ramiro et al., 2006).

Under physiological conditions, AID rarely induces c-myc/IgH translocations (Ramiro et al., 2006; Roschke et al., 1997), suggesting the existence of surveillance mechanisms that detect DNA damage and prevent DSBs from being channeled to translocations or that kill cells that overexpress translocated c-myc. Interestingly, ATM deficiency but not deficiency in H2AX or 53BP1 results in accumulation of translocation events (Ramiro et al., 2006). In addition, mutations in the tumor suppressor genes p53 and p19 (ARF) also increase the observed frequency of c-myc/IgH translocations (Ramiro et al., 2006). Together these results are consistent with two independent mechanisms converging on p53 and protecting B cells against chromosome translocations namely, the DNA damage response checkpoint through ATM activation and the oncogenic stress pathway triggered by translocated c-myc and p19 activation. These pathways may overlap since myc overexpression also induces an ATM-p53 dependent DNA damage response (Pusapati et al., 2006). Interestingly, defective CSR, even if it results in an accumulation of IgH associated DSBs, as in the case of H2AX or 53BP1 (Franco et al., 2006; Ramiro et al., 2006) is not sufficient to increase susceptibility to c-myc/IgH translocations (Ramiro et al., 2006). Instead, it seems that translocation susceptibility is related both to the frequency of unresolved breaks and to the degree of impairment of p53 signaling (Ramiro et al., 2006).

A translocation reaction involves the generation of DSBs at both chromosomal partners. While it is established that breaks at the Ig locus are initiated by AID (see above), there is no direct proof that DSBs at proto-oncogenes are also

AID dependent or that transcription of the partner is required. The observations that AID can target genes other than Ig (see above) and that AID can localize with the myc locus in activated B cells (Duquette et al., 2005) are compatible with AID mediating these breaks. Alternatively, or additionally, some of the genes involved in chromosome translocations to the Ig locus may contain fragile sites prone to breakage under replicative stress.

Translocations to the Ig light chain loci, which undergo SHM but not CSR, can also occur in B-cell lymphomas (reviewed in Kuppers and Dalla-Favera, 2001). Some of these are likely to involve lesions produced during V(D)J recombination (Lieber et al., 2006; Reddy et al., 2006), but they could also be products of SHM. DSBs have been detected on Ig loci during SHM, but they are not obligate intermediates in this reaction, as shown by direct analysis of breaks and by the fact that DSB response proteins are dispensable for SHM (Bross et al., 2002; Chua et al., 2002; Papavasiliou and Schatz, 2002; Petersen et al., 2001; Reina-San-Martin et al., 2003). Nevertheless, these broken DNA ends could serve as intermediates in the translocation reaction.

6. Conclusions and Perspectives

AID triggers all B-cell specific DNA modifications reactions that shape the antibody repertoire and can also initiate chromosome translocations. How the initial AID-induced DNA lesion is processed determines the outcome of the reaction and different factors are involved in these processes. ATM is an interesting example, because it is not required for SHM, but is required for CSR and in its absence c-myc/IgH translocations are increased.

Why CSR should be preferred to a translocation once a DSB is generated in the switch regions of the heavy chain locus is an important question that lacks a complete mechanistic explanation. Local availability of DSBs and limited off target lesions by AID may be part of the answer, but additional mechanisms involving local chromatin modification by factors such as H2AX and 53BP1 must also play a role. Finally, as a failsafe mechanism, cells that do undergo translocation appear to be deleted by the oncogenic stress response. Understanding how each of these contributes to maintaining genomic stability and preventing translocations is an important area for future research.

References

Ahnesorg, P., Smith, P., and Jackson, S. P. (2006). XLF interacts with the XRCC4-DNA ligase IV complex to promote DNA nonhomologous end-joining. *Cell* **124**, 301–313.

Anderson, L., Henderson, C., and Adachi, Y. (2001). Phosphorylation and rapid relocalization of 53BP1 to nuclear foci upon DNA damage. *Mol. Cell. Biol.* **21**, 1719–1729.

Bachl, J., Carlson, C., Gray-Schopfer, V., Dessing, M., and Olsson, C. (2001). Increased transcription levels induce higher mutation rates in a hypermutating cell line. *J. Immunol.* **166,** 5051–5057.

Bakkenist, C. J., and Kastan, M. B. (2003). DNA damage activates ATM through intermolecular autophosphorylation and dimer dissociation. *Nature* **421,** 499–506.

Barlow, C., Hirotsune, S., Paylor, R., Liyanage, M., Eckhaus, M., Collins, F., Shiloh, Y., Crawley, J. N., Ried, T., Tagle, D., and Wynshaw-Boris, A. (1996). Atm-deficient mice: A paradigm of ataxia telangiectasia. *Cell* **86,** 159–171.

Barnes, D. E., Stamp, G., Rosewell, I., Denzel, A., and Lindahl, T. (1998). Targeted disruption of the gene encoding DNA ligase IV leads to lethality in embryonic mice. *Curr. Biol.* **8,** 1395–1398.

Barreto, V., Reina-San-Martin, B., Ramiro, A. R., McBride, K. M., and Nussenzweig, M. C. (2003). C-terminal deletion of AID uncouples class switch recombination from somatic hypermutation and gene conversion. *Mol. Cell* **12,** 501–508.

Barreto, V. M., Pan-Hammarstrom, Q., Zhao, Y., Hammarstrom, L., Misulovin, Z., and Nussenzweig, M. C. (2005a). AID from bony fish catalyzes class switch recombination. *J. Exp. Med.* **202,** 733–738.

Barreto, V. M., Ramiro, A. R., and Nussenzweig, M. C. (2005b). Activation-induced deaminase: Controversies and open questions. *Trends Immunol.* **26,** 90–96.

Bassing, C. H., and Alt, F. W. (2004). H2AX may function as an anchor to hold broken chromosomal DNA ends in close proximity. *Cell Cycle* **3,** 149–153.

Basu, U., Chaudhuri, J., Alpert, C., Dutt, S., Ranganath, S., Li, G., Schrum, J. P., Manis, J. P., and Alt, F. W. (2005). The AID antibody diversification enzyme is regulated by protein kinase A phosphorylation. *Nature* **438,** 508–511.

Begum, N. A., Kinoshita, K., Kakazu, N., Muramatsu, M., Nagaoka, H., Shinkura, R., Biniszkiewicz, D., Boyer, L. A., Jaenisch, R., and Honjo, T. (2004). Uracil DNA glycosylase activity is dispensable for immunoglobulin class switch. *Science* **305,** 1160–1163.

Besmer, E., Market, E., and Papavasiliou, F. N. (2006). The transcription elongation complex directs activation-induced cytidine deaminase-mediated DNA deamination. *Mol. Cell. Biol.* **26,** 4378–4385.

Borghesani, P. R., Alt, F. W., Bottaro, A., Davidson, L., Aksoy, S., Rathbun, G. A., Roberts, T. M., Swat, W., Segal, R. A., and Gu, Y. (2000). Abnormal development of Purkinje cells and lymphocytes in Atm mutant mice. *Proc. Natl. Acad. Sci. USA* **97,** 3336–3341.

Bosma, G. C., Kim, J., Urich, T., Fath, D. M., Cotticelli, M. G., Ruetsch, N. R., Radic, M. Z., and Bosma, M. J. (2002). DNA-dependent protein kinase activity is not required for immunoglobulin class switching. *J. Exp. Med.* **196,** 1483–1495.

Bransteitter, R., Pham, P., Scharff, M. D., and Goodman, M. F. (2003). Activation-induced cytidine deaminase deaminates deoxycytidine on single-stranded DNA but requires the action of RNase. *Proc. Natl. Acad. Sci. USA* **100,** 4102–4107.

Brar, S. S., Watson, M., and Diaz, M. (2004). Activation-induced cytosine deaminase (AID) is actively exported out of the nucleus but retained by the induction of DNA breaks. *J. Biol. Chem.* **279,** 26395–26401.

Bross, L., Muramatsu, M., Kinoshita, K., Honjo, T., and Jacobs, H. (2002). DNA double-strand breaks: Prior to but not sufficient in targeting hypermutation. *J. Exp. Med.* **195,** 1187–1192.

Brown, E. J., and Baltimore, D. (2003). Essential and dispensable roles of ATR in cell cycle arrest and genome maintenance. *Genes Dev.* **17,** 615–628.

Buck, D., Malivert, L., de Chasseval, R., Barraud, A., Fondaneche, M. C., Sanal, O., Plebani, A., Stephan, J. L., Hufnagel, M., le Deist, F., Fischer, A., Durandy, A., et al. (2006). Cernunnos, a novel nonhomologous end-joining factor, is mutated in human immunodeficiency with microcephaly. Cell **124**, 287–299.

Burma, S., Chen, B. P., Murphy, M., Kurimasa, A., and Chen, D. J. (2001). ATM phosphorylates histone H2AX in response to DNA double-strand breaks. J. Biol. Chem. **276**, 42462–42467.

Carney, J. P., Maser, R. S., Olivares, H., Davis, E. M., Le Beau, M., Yates, J. R., III, Hays, L., Morgan, W. F., and Petrini, J. H. (1998). The hMre11/hRad50 protein complex and Nijmegen breakage syndrome: Linkage of double-strand break repair to the cellular DNA damage response. Cell **93**, 477–486.

Casellas, R., Nussenzweig, A., Wuerffel, R., Pelanda, R., Reichlin, A., Suh, H., Qin, X. F., Besmer, E., Kenter, A., Rajewsky, K., and Nussenzweig, M. C. (1998). Ku80 is required for immunoglobulin isotype switching. EMBO J. **17**, 2404–2411.

Celeste, A., Petersen, S., Romanienko, P. J., Fernandez-Capetillo, O., Chen, H. T., Sedelnikova, O. A., Reina-San-Martin, B., Coppola, V., Meffre, E., Difilippantonio, M. J., Redon, C., Pilch, D. R., et al. (2002). Genomic instability in mice lacking histone H2AX. Science **296**, 922–927.

Celeste, A., Fernandez-Capetillo, O., Kruhlak, M. J., Pilch, D. R., Staudt, D. W., Lee, A., Bonner, R. F., Bonner, W. M., and Nussenzweig, A. (2003). Histone H2AX phosphorylation is dispensable for the initial recognition of DNA breaks. Nat. Cell Biol. **5**, 675–679.

Chaudhuri, J., Tian, M., Khuong, C., Chua, K., Pinaud, E., and Alt, F. W. (2003). Transcription-targeted DNA deamination by the AID antibody diversification enzyme. Nature **422**, 726–730.

Chaudhuri, J., Khuong, C., and Alt, F. W. (2004). Replication protein A interacts with AID to promote deamination of somatic hypermutation targets. Nature **430**, 992–998.

Chua, K. F., Alt, F. W., and Manis, J. P. (2002). The function of AID in somatic mutation and class switch recombination: Upstream or downstream of DNA breaks. J. Exp. Med. **195**, F37–F41.

Conticello, S. G., Thomas, C. J., Petersen-Mahrt, S. K., and Neuberger, M. S. (2005). Evolution of the AID/APOBEC family of polynucleotide (deoxy)cytidine deaminases. Mol. Biol. Evol. **22**, 367–377.

Cook, A. J., Oganesian, L., Harumal, P., Basten, A., Brink, R., and Jolly, C. J. (2003). Reduced switching in SCID B cells is associated with altered somatic mutation of recombined S regions. J. Immunol. **171**, 6556–6564.

D'Amours, D., and Jackson, S. P. (2002). The Mre11 complex: At the crossroads of DNA repair and checkpoint signalling. Nat. Rev. Mol. Cell Biol. **3**, 317–327.

de Villartay, J. P., Fischer, A., and Durandy, A. (2003). The mechanisms of immune diversification and their disorders. Nat. Rev. Immunol. **3**, 962–972.

de Yebenes, V. G., and Ramiro, A. R. (2006). Activation-induced deaminase: Light and dark sides. Trends Mol. Med. **12**, 432–439.

Dedeoglu, F., Horwitz, B., Chaudhuri, J., Alt, F. W., and Geha, R. S. (2004). Induction of activation-induced cytidine deaminase gene expression by IL-4 and CD40 ligation is dependent on STAT6 and NFkappaB. Int. Immunol. **16**, 395–404.

Di Noia, J., and Neuberger, M. S. (2002). Altering the pathway of immunoglobulin hypermutation by inhibiting uracil-DNA glycosylase. Nature **419**, 43–48.

Dickerson, S. K., Market, E., Besmer, E., and Papavasiliou, F. N. (2003). AID mediates hypermutation by deaminating single stranded DNA. J. Exp. Med. **197**, 1291–1296.

DiTullio, R. A., Jr., Mochan, T. A., Venere, M., Bartkova, J., Sehested, M., Bartek, J., and Halazonetis, T. D. (2002). 53BP1 functions in an ATM-dependent checkpoint pathway that is constitutively activated in human cancer. *Nat. Cell Biol.* **4,** 998–1002.

Dudley, D. D., Manis, J. P., Zarrin, A. A., Kaylor, L., Tian, M., and Alt, F. W. (2002). Internal IgH class switch region deletions are position-independent and enhanced by AID expression. *Proc. Natl. Acad. Sci. USA* **99,** 9984–9989.

Duquette, M. L., Pham, P., Goodman, M. F., and Maizels, N. (2005). AID binds to transcription-induced structures in c-MYC that map to regions associated with translocation and hypermutation. *Oncogene* **24,** 5791–5798.

Durandy, A., Peron, S., and Fischer, A. (2006). Hyper-IgM syndromes. *Curr. Opin. Rheumatol.* **18,** 369–376.

Elson, A., Wang, Y., Daugherty, C. J., Morton, C. C., Zhou, F., Campos-Torres, J., and Leder, P. (1996). Pleiotropic defects in ataxia-telangiectasia protein-deficient mice. *Proc. Natl. Acad. Sci. USA* **93,** 13084–13089.

Fernandez-Capetillo, O., Chen, H. T., Celeste, A., Ward, I., Romanienko, P. J., Morales, J. C., Naka, K., Xia, Z., Camerini-Otero, R. D., Motoyama, N., Carpenter, P. B., Bonner, W. M., *et al.* (2002). DNA damage-induced G2-M checkpoint activation by histone H2AX and 53BP1. *Nat. Cell Biol.* **4,** 993–997.

Fernandez-Capetillo, O., Mahadevaiah, S. K., Celeste, A., Romanienko, P. J., Camerini-Otero, R. D., Bonner, W. M., Manova, K., Burgoyne, P., and Nussenzweig, A. (2003). H2AX is required for chromatin remodeling and inactivation of sex chromosomes in male mouse meiosis. *Dev. Cell* **4,** 497–508.

Fernandez-Capetillo, O., Lee, A., Nussenzweig, M., and Nussenzweig, A. (2004). H2AX: The histone guardian of the genome. *DNA Repair (Amst.)* **3,** 959–967.

Franco, S., Gostissa, M., Zha, S., Lombard, D. B., Murphy, M. M., Zarrin, A. A., Yan, C., Tepsuporn, S., Morales, J. C., Adams, M. M., Lou, Z., Bassing, C. H., *et al.* (2006). H2AX prevents DNA breaks from progressing to chromosome breaks and translocations. *Mol. Cell* **21,** 201–214.

Frank, K. M., Sekiguchi, J. M., Seidl, K. J., Swat, W., Rathbun, G. A., Cheng, H. L., Davidson, L., Kangaloo, L., and Alt, F. W. (1998). Late embryonic lethality and impaired V(D)J recombination in mice lacking DNA ligase IV. *Nature* **396,** 173–177.

Fukita, Y., Jacobs, H., and Rajewsky, K. (1998). Somatic hypermutation in the heavy chain locus correlates with transcription. *Immunity* **9,** 105–114.

Gao, Y., Sun, Y., Frank, K. M., Dikkes, P., Fujiwara, Y., Seidl, K. J., Sekiguchi, J. M., Rathbun, G. A., Swat, W., Wang, J., Bronson, R. T., Malynn, B. A., *et al.* (1998). A critical role for DNA end-joining proteins in both lymphogenesis and neurogenesis. *Cell* **95,** 891–902.

Gonda, H., Sugai, M., Nambu, Y., Katakai, T., Agata, Y., Mori, K. J., Yokota, Y., and Shimizu, A. (2003). The balance between Pax5 and Id2 activities is the key to AID gene expression. *J. Exp. Med.* **198,** 1427–1437.

Gordon, M. S., Kanegai, C. M., Doerr, J. R., and Wall, R. (2003). Somatic hypermutation of the B cell receptor genes B29 (Igbeta, CD79b) and mb1 (Igalpha, CD79a). *Proc. Natl. Acad. Sci. USA* **100,** 4126–4131.

Honjo, T., Kinoshita, K., and Muramatsu, M. (2002). Molecular mechanism of class switch recombination: Linkage with somatic hypermutation. *Annu. Rev. Immunol.* **20,** 165–196.

Honjo, T., Nagaoka, H., Shinkura, R., and Muramatsu, M. (2005). AID to overcome the limitations of genomic information. *Nat. Immunol.* **6,** 655–661.

Huyen, Y., Zgheib, O., DiTullio, R. A., Jr., Gorgoulis, V. G., Zacharatos, P., Petty, T. J., Sheston, E. A., Mellert, H. S., Stavridi, E. S., and Halazonetis, T. D. (2004). Methylated lysine 79 of histone H3 targets 53BP1 to DNA double-strand breaks. *Nature* **432**, 406–411.

Ichikawa, H. T., Sowden, M. P., Torelli, A. T., Bachl, J., Huang, P., Dance, G. S., Marr, S. H., Robert, J., Wedekind, J. E., Smith, H. C., and Bottaro, A. (2006). Structural phylogenetic analysis of activation-induced deaminase function. *J. Immunol.* **177**, 355–361.

Imai, K., Slupphaug, G., Lee, W. I., Revy, P., Nonoyama, S., Catalan, N., Yel, L., Forveille, M., Kavli, B., Krokan, H. E., Ochs, H. D., Fischer, A., *et al.* (2003). Human uracil-DNA glycosylase deficiency associated with profoundly impaired immunoglobulin class-switch recombination. *Nat. Immunol.* **4**, 1023–1028.

Imai, K., Zhu, Y., Revy, P., Morio, T., Mizutani, S., Fischer, A., Nonoyama, S., and Durandy, A. (2005). Analysis of class switch recombination and somatic hypermutation in patients affected with autosomal dominant hyper-IgM syndrome type 2. *Clin. Immunol.* **115**, 277–285.

Ito, S., Nagaoka, H., Shinkura, R., Begum, N., Muramatsu, M., Nakata, M., and Honjo, T. (2004). Activation-induced cytidine deaminase shuttles between nucleus and cytoplasm like apolipoprotein B mRNA editing catalytic polypeptide 1. *Proc. Natl. Acad. Sci. USA* **101**, 1975–1980.

Jung, S., Rajewsky, K., and Radbruch, A. (1993). Shutdown of class switch recombination by deletion of a switch region control element. *Science* **259**, 984–987.

Klein, U., Goossens, T., Fischer, M., Kanzler, H., Braeuninger, A., Rajewsky, K., and Kuppers, R. (1998). Somatic hypermutation in normal and transformed human B cells. *Immunol. Rev.* **162**, 261–280.

Klein, U., Casola, S., Cattoretti, G., Shen, Q., Lia, M., Mo, T., Ludwig, T., Rajewsky, K., and Dalla-Favera, R. (2006). Transcription factor IRF4 controls plasma cell differentiation and class-switch recombination. *Nat. Immunol.* **7**, 773–782.

Kotani, A., Okazaki, I. M., Muramatsu, M., Kinoshita, K., Begum, N. A., Nakajima, T., Saito, H., and Honjo, T. (2005). A target selection of somatic hypermutations is regulated similarly between T and B cells upon activation-induced cytidine deaminase expression. *Proc. Natl. Acad. Sci. USA* **102**, 4506–4511.

Kracker, S., Bergmann, Y., Demuth, I., Frappart, P. O., Hildebrand, G., Christine, R., Wang, Z. Q., Sperling, K., Digweed, M., and Radbruch, A. (2005). Nibrin functions in Ig class-switch recombination. *Proc. Natl. Acad. Sci. USA* **102**, 1584–1589.

Kuppers, R. (2005). Mechanisms of B-cell lymphoma pathogenesis. *Nat. Rev. Cancer* **5**, 251–262.

Kuppers, R., and Dalla-Favera, R. (2001). Mechanisms of chromosomal translocations in B cell lymphomas. *Oncogene* **20**, 5580–5594.

Lahdesmaki, A., Taylor, A. M., Chrzanowska, K. H., and Pan-Hammarstrom, Q. (2004). Delineation of the role of the Mre11 complex in class switch recombination. *J. Biol. Chem.* **279**, 16479–16487.

Li, Z., Luo, Z., and Scharff, M. D. (2004a). Differential regulation of histone acetylation and generation of mutations in switch regions is associated with Ig class switching. *Proc. Natl. Acad. Sci. USA* **101**, 15428–15433.

Li, Z., Scherer, S. J., Ronai, D., Iglesias-Ussel, M. D., Peled, J. U., Bardwell, P. D., Zhuang, M., Lee, K., Martin, A., Edelmann, W., and Scharff, M. D. (2004b). Examination of Msh6- and Msh3-deficient mice in class switching reveals overlapping and distinct roles of MutS homologues in antibody diversification. *J. Exp. Med.* **200**, 47–59.

Li, Z., Woo, C. J., Iglesias-Ussel, M. D., Ronai, D., and Scharff, M. D. (2004c). The generation of antibody diversity through somatic hypermutation and class switch recombination. *Genes Dev.* **18**, 1–11.

Li, Z., Zhao, C., Iglesias-Ussel, M. D., Polonskaya, Z., Zhuang, M., Yang, G., Luo, Z., Edelmann, W., and Scharff, M. D. (2006). The mismatch repair protein Msh6 influences the *in vivo* AID targeting to the Ig locus. *Immunity* **24**, 393–403.

Lieber, M. R., Yu, K., and Raghavan, S. C. (2006). Roles of nonhomologous DNA end joining, V(D)J recombination, and class switch recombination in chromosomal translocations. *DNA Repair (Amst.)* **5**, 1234–1245.

Lin, K. I., Angelin-Duclos, C., Kuo, T. C., and Calame, K. (2002). Blimp-1-dependent repression of Pax-5 is required for differentiation of B cells to immunoglobulin M-secreting plasma cells. *Mol. Cell Biol.* **22**, 4771–4780.

Lumsden, J. M., McCarty, T., Petiniot, L. K., Shen, R., Barlow, C., Wynn, T. A., Morse, H. C., III, Gearhart, P. J., Wynshaw-Boris, A., Max, E. E., and Hodes, R. J. (2004). Immunoglobulin class switch recombination is impaired in Atm-deficient mice. *J. Exp. Med.* **200**, 1111–1121.

Luo, Z., Ronai, D., and Scharff, M. D. (2004). The role of activation-induced cytidine deaminase in antibody diversification, immunodeficiency, and B-cell malignancies. *J. Allergy Clin. Immunol.* **114**, 726–735; quiz 736.

Manis, J. P., Gu, Y., Lansford, R., Sonoda, E., Ferrini, R., Davidson, L., Rajewsky, K., and Alt, F. W. (1998). Ku70 is required for late B cell development and immunoglobulin heavy chain class switching. *J. Exp. Med.* **187**, 2081–2089.

Manis, J. P., Dudley, D., Kaylor, L., and Alt, F. W. (2002). IgH class switch recombination to IgG1 in DNA-PKcs-deficient B cells. *Immunity* **16**, 607–617.

Manis, J. P., Morales, J. C., Xia, Z., Kutok, J. L., Alt, F. W., and Carpenter, P. B. (2004). 53BP1 links DNA damage-response pathways to immunoglobulin heavy chain class-switch recombination. *Nat. Immunol.* **5**, 481–487.

Martin, A., and Scharff, M. D. (2002). Somatic hypermutation of the AID transgene in B and non-B cells. *Proc. Natl. Acad. Sci. USA* **99**, 12304–12308.

Martomo, S. A., Yang, W. W., and Gearhart, P. J. (2004). A role for Msh6 but not Msh3 in somatic hypermutation and class switch recombination. *J. Exp. Med.* **200**, 61–68.

McBride, K. M., Barreto, V., Ramiro, A. R., Stavropoulos, P., and Nussenzweig, M. C. (2004). Somatic hypermutation is limited by CRM1-dependent nuclear export of activation-induced deaminase. *J. Exp. Med.* **199**, 1235–1244.

McBride, K. M., Gazumyan, A., Woo, E. M., Barreto, V. M., Robbiani, D. F., Chait, B. T., and Nussenzweig, M. C. (2006). Regulation of hypermutation by activation-induced cytidine deaminase phosphorylation. *Proc. Natl. Acad. Sci. USA* **103**, 8798–8803.

McKean, D., Huppi, K., Bell, M., Staudt, L., Gerhard, W., and Weigert, M. (1984). Generation of antibody diversity in the immune response of BALB/c mice to influenza virus hemagglutinin. *Proc. Natl. Acad. Sci. USA* **81**, 3180–3184.

Meffre, E., Casellas, R., and Nussenzweig, M. C. (2000). Antibody regulation of B cell development. *Nat. Immunol.* **1**, 379–385.

Migliazza, A., Martinotti, S., Chen, W., Fusco, C., Ye, B. H., Knowles, D. M., Offit, K., Chaganti, R. S., and Dalla-Favera, R. (1995). Frequent somatic hypermutation of the 5' noncoding region of the BCL6 gene in B-cell lymphoma. *Proc. Natl. Acad. Sci. USA* **92**, 12520–12524.

Mochan, T. A., Venere, M., DiTullio, R. A., Jr., and Halazonetis, T. D. (2004). 53BP1, an activator of ATM in response to DNA damage. *DNA Repair (Amst.)* **3**, 945–952.

Morales, J. C., Xia, Z., Lu, T., Aldrich, M. B., Wang, B., Rosales, C., Kellems, R. E., Hittelman, W. N., Elledge, S. J., and Carpenter, P. B. (2003). Role for the BRCA1 C-terminal repeats (BRCT) protein 53BP1 in maintaining genomic stability. *J. Biol. Chem.* **278**, 14971–14977.

Moshous, D., Callebaut, I., de Chasseval, R., Corneo, B., Cavazzana-Calvo, M., Le Deist, F., Tezcan, I., Sanal, O., Bertrand, Y., Philippe, N., Fischer, A., and de Villartay, J. P. (2001). Artemis, a novel DNA double-strand break repair/V(D)J recombination protein, is mutated in human severe combined immune deficiency. *Cell* **105**, 177-186.

Muramatsu, M., Sankaranand, V. S., Anant, S., Sugai, M., Kinoshita, K., Davidson, N. O., and Honjo, T. (1999). Specific expression of activation-induced cytidine deaminase (AID), a novel member of the RNA-editing deaminase family in germinal center B cells. *J. Biol. Chem.* **274**, 18470-18476.

Muschen, M., Re, D., Jungnickel, B., Diehl, V., Rajewsky, K., and Kuppers, R. (2000). Somatic mutation of the CD95 gene in human B cells as a side-effect of the germinal center reaction. *J. Exp. Med.* **192**, 1833-1840.

Muto, T., Okazaki, I. M., Yamada, S., Tanaka, Y., Kinoshita, K., Muramatsu, M., Nagaoka, H., and Honjo, T. (2006). Negative regulation of activation-induced cytidine deaminase in B cells. *Proc. Natl. Acad. Sci. USA.* **103**, 2752-2757.

Nagaoka, H., Muramatsu, M., Yamamura, N., Kinoshita, K., and Honjo, T. (2002). Activation-induced deaminase (AID)-directed hypermutation in the immunoglobulin Smu region: Implication of AID involvement in a common step of class switch recombination and somatic hypermutation. *J. Exp. Med.* **195**, 529-534.

Nambu, Y., Sugai, M., Gonda, H., Lee, C. G., Katakai, T., Agata, Y., Yokota, Y., and Shimizu, A. (2003). Transcription-coupled events associating with immunoglobulin switch region chromatin. *Science* **302**, 2137-2140.

Neuberger, M. S., Di Noia, J. M., Beale, R. C., Williams, G. T., Yang, Z., and Rada, C. (2005). Somatic hypermutation at A.T pairs: Polymerase error versus dUTP incorporation. *Nat. Rev. Immunol.* **5**, 171-178.

Odegard, V. H., Kim, S. T., Anderson, S. M., Shlomchik, M. J., and Schatz, D. G. (2005). Histone modifications associated with somatic hypermutation. *Immunity* **23**, 101-110.

Okazaki, I. M., Kinoshita, K., Muramatsu, M., Yoshikawa, K., and Honjo, T. (2002). The AID enzyme induces class switch recombination in fibroblasts. *Nature* **416**, 340-345.

Okazaki, I. M., Hiai, H., Kakazu, N., Yamada, S., Muramatsu, M., Kinoshita, K., and Honjo, T. (2003). Constitutive expression of AID leads to tumorigenesis. *J. Exp. Med.* **197**, 1173-1181.

Pan-Hammarstrom, Q., Dai, S., Zhao, Y., van Dijk-Hard, I. F., Gatti, R. A., Borresen-Dale, A. L., and Hammarstrom, L. (2003). ATM is not required in somatic hypermutation of VH, but is involved in the introduction of mutations in the switch mu region. *J. Immunol.* **170**, 3707-3716.

Pan-Hammarstrom, Q., Jones, A. M., Lahdesmaki, A., Zhou, W., Gatti, R. A., Hammarstrom, L., Gennery, A. R., and Ehrenstein, M. R. (2005). Impact of DNA ligase IV on nonhomologous end joining pathways during class switch recombination in human cells. *J. Exp. Med.* **201**, 189-194.

Papavasiliou, F. N., and Schatz, D. G. (2002). The activation-induced deaminase functions in a postcleavage step of the somatic hypermutation process. *J. Exp. Med.* **195**, 1193-1198.

Parsa, J. Y., Basit, W., Wang, C. L., Gommerman, J. L., Carlyle, J. R., and Martin, A. (2006). AID mutates a non-immunoglobulin transgene independent of chromosomal position. *Mol. Immunol.* **44**, 567-575.

Pasqualucci, L., Migliazza, A., Fracchiolla, N., William, C., Neri, A., Baldini, L., Chaganti, R. S., Klein, U., Kuppers, R., Rajewsky, K., and Dalla-Favera, R. (1998). BCL-6 mutations in normal germinal center B cells: Evidence of somatic hypermutation acting outside Ig loci. *Proc. Natl. Acad. Sci. USA* **95**, 11816-11821.

Pasqualucci, L., Neumeister, P., Goossens, T., Nanjangud, G., Chaganti, R. S., Kuppers, R., and Dalla-Favera, R. (2001). Hypermutation of multiple proto-oncogenes in B-cell diffuse large-cell lymphomas. *Nature* **412**, 341–346.

Pasqualucci, L., Migliazza, A., Basso, K., Houldsworth, J., Chaganti, R. S., and Dalla-Favera, R. (2003). Mutations of the BCL6 proto-oncogene disrupt its negative autoregulation in diffuse large B-cell lymphoma. *Blood* **101**, 2914–2923.

Pasqualucci, L., Kitaura, Y., Gu, H., and Dalla-Favera, R. (2006). PKA-mediated phosphorylation regulates the function of activation-induced deaminase (AID) in B cells. *Proc. Natl. Acad. Sci. USA* **103**, 395–400.

Paull, T. T., Rogakou, E. P., Yamazaki, V., Kirchgessner, C. U., Gellert, M., and Bonner, W. M. (2000). A critical role for histone H2AX in recruitment of repair factors to nuclear foci after DNA damage. *Curr. Biol.* **10**, 886–895.

Pellegrini, M., Celeste, A., Difilippantonio, S., Guo, R., Wang, W., Feigenbaum, L., and Nussenzweig, A. (2006). Autophosphorylation at serine 1987 is dispensable for murine Atm activation *in vivo*. *Nature* **443**, 222–225.

Petersen, S., Casellas, R., Reina-San-Martin, B., Chen, H. T., Difilippantonio, M. J., Wilson, P. C., Hanitsch, L., Celeste, A., Muramatsu, M., Pilch, D. R., Redon, C., Ried, T., *et al*. (2001). AID is required to initiate Nbs1/gamma-H2AX focus formation and mutations at sites of class switching. *Nature* **414**, 660–665.

Petersen-Mahrt, S. K., and Neuberger, M. S. (2003). *In vitro* deamination of cytosine to uracil in single-stranded DNA by apolipoprotein B editing complex catalytic subunit 1 (APOBEC1). *J. Biol. Chem.* **278**, 19583–19586.

Petersen-Mahrt, S. K., Harris, R. S., and Neuberger, M. S. (2002). AID mutates *E. coli* suggesting a DNA deamination mechanism for antibody diversification. *Nature* **418**, 99–103.

Pham, P., Bransteitter, R., Petruska, J., and Goodman, M. F. (2003). Processive AID-catalysed cytosine deamination on single-stranded DNA simulates somatic hypermutation. *Nature* **424**, 103–107.

Poltoratsky, V. P., Wilson, S. H., Kunkel, T. A., and Pavlov, Y. I. (2004). Recombinogenic phenotype of human activation-induced cytosine deaminase. *J. Immunol.* **172**, 4308–4313.

Potter, M. (2003). Neoplastic development in plasma cells. *Immunol. Rev.* **194**, 177–195.

Pusapati, R. V., Rounbehler, R. J., Hong, S., Powers, J. T., Yan, M., Kiguchi, K., McArthur, M. J., Wong, P. K., and Johnson, D. G. (2006). ATM promotes apoptosis and suppresses tumorigenesis in response to Myc. *Proc. Natl. Acad. Sci. USA* **103**, 1446–1451.

Quartier, P., Bustamante, J., Sanal, O., Plebani, A., Debre, M., Deville, A., Litzman, J., Levy, J., Fermand, J. P., Lane, P., Horneff, G., Aksu, G., *et al*. (2004). Clinical, immunologic and genetic analysis of 29 patients with autosomal recessive hyper-IgM syndrome due to activation-induced cytidine deaminase deficiency. *Clin. Immunol.* **110**, 22–29.

Rada, C., Ehrenstein, M. R., Neuberger, M. S., and Milstein, C. (1998). Hot spot focusing of somatic hypermutation in MSH2-deficient mice suggests two stages of mutational targeting. *Immunity* **9**, 135–141.

Rada, C., Jarvis, J. M., and Milstein, C. (2002a). AID-GFP chimeric protein increases hypermutation of Ig genes with no evidence of nuclear localization. *Proc. Natl. Acad. Sci. USA* **99**, 7003–7008.

Rada, C., Williams, G. T., Nilsen, H., Barnes, D. E., Lindahl, T., and Neuberger, M. S. (2002b). Immunoglobulin isotype switching is inhibited and somatic hypermutation perturbed in UNG-deficient mice. *Curr. Biol.* **12**, 1748–1755.

Rada, C., Di Noia, J. M., and Neuberger, M. S. (2004). Mismatch recognition and uracil excision provide complementary paths to both Ig switching and the A/T-focused phase of somatic mutation. *Mol. Cell* **16**, 163–171.

Rajewsky, K. (1996). Clonal selection and learning in the antibody system. *Nature* **381**, 751–758.

Ramiro, A. R., Stavropoulos, P., Jankovic, M., and Nussenzweig, M. C. (2003). Transcription enhances AID-mediated cytidine deamination by exposing single-stranded DNA on the nontemplate strand. *Nat. Immunol.* **4**, 452–456.

Ramiro, A. R., Jankovic, M., Eisenreich, T., Difilippantonio, S., Chen-Kiang, S., Muramatsu, M., Honjo, T., Nussenzweig, A., and Nussenzweig, M. C. (2004). AID is required for c-myc/IgH chromosome translocations *in vivo*. *Cell* **118**, 431–438.

Ramiro, A. R., Jankovic, M., Callen, E., Difilippantonio, S., Chen, H. T., McBride, K. M., Eisenreich, T. R., Chen, J., Dickins, R. A., Lowe, S. W., Nussenzweig, A., and Nussenzweig, M. C. (2006). Role of genomic instability and p53 in AID-induced c-myc-Igh translocations. *Nature* **440**, 105–109.

Rappold, I., Iwabuchi, K., Date, T., and Chen, J. (2001). Tumor suppressor p53 binding protein 1 (53BP1) is involved in DNA damage-signaling pathways. *J. Cell Biol.* **153**, 613–620.

Reddy, Y. V., Perkins, E. J., and Ramsden, D. A. (2006). Genomic instability due to V(D)J recombination-associated transposition. *Genes Dev.* **20**, 1575–1582.

Reina-San-Martin, B., Difilippantonio, S., Hanitsch, L., Masilamani, R. F., Nussenzweig, A., and Nussenzweig, M. C. (2003). H2AX is required for recombination between immunoglobulin switch regions but not for intra-switch region recombination or somatic hypermutation. *J. Exp. Med.* **197**, 1767–1778.

Reina-San-Martin, B., Chen, H. T., Nussenzweig, A., and Nussenzweig, M. C. (2004). ATM is required for efficient recombination between immunoglobulin switch regions. *J. Exp. Med.* **200**, 1103–1110.

Reina-San-Martin, B., Nussenzweig, M. C., Nussenzweig, A., and Difilippantonio, S. (2005). Genomic instability, endoreduplication, and diminished Ig class-switch recombination in B cells lacking Nbs1. *Proc. Natl. Acad. Sci. USA* **102**, 1590–1595.

Reina-San-Martin, B., Chen, J., Nussenzweig, A., and Nussenzweig, M. C. (2007). Enhanced intra-switch region recombination during immunoglobulin class switch recombination in 53BP1(−/−) B cells. *Eur. J. Immunol.* **37**, 235–239.

Revy, P., Muto, T., Levy, Y., Geissmann, F., Plebani, A., Sanal, O., Catalan, N., Forveille, M., Dufourcq-Labelouse, R., Gennery, A., Tezcan, I., Ersoy, F., *et al.* (2000). Activation-induced cytidine deaminase (AID) deficiency causes the autosomal recessive form of the Hyper-IgM syndrome (HIGM2). *Cell* **102**, 565–575.

Rogakou, E. P., Pilch, D. R., Orr, A. H., Ivanova, V. S., and Bonner, W. M. (1998). DNA double-stranded breaks induce histone H2AX phosphorylation on serine 139. *J. Biol. Chem.* **273**, 5858–5868.

Rolink, A., Melchers, F., and Andersson, J. (1996). The SCID but not the RAG-2 gene product is required for S mu-S epsilon heavy chain class switching. *Immunity* **5**, 319–330.

Rooney, S., Alt, F. W., Sekiguchi, J., and Manis, J. P. (2005). Artemis-independent functions of DNA-dependent protein kinase in Ig heavy chain class switch recombination and development. *Proc. Natl. Acad. Sci. USA* **102**, 2471–2475.

Roschke, V., Kopantzev, E., Dertzbaugh, M., and Rudikoff, S. (1997). Chromosomal translocations deregulating c-myc are associated with normal immune responses. *Oncogene* **14**, 3011–3016.

Rucci, F., Cattaneo, L., Marrella, V., Sacco, M. G., Sobacchi, C., Lucchini, F., Nicola, S., Della Bella, S., Villa, M. L., Imberti, L., Gentili, F., Montagna, C., *et al.* (2006). Tissue-specific sensitivity to AID expression in transgenic mouse models. *Gene* **377**, 150–158.

Sancar, A., Lindsey-Boltz, L. A., Unsal-Kacmaz, K., and Linn, S. (2004). Molecular mechanisms of mammalian DNA repair and the DNA damage checkpoints. *Annu. Rev. Biochem.* **73**, 39–85.

Savitsky, K., Bar-Shira, A., Gilad, S., Rotman, G., Ziv, Y., Vanagaite, L., Tagle, D. A., Smith, S., Uziel, T., Sfez, S., *et al.* (1995). A single ataxia telangiectasia gene with a product similar to PI-3 kinase. *Science* **268**, 1749–1753.

Sayegh, C. E., Quong, M. W., Agata, Y., and Murre, C. (2003). E-proteins directly regulate expression of activation-induced deaminase in mature B cells. *Nat. Immunol.* **4**, 586–593.

Schrader, C. E., Edelmann, W., Kucherlapati, R., and Stavnezer, J. (1999). Reduced isotype switching in splenic B cells from mice deficient in mismatch repair enzymes. *J. Exp. Med.* **190**, 323–330.

Schrader, C. E., Linehan, E. K., Mochegova, S. N., Woodland, R. T., and Stavnezer, J. (2005). Inducible DNA breaks in Ig S regions are dependent on AID and UNG. *J. Exp. Med.* **202**, 561–568.

Sciammas, R., Shaffer, A. L., Schatz, J. H., Zhao, H., Staudt, L. M., and Singh, H. (2006). Graded expression of interferon regulatory factor-4 coordinates isotype switching with plasma cell differentiation. *Immunity* **25**, 225–236.

Shaffer, A. L., Lin, K. I., Kuo, T. C., Yu, X., Hurt, E. M., Rosenwald, A., Giltnane, J. M., Yang, L., Zhao, H., Calame, K., and Staudt, L. M. (2002). Blimp-1 orchestrates plasma cell differentiation by extinguishing the mature B cell gene expression program. *Immunity* **17**, 51–62.

Shen, H. M., and Storb, U. (2004). Activation-induced cytidine deaminase (AID) can target both DNA strands when the DNA is supercoiled. *Proc. Natl. Acad. Sci. USA* **101**, 12997–13002.

Shen, H. M., Peters, A., Baron, B., Zhu, X., and Storb, U. (1998). Mutation of BCL-6 gene in normal B cells by the process of somatic hypermutation of Ig genes. *Science* **280**, 1750–1752.

Shen, H. M., Ratnam, S., and Storb, U. (2005). Targeting of the activation-induced cytosine deaminase is strongly influenced by the sequence and structure of the targeted DNA. *Mol. Cell. Biol.* **25**, 10815–10821.

Shiloh, Y. (2003). ATM and related protein kinases: Safeguarding genome integrity. *Nat. Rev. Cancer* **3**, 155–168.

Shinkura, R., Tian, M., Smith, M., Chua, K., Fujiwara, Y., and Alt, F. W. (2003). The influence of transcriptional orientation on endogenous switch region function. *Nat. Immunol.* **4**, 435–441.

Shinkura, R., Ito, S., Begum, N. A., Nagaoka, H., Muramatsu, M., Kinoshita, K., Sakakibara, Y., Hijikata, H., and Honjo, T. (2004). Separate domains of AID are required for somatic hypermutation and class-switch recombination. *Nat. Immunol.* **5**, 707–712.

Sohail, A., Klapacz, J., Samaranayake, M., Ullah, A., and Bhagwat, A. S. (2003). Human activation-induced cytidine deaminase causes transcription-dependent, strand-biased C to U deaminations. *Nucleic Acids Res.* **31**, 2990–2994.

Stavnezer, J. (1996). Antibody class switching. *Adv. Immunol.* **61**, 79–146.

Stavnezer, J. (2000). Molecular processes that regulate class switching. *Curr. Top. Microbiol. Immunol.* **245**, 127–168.

Stewart, G. S., Maser, R. S., Stankovic, T., Bressan, D. A., Kaplan, M. I., Jaspers, N. G., Raams, A., Byrd, P. J., Petrini, J. H., and Taylor, A. M. (1999). The DNA double-strand break repair gene hMRE11 is mutated in individuals with an ataxia-telangiectasia-like disorder. *Cell* **99**, 577–587.

Stracker, T. H., Theunissen, J. W., Morales, M., and Petrini, J. H. (2004). The Mre11 complex and the metabolism of chromosome breaks: The importance of communicating and holding things together. *DNA Repair (Amst.)* **3**, 845–854.

Ta, V. T., Nagaoka, H., Catalan, N., Durandy, A., Fischer, A., Imai, K., Nonoyama, S., Tashiro, J., Ikegawa, M., Ito, S., Kinoshita, K., Muramatsu, M., et al. (2003). AID mutant analyses indicate requirement for class-switch-specific cofactors. *Nat. Immunol.* **4**, 843–848.

Tian, M., and Alt, F. W. (2000). Transcription-induced cleavage of immunoglobulin switch regions by nucleotide excision repair nucleases *in vitro*. *J. Biol. Chem.* **275**, 24163–24172.

Unniraman, S., Zhou, S., and Schatz, D. G. (2004). Identification of an AID-independent pathway for chromosomal translocations between the Igh switch region and Myc. *Nat. Immunol.* **5**, 1117–1123.

Varon, R., Vissinga, C., Platzer, M., Cerosaletti, K. M., Chrzanowska, K. H., Saar, K., Beckmann, G., Seemanova, E., Cooper, P. R., Nowak, N. J., Stumm, M., Weemaes, C. M., et al. (1998). Nibrin, a novel DNA double-strand break repair protein, is mutated in Nijmegen breakage syndrome. *Cell* **93**, 467–476.

Wakae, K., Magor, B. G., Saunders, H., Nagaoka, H., Kawamura, A., Kinoshita, K., Honjo, T., and Muramatsu, M. (2006). Evolution of class switch recombination function in fish activation-induced cytidine deaminase, AID. *Int. Immunol.* **18**, 41–47.

Wang, B., Matsuoka, S., Carpenter, P. B., and Elledge, S. J. (2002). 53BP1, a mediator of the DNA damage checkpoint. *Science* **298**, 1435–1438.

Wang, C. L., Harper, R. A., and Wabl, M. (2004). Genome-wide somatic hypermutation. *Proc. Natl. Acad. Sci. USA* **101**, 7352–7356.

Wang, J., Shinkura, R., Muramatsu, M., Nagaoka, H., Kinoshita, K., and Honjo, T. (2006a). Identification of a specific domain required for dimerization of activation-induced cytidine deaminase. *J. Biol. Chem.* **281**, 19115–19123.

Wang, L., Whang, N., Wuerffel, R., and Kenter, A. L. (2006b). AID-dependent histone acetylation is detected in immunoglobulin S regions. *J. Exp. Med.* **203**, 215–226.

Ward, I. M., and Chen, J. (2001). Histone H2AX is phosphorylated in an ATR-dependent manner in response to replicational stress. *J. Biol. Chem.* **276**, 47759–47762.

Ward, I. M., Minn, K., Jorda, K. G., and Chen, J. (2003a). Accumulation of checkpoint protein 53BP1 at DNA breaks involves its binding to phosphorylated histone H2AX. *J. Biol. Chem.* **278**, 19579–19582.

Ward, I. M., Minn, K., van Deursen, J., and Chen, J. (2003b). p53 binding protein 53BP1 is required for DNA damage responses and tumor suppression in mice. *Mol. Cell. Biol.* **23**, 2556–2563.

Ward, I. M., Reina-San-Martin, B., Olaru, A., Minn, K., Tamada, K., Lau, J. S., Cascalho, M., Chen, L., Nussenzweig, A., Livak, F., Nussenzweig, M. C., and Chen, J. (2004). 53BP1 is required for class switch recombination. *J. Cell Biol.* **165**, 459–464.

Wardemann, H., Yurasov, S., Schaefer, A., Young, J. W., Meffre, E., and Nussenzweig, M. C. (2003). Predominant autoantibody production by early human B cell precursors. *Science* **301**, 1374–1377.

Wiesendanger, M., Kneitz, B., Edelmann, W., and Scharff, M. D. (2000). Somatic hypermutation in MutS homologue (MSH)3-, MSH6-, and MSH3/MSH6-deficient mice reveals a role for the MSH2-MSH6 heterodimer in modulating the base substitution pattern. *J. Exp. Med.* **191**, 579–584.

Woo, C. J., Martin, A., and Scharff, M. D. (2003). Induction of somatic hypermutation is associated with modifications in immunoglobulin variable region chromatin. *Immunity* **19**, 479–489.

Xiao, Y., and Weaver, D. T. (1997). Conditional gene targeted deletion by Cre recombinase demonstrates the requirement for the double-strand break repair Mre11 protein in murine embryonic stem cells. *Nucleic Acids Res.* **25**, 2985–2991.

Xie, K., Sowden, M. P., Dance, G. S., Torelli, A. T., Smith, H. C., and Wedekind, J. E. (2004). The structure of a yeast RNA-editing deaminase provides insight into the fold and function of activation-induced deaminase and APOBEC-1. *Proc. Natl. Acad. Sci. USA* **101**, 8114–8119.

Xu, Y., Ashley, T., Brainerd, E. E., Bronson, R. T., Meyn, M. S., and Baltimore, D. (1996). Targeted disruption of ATM leads to growth retardation, chromosomal fragmentation during meiosis, immune defects, and thymic lymphoma. *Genes Dev.* **10**, 2411–2422.

Xue, K., Rada, C., and Neuberger, M. S. (2006). The *in vivo* pattern of AID targeting to immunoglobulin switch regions deduced from mutation spectra in msh2$-/-$ ung$-/-$ mice. *J. Exp. Med.* **203**, 2085–2094.

Yang, Y., Sowden, M. P., Yang, Y., and Smith, H. C. (2001). Intracellular trafficking determinants in APOBEC-1, the catalytic subunit for cytidine to uridine editing of apolipoprotein B mRNA. *Exp. Cell Res.* **267**, 153–164.

Yoshikawa, K., Okazaki, I. M., Eto, T., Kinoshita, K., Muramatsu, M., Nagaoka, H., and Honjo, T. (2002). AID enzyme-induced hypermutation in an actively transcribed gene in fibroblasts. *Science* **296**, 2033–2036.

Yu, K., Chedin, F., Hsieh, C. L., Wilson, T. E., and Lieber, M. R. (2003). R-loops at immunoglobulin class switch regions in the chromosomes of stimulated B cells. *Nat. Immunol.* **4**, 442–451.

Yu, K., Roy, D., Bayramyan, M., Haworth, I. S., and Lieber, M. R. (2005). Fine-structure analysis of activation-induced deaminase accessibility to class switch region R-loops. *Mol. Cell. Biol.* **25**, 1730–1736.

Zaim, J., and Kierzek, A. M. (2003). Domain organization of activation-induced cytidine deaminase. *Nat. Immunol.* **4**, 1153; author reply 1154.

Zhang, J., Bottaro, A., Li, S., Stewart, V., and Alt, F. W. (1993). A selective defect in IgG2b switching as a result of targeted mutation of the I gamma 2b promoter and exon. *EMBO J.* **12**, 3529–3537.

Zhao, Y., Pan-Hammarstrom, Q., Zhao, Z., and Hammarstrom, L. (2005). Identification of the activation-induced cytidine deaminase gene from zebrafish: An evolutionary analysis. *Dev. Comp. Immunol.* **29**, 61–71.

Zhou, C., Saxon, A., and Zhang, K. (2003). Human activation-induced cytidine deaminase is induced by IL-4 and negatively regulated by CD45: Implication of CD45 as a Janus kinase phosphatase in antibody diversification. *J. Immunol.* **170**, 1887–1893.

Zhu, J., Petersen, S., Tessarollo, L., and Nussenzweig, A. (2001). Targeted disruption of the Nijmegen breakage syndrome gene NBS1 leads to early embryonic lethality in mice. *Curr. Biol.* **11**, 105–109.

Targeting of AID-Mediated Sequence Diversification by cis-Acting Determinants

Shu Yuan Yang* and David G. Schatz*,†

*Section of Immunobiology, Yale University School of Medicine,
New Haven, Connecticut
†Howard Hughes Medical Institute, Yale University School of Medicine,
New Haven, Connecticut

Abstract 109
1. Introduction 109
2. The Link Between Transcription and AID-Mediated Sequence Diversification 111
3. Other cis-Acting Determinants Involved in the Targeting of AID 116
4. Future Outlook 120
References 120

Abstract

After their assembly by V(D)J recombination, immunoglobulin (Ig) genes undergo somatic hypermutation, gene conversion, and class switch recombination to generate additional antibody diversity. The three diversification processes depend on activation-induced cytidine deaminase (AID) and are tightly linked to transcription. The reactions occur primarily on Ig genes and the molecular mechanisms that underlie their targeting to Ig loci have been of intense interest. In this chapter, we discuss the evidence linking transcription and transcriptional control elements to the three diversification pathways, and we consider how various features of chromatin could render parts of the genome permissive for AID-mediated sequence diversification.

1. Introduction

Antigen receptor diversification in B cells is an integral part of potent immune responses, with a wide variety in antigen receptor-binding specificities allowing for recognition of almost all foreign antigens entering the body. Sequence variations are introduced at the level of genomic DNA in the immunoglobulin (Ig) genes that encode for the B-cell antigen receptor. Such diversification is first generated via V(D)J recombination; subsequently, three additional processes can occur to further diversify Ig genes: somatic hypermutation (SHM), gene conversion (GCV), and class switch recombination (CSR). All three postrearrangement diversification processes are dependent on activation-induced cytidine deaminase (AID) (Arakawa *et al.*, 2002; Harris *et al.*, 2002; Muramatsu *et al.*, 2000; Revy *et al.*, 2000). It is thought that SHM, GCV, and

CSR are initiated through deamination of cytosine residues in DNA by AID (Chaudhuri et al., 2003; Dickerson et al., 2003; Petersen-Mahrt et al., 2002; Sohail et al., 2003). Resulting uracil residues in DNA are either replicated over directly or recognized and processed by various DNA repair mechanisms to give rise to SHM, GCV, or CSR events (Di Noia and Neuberger, 2002, 2004; Rada et al., 2002, 2004; Saribasak et al., 2006).

The three AID-mediated diversification events are thought to be restricted primarily to Ig genes. On the basis of genealogical trees of mutations found in mouse germinal center B cells, the rate of SHM in Ig genes has been estimated to be 10^{-3}–10^{-4} mutations per bp per cell division (Kleinstein et al., 2003; McKean et al., 1984; Sablitzky et al., 1985), 10^5- to 10^6-fold higher than spontaneous mutation rates calculated for somatic cells. Analyses of several non-Ig genes in hypermutating B cells revealed very low mutation frequencies. Fluctuation analyses of mouse myeloma B cells and the human Burkitt's lymphoma B-cell line Ramos reported rates for acquiring various drug resistances through mutations in housekeeping genes to be 10^3- to 10^4-fold lower than mutation rates in Ig genes (Baumal et al., 1973; Sale and Neuberger, 1998). Direct sequencing of non-Ig genes confirmed that many of them do not mutate above background levels, corroborating the idea that SHM occurs specifically at Ig genes (Shen et al., 1998, 2000).

Nonetheless, it is important to note that a number of non-Ig genes exhibit elevated mutation levels in hypermutating B cells or B lymphoma cells compared to other non-Ig genes as well as their counterparts in B cells that do not hypermutate (Gordon et al., 2003; Landowski et al., 1997; Muschen et al., 2000; Pasqualucci et al., 1998; Shen et al., 1998, 2000). While the non-Ig genes that do mutate do so at rates more than 50-fold lower than those in Ig genes, these results indicate that SHM does take place outside of Ig loci. As SHM at non-Ig loci exhibits key features observed in Ig diversification such as a preference for similar hot spot motifs, it is reasonable to think that "mistargeting" of SHM to non-Ig loci is directed by mechanisms that resemble those involved in targeting to Ig loci.

As AID-dependent diversification processes have the potential to introduce deleterious mutations and have been linked to chromosomal translocations and tumorigenesis, it is crucial to understand the molecular basis of targeting specificity (Franco et al., 2006; Gordon et al., 2003; Kuppers and Dalla-Favera, 2001; Landowski et al., 1997; Pasqualucci et al., 2001; Ramiro et al., 2006). Targeting of SHM to specific regions of the genome is likely to be enforced at the step of AID-mediated deamination but it could also be established in part at the repair phase of the reaction. Despite extensive efforts devoted to the targeting problem, a clear answer has yet to emerge. In this chapter, we will discuss the recent advances made in our understanding of how transcription and *cis*-acting determinants contribute to the targeting of AID to Ig genes. In addition, we would like to put forth ideas concerning the molecular features of Ig genes that render them specific targets of AID in light of some of our new results.

2. The Link Between Transcription and AID-Mediated Sequence Diversification

2.1. Transcription Is Necessary for SHM, GCV, and CSR

Transcription is one of the best established characteristics central to Ig gene diversification. In mouse and human SHM, mutations first appear 100- to 200-bp downstream of the transcription start site, peak at 400–500 bp past the start site of transcription, and decline gradually as the distance from the promoter increases further, reducing to background levels 1- to 2-kb downstream of the promoter (Lebecque and Gearhart, 1990; Rada and Milstein, 2001; Rada *et al.*, 1994; Winter *et al.*, 1997). This profile maximizes mutations in the variable regions of Ig genes and spares the Ig constant regions that are situated further downstream. This window of mutation is defined by the promoter; changing the position of the promoter in an Igκ transgene moved the mutation region correspondingly, and addition of an Ig promoter immediately upstream of the constant region in another transgene created a new mutation window downstream of the inserted promoter (Peters and Storb, 1996; Winter *et al.*, 1997). Moreover, an active promoter is essential for SHM, as illustrated by the finding that deletion of the endogenous murine IgH promoter abrogated SHM (Fukita *et al.*, 1998). Such a relationship has also been found in other AID-dependent diversification processes. Deletion of the promoter upstream of the mouse Ig heavy chain (IgH) switch μ (Sμ) region led to ablation of CSR (Bottaro *et al.*, 1994). We showed that replacement of the endogenous Ig light chain (IgL) promoter with a silent promoter in DT40 cells, a chicken B-cell line, abrogated both GCV and SHM (Yang *et al.*, 2006). These results suggest a common role for transcription in the three diversification processes and they establish a clear requirement for active transcription in AID-mediated diversification pathways.

2.2. Heterologous Promoters Can Substitute for Ig Promoters to Direct SHM and CSR in Mammalian Cells

Interestingly, the endogenous Ig promoters have been found not to be required for SHM and CSR in mammalian cells. In a mouse study in which a transgene formed a hybrid chromosome with the endogenous IgH locus, the B29 promoter successfully substituted for the endogenous IgH promoter to support SHM (Tumas-Brundage and Manser, 1997). Several other mouse transgenic studies indicated that the chicken β-globin and CMV promoters are able to substitute for endogenous Ig promoters (Betz et al., 1994; Papavasiliou and Schatz, 2000; Yelamos et al., 1995). In addition, in cell lines expressing AID endogenously or ectopically, transcription cassettes driven by non-Ig promoters can be mutated (Bachl et al., 2001; Martin and Scharff, 2002; Parsa et al., 2007; Ruckerl and Bachl, 2005; Ruckerl et al., 2004, 2006; Wang et al., 2004; Yoshikawa et al., 2002). Similarly, CSR can take place when transcription is driven by a heterologous promoter (Bottaro et al., 1994; Okazaki et al., 2002).

Attempts have also been made to drive SHM with non-RNA polymerase II (RNA pol II) promoters. RNA polymerase I (RNA pol I) and polymerase III (RNA pol III) promoters have been tested using IgH knockin mice and transgenic mice, respectively (Fukita et al., 1998, Shen et al., 2001). In these studies, however, RNA pol II continued to drive transcription at the Ig loci under study and thus it is yet unclear if non-pol II promoters are able to support SHM. Nevertheless, the IgH RNA pol I promoter knockin mice (Fukita et al., 1998) were able to support IgH SHM, demonstrating again the ability of non-Ig promoters to substitute for Ig promoters.

The dispensability of the endogenous Ig promoters indicates that the specificity determinants for SHM and CSR do not reside in the promoter region. These results also suggest that the primary, or perhaps only, function of the promoter is to drive the transcription necessary for Ig sequence diversification. Consequently, it has been proposed that the mutation machinery, likely including AID, can load onto elongating transcription complexes and be deposited along the transcription unit to initiate SHM (Longerich et al., 2006; Peters and Storb, 1996). Moreover, as AID is now thought to initiate the diversification processes through deamination of single-stranded DNA, transcription has become an appealing candidate for the process that generates substrates for AID deamination at least on the nontemplate strand.

An important prediction of this model is that transcription elongation *per se* through particular sequences is required for the actions of AID at those sequences. However, RNA pol II termination mechanisms are not yet sufficiently well understood for a direct experimental test of this to be possible (Bentley, 2005). One result consistent with such a requirement is the coimmunoprecipitation of AID with RNA pol II in B cells stimulated to undergo CSR *ex vivo* (Nambu et al., 2003). Experiments performed with AID *in vitro* and in bacteria have provided additional support for the prediction (discussed below).

The fact that SHM is biased toward the promoter-proximal end of the gene might be explained by an important role for transcription initiation in the loading of the mutation machinery. An alternative explanation is that the transition from transcription initiation to elongation (promoter clearance) plays this role. Transcription pausing immediately downstream of Ig promoters has been reported (Raschke et al., 1999). Another possibility, not yet tested, is that RNA pol II is most densely arrayed at the 5' end of Ig genes (Schroeder et al., 2000), localizing a higher concentration of AID in the promoter-proximal regions. A study performed with the human Burkitt's lymphoma B-cell line BL2 showed that inhibition of transcription with actinomycin D for 2 h did not affect Ig SHM, suggesting that *de novo* RNA synthesis was not necessary (Faili et al., 2002). However, it is unclear exactly how much Ig transcription was affected by the drug treatment, as this parameter was not examined directly.

2.3. Not All Heterologous Promoters Support Efficient GCV/SHM in DT40 Cells

Our recent experiments replacing the endogenous IgL promoter in DT40 cells with heterologous RNA pol II promoters yielded results different from those of studies performed in mammalian B cells. The two promoters tested, chicken β-actin and human EF1-α, were able to drive transcription at levels higher than that of the endogenous IgL promoter (Yang et al., 2006). However, while the β-actin promoter was able to support GCV/SHM at levels comparable to the endogenous IgL promoter, the EF1-α promoter was not. These results were unexpected given the well-accepted notion that strong, heterologous promoters are capable of substituting for the endogenous Ig promoters in supporting AID-mediated sequence diversification in mammalian cells, and they indicate that the promoter provides additional information to facilitate GCV and SHM beyond simply driving transcription. In mammalian cells, most promoter-swapping experiments have been performed using transgenes that typically mutate at frequencies much lower than endogenous Ig genes (Betz et al., 1994; Papavasiliou and Schatz, 2000; Yelamos et al., 1995). Transgenes are also subject to integration site effects and interactions between multiple integrated copies of the transgene. In the two studies in which targeted replacement of an endogenous Ig promoter was achieved in mice, both SHM and transcription levels appeared to be reduced (Fukita et al., 1998; Shen et al., 2001). Therefore, it is possible that negative effects of the promoter substitutions were masked by the reduction in transcription levels. Another explanation for the discrepancy might be that the roles of promoters in GCV/SHM in chicken B cells are not identical to those in mammalian cells.

Our finding that not all strong, heterologous promoters can support efficient GCV/SHM does not contradict current models for the role of transcription in AID-dependent diversification pathways. Instead, we think that the promoter makes an additional contribution to targeting of AID, and there are several ways by which this could happen. Transcription factors present at the Ig promoters could be involved in the formation of an interaction surface that recruits AID or that localizes Ig loci to specific nuclear compartments accessible to AID. Certain promoters, such as EF1-α, might fail to contribute to the interaction surface and result in reduced efficiencies in targeting of AID. Alternatively, GCV and SHM could have specific temporal (e.g., cell cycle) requirements, and thus other features of transcription driven by the EF1-α promoter could preclude participation in robust GCV/SHM. Different DNA repair mechanisms prevail in different stages of the cell cycle and it has been suggested that the pathway used to process a DNA deamination event could be significantly influenced by when it occurs in the cell cycle (Di Noia *et al.*, 2006). The finding that the EF1-α promoter shows a defect in supporting GCV/SHM has opened doors to addressing these possibilities.

2.4. Can Non-Ig Transcription Cassettes Be Targeted for AID-Mediated Sequence Diversification?

Several studies have showed that transcription cassettes with no Ig sequences can undergo AID-dependent mutagenesis in various cell lines expressing AID endogenously or ectopically (Bachl *et al.*, 2001; Martin and Scharff, 2002; Parsa *et al.*, 2007; Ruckerl and Bachl, 2005; Ruckerl *et al.*, 2004, 2006; Wang *et al.*, 2004; Yoshikawa *et al.*, 2002). On the basis of those results, it has been proposed that high-level transcription is one of the few key characteristics of Ig genes that render them efficient targets of AID-mediated diversification processes (Wang *et al.*, 2004). Several different non-Ig mutation cassettes have been tested, and the most popular design has been the one composed of non-Ig promoters (CMV promoter, thymidine kinase promoter, or retroviral 5′ LTR) driving expression of an enhanced green fluorescence protein (EGFP) gene bearing a premature stop codon. The mutated EGFP construct allows for a convenient flow cytometric assay of mutations at the stop codon that causes reversion to a functional GFP protein. Most studies were able to detect higher levels of GFP reversion when cells express AID. However, the GFP^+ percentages are typically low even when AID is present, ranging between 0.02% and 0.1% of GFP^+ cells accumulated over 5–30 days, and some studies did not report corresponding sequencing data. The GFP reversion assay is arguably more sensitive than direct sequencing and it is possible that mutation rates in the non-Ig constructs are too low to be detected by direct sequencing. It is also difficult in such studies to compare mutation frequencies in the non-Ig cassettes to those of Ig genes. Hence, although these studies indicate that AID can act as a mutator of non-Ig cassettes, it is not always clear how efficient the process is.

Recently, we tested the ability of a transfected non-Ig transcription cassette, containing the human EF1-α promoter, to be mutated in non-Ig loci of DT40 cells (Yang et al., submitted for publication). We found that the cassette was mutated at frequencies similar to the combined frequency of GCV and SHM at the endogenous Ig genes but that mutagenesis of the non-Ig construct occurred only transiently and was lost by 3 weeks postintegration. In contrast, the endogenous IgL locus performed GCV/SHM robustly at all time points and provided a critical internal control for the activity of the mutation machinery in these cells. Curiously, the cassette also mutated only transiently when integrated into the IgL locus. These results indicate that, despite its robust transcription, the non-Ig construct lacks information to confer stable targeting of AID. Together with the finding discussed earlier that the EF1-α promoter supported robust transcription but poor GCV/SHM of the IgL locus, these results provide a strong argument against the model that high levels of transcription act as the primary targeting parameter in AID-mediated sequence diversification. While AID can act as an ectopic mutator at highly transcribed non-Ig genes, additional mechanisms, perhaps involving several *cis*-acting elements, exist to ensure tight regulation and targeting of AID to Ig substrates in B cells.

2.5. Correlation Between Transcription Levels and Frequencies of AID-Mediated Sequence Diversification

Using the GFP reversion assay with constructs driven by inducible promoters in either a B-cell line or a fibroblast cell line overexpressing AID, a positive correlation was found between transcription levels and SHM (Bachl et al., 2001; Yoshikawa et al., 2002). Such a correlation is not difficult to imagine if transcription is responsible for generating the single-stranded DNA substrates for AID deamination. However, our experiments replacing the endogenous IgL promoter with non-Ig counterparts in DT40 cells revealed that GCV/SHM efficiencies were not proportional to promoter strength (Yang et al., 2006). The β-actin promoter, which drove levels of transcription more than three times higher than those of the endogenous IgL promoter, was no more efficient in supporting GCV/SHM than the endogenous promoter. The EF1-α promoter was at least 1.5-fold stronger than the endogenous promoter but supported GCV/SHM ≈3-fold less efficiently. It is possible that Ig promoters are driving levels of transcription that are saturating for the action of the mutation machinery, and therefore that levels of transcription higher than that directed by Ig promoters do not result in increased levels of GCV/SHM. However, these results could also reflect a lack of a correlation between transcription rates and GCV/SHM in endogenous Ig loci, or the possibility that the β-actin promoter, like the EF1-α promoter, has a defect in supporting GCV/SHM that is compensated for by its strong transcription activity. To resolve this issue, the DT40 IgL promoter could be replaced with an inducible promoter and frequencies of GCV/SHM determined at different levels of transcription.

2.6. Transcription and AID Deamination *In Vitro*

Many aspects of the requirement for transcription in SHM have been recapitulated in *Escherichia coli* expressing AID and also in AID-directed plasmid deamination assays *in vitro*. Transcription is needed for AID-dependent mutagenesis in bacteria and increased transcription is associated with higher levels of mutations (Ramiro *et al.*, 2003). In biochemical assays, plasmid deamination by AID has been demonstrated with transcription driven by bacteriophage RNA polymerases and by *E. coli* RNA polymerase (Besmer *et al.*, 2006; Chaudhuri *et al.*, 2003; Pham *et al.*, 2003; Shen *et al.*, 2005; Sohail *et al.*, 2003). In addition, RNA polymerase and AID could be UV-crosslinked to each other in an *in vitro* AID-deamination assay with *E. coli* proteins driving transcription (Besmer *et al.*, 2006). These results provide support for the model that the act of transcription produces single-stranded DNA substrates for AID deamination. In addition, the mutation pattern was largely biased toward the nontemplate strand, suggesting that AID deamination occurs primarily in a strand-biased manner on the nontemplate strand exposed as single-stranded DNA during transcription. However, a study showed that such a bias could be due in part to the drug selection scheme employed in the deamination assays (Besmer *et al.*, 2006).

In summary, although high-level transcription is not sufficient to confer accessibility to AID, the promoter is a key element in AID-mediated sequence diversification, not only for driving transcription but also for regulating the recruitment of AID via as yet unknown mechanisms. Further experiments will be required to elucidate the precise role of transcription in SHM, GCV, and CSR and results from the last few years suggest that *in vivo* analyses of this issue should focus on the endogenous Ig loci.

3. Other *cis*-Acting Determinants Involved in the Targeting of AID

3.1. Targeting DNA Elements in Ig Loci

If high-level transcription by itself does not explain what directs AID to certain genes and not others, what does? A popular concept has been that DNA motifs within Ig genes serve as targeting elements. Transcriptional enhancers in mouse Ig loci have been examined extensively for their potential roles as such targeting elements, as detailed in a review (Odegard and Schatz, 2006). To summarize a large body of work, the mouse Ig enhancers that have been analyzed are not sufficient to explain how AID is recruited to the Ig genes. In fact, in no case has deletion of an endogenous mouse Ig enhancer revealed an essential, nonredundant role for these elements in the targeting of SHM. We have investigated the IgL enhancer in DT40 cells and found that, as in mammalian cells, the enhancer was largely dispensable for GCV/SHM (Yang *et al.*, 2006).

Conversely, E-box motifs appear to be a positive *cis*-acting regulator for AID-mediated diversification pathways. These motifs are found in multiple locations in Ig genes, including enhancers, and serve as binding sites for a family of transcription factors that includes the *E2A*-encoded proteins E12 and E47. E12 and E47 play important roles at several stages of B-cell development (Kee *et al.*, 2000), and a number of studies have implicated them as stimulators of SHM and GCV (Conlon and Meyer, 2006; Michael *et al.*, 2003; Schoetz *et al.*, 2006). They are also potent stimulators of CSR (Goldfarb *et al.*, 1996; Quong *et al.*, 1999), which is due at least in part to their ability to stimulate expression of AID (Sayegh *et al.*, 2003). The mechanism by which the *E2A*-encoded proteins increase SHM/GCV is unknown but cannot be explained solely on the basis of enhanced Ig transcription or AID expression. However, as *E2A*-deficient DT40 cells show a significant reduction rather than complete abrogation of Ig gene diversification (Schoetz *et al.*, 2006), it is unlikely that E-box motifs are the sole targeting elements in the recruitment of AID. Our finding that the IgL enhancer is dispensable for Ig GCV/SHM in DT40 cells suggests that *E2A*-encoded proteins exert their effects through some other DNA element. A direct link between the *E2A*-encoded proteins and the targeting of AID has yet to be demonstrated.

3.2. DNA Newly Incorporated into the Genome Can Undergo a Transient Phase of Mutability

A simple mechanism by which *cis*-acting targeting elements could act is through the recruitment of AID to Ig loci (either directly or indirectly via other DNA binding factors). However, another (not mutually exclusive) possibility is that the targeting elements recruit an activity that promotes an Ig locus organization/structure that is highly accessible to AID. This idea was suggested by our recent finding, described above, that a non-Ig transcription cassette undergoes mutation for a short period of time postintegration regardless of its integration site (Yang *et al.*, submitted for publication). These results show that while the non-Ig cassette did not contain sufficient targeting information to be mutated stably over time, this could be overcome by the cassette being recently incorporated into the genome.

It is possible that the processes that lead to mutation of Ig loci and of newly integrated DNA by AID are entirely unrelated. An appealing alternative, however, is that the two types of DNA are accessed by AID via convergent mechanisms, which would suggest that newly integrated DNA possesses molecular properties that mimic those of Ig loci which render them particularly suitable substrates of AID. The identity of the common molecular characteristics is currently unknown, but the ability of AID to act on newly integrated DNA could reflect AID's membership in a family of ancient deaminases, some of which possess host-defense capabilities (Gourzi et al., 2006; Harris and Liddament, 2004). Curiously, AID expression has been reported in mouse germ cells (Morgan et al., 2004; Schreck et al., 2006) and while no genes have yet been shown to mutate as a result of AID expression in those cells, it is tempting to hypothesize that AID can influence evolution by generating germ line sequence diversity, perhaps by mechanisms similar to those used in Ig gene diversification. In the following sections, we discuss several parameters that might explain how DNA newly incorporated into the genome becomes transiently accessible to AID, with implications for how targeting of AID to Ig genes is achieved.

3.2.1. Histone and DNA Structure

A notable difference between newly integrated DNA and genomic DNA is chromatin packaging. As unpackaged DNA inserted into the genome will become packaged in chromatin over time, chromatin structure is an appealing explanation for the transient mutation phenomenon we observe. Several core histone modifications have been analyzed for their potential involvement in SHM and CSR in mammalian cells. A study performed in human BL2 cells found that hyperacetylation of histones H3 and H4 is associated with the IgH variable region and not the constant region, suggesting a correlation between acetylated histones H3/H4 and SHM (Woo et al., 2003). However, experiments performed on primary mouse B cells showed that while such a distinction is observed in the heavy chain locus, it is not present in the Igλ light chain locus (Odegard et al., 2005). Therefore, while these histone modifications might be important for SHM, they are not specific markers for hypermutating regions. Conversely, a correlation was observed between SHM/CSR and phosphorylation of serine 14 of histone H2B at Ig variable and switch regions (Odegard et al., 2005). However, because detectable H2B phosphorylation was AID dependent, the simplest interpretation is that it occurs post-AID recruitment and is not responsible for AID targeting. Hyperacetylated histones H3 and H4 are found in the appropriate downstream switch regions when cells are stimulated to undergo CSR (Li et al., 2004; Nambu et al., 2003), and H4 acetylation is stimulated by AID (Wang et al., 2006). However, there is as yet no direct link between histone modifications and the targeting of AID to switch regions during CSR.

While no core histone modifications examined to date have been strongly implicated in the targeting of AID, the search has not been exhaustive and it remains possible that other core histone modifications play a role in AID recruitment. In addition, other possibilities such as nucleosome positioning and distribution of histone variants could influence AID recruitment and have yet to be investigated.

Linker histones are interesting candidates that have not yet been investigated for a contribution to Ig gene diversification. Linker histones are known to be important in compacting chromatin and regulating accessibility of DNA to protein factors and have also been implicated in the maintenance of genomic integrity (Harvey and Downs, 2004). Like core histones, there are many variants of linker histones, and their differential usage could help distinguish regions accessible to AID from those that are not.

Another difference between newly integrated DNA and genomic DNA is cytosine methylation, a hallmark of inactive regions of chromatin. Newly integrated DNA, being bacterial in origin, would completely lack CpG methylation and hence might be a readily accessed target for AID. Conflicting results have been reported as to whether methylated cytidine residues could be deaminated by AID (Larijani et al., 2005; Morgan et al., 2004). If methylation protects cytidines from AID deamination, lack of methylation could facilitate the action of AID on newly integrated DNA and the accumulation of methylation over time could contribute to the loss of accessibility to AID.

3.2.2. Subnuclear Compartmentalization

A different basis for how newly incorporated non-Ig cassettes are accessed by AID could be subnuclear compartmentalization. The eukaryotic nucleus is not a homogeneous mass in which DNA, RNA, and protein factors are distributed and localized randomly. Subnuclear compartmentalization of transcription factors is well established (Zaidi et al., 2005) and coregulation of different genomic loci through coordinated subnuclear localization has also been documented (Lomvardas et al., 2006; Spilianakis et al., 2005). Therefore, an interesting possibility is that new DNA in the genome is brought to the vicinity of hypothetical subnuclear compartments where AID and Ig genes are localized; over time, assimilation of newly integrated DNA into surrounding DNA might lead to relocalization within the nucleus and its separation from AID activity. It is not known yet if AID exhibits unique spatial patterning in the nucleus and if genomic loci targeted for the diversification processes are clustered in the same region of the nucleus. A study indicates that phosphorylated (and hence presumably activated) AID is preferentially associated with chromatin (McBride *et al.*, 2006), thus a variation of this model would be that phosphorylated AID and Ig genes colocalize in specific parts of the nucleus. It would be interesting to test if an SHM hub consisting of Ig genes, AID, and DNA repair molecules exists in the nucleus of hypermutating B cells, and if so, whether there is a correlation between SHM frequencies of non-Ig loci and their proximity to this hub.

4. Future Outlook

Numerous mysteries remain in our understanding of how *cis*-acting determinants promote targeting specificity in AID-mediated sequence diversification pathways. A complex network of elements might be essential for the specificity observed in the diversification processes, but it is unclear what these elements are or how they act together. It is possible that several *cis*-acting elements contribute substantially to the efficiencies of the processes without being absolutely required. It is important to note that contributions of different *cis*-acting components to the targeting of Ig gene diversification do not have to act in a mutually exclusive manner. Conversely, possessing only a subset of the targeting requirements (e.g., high levels of transcription, the presence of Ig enhancers, and/or E-box motifs) also does not support optimal sequence diversification by AID. This could explain why transgenes can be mutated but at levels lower than those of Ig loci; similarly, this could underlie how certain non-Ig genes in mutating B cells become targeted for SHM, albeit inefficiently. By carefully analyzing the effects of endogenous Ig locus manipulations and molecular similarities between Ig genes and non-Ig sequences targeted for diversification, it should be possible to dissect and reconstruct the map of *cis*-acting components involved in determining target specificity in SHM, GCV, and CSR.

Acknowledgments

The authors would like to thank Sebastian Fugmann, Shyam Unniraman, and Monalisa Chatterji for helpful discussions and critical reading of the chapter. The authors acknowledge support from the National Institutes of Health and the Howard Hughes Medical Institute.

References

Arakawa, H., Hauschild, J., and Buerstedde, J. M. (2002). Requirement of the activation-induced deaminase (AID) gene for immunoglobulin gene conversion. *Science* **295**, 1301–1306.

Bachl, J., Carlson, C., Gray-Schopfer, V., Dessing, M., and Olsson, C. (2001). Increased transcription levels induce higher mutation rates in a hypermutating cell line. *J. Immunol.* **166,** 5051–5057.

Baumal, R., Birshtein, B. K., Coffino, P., and Scharff, M. D. (1973). Mutations in immunoglobulin-producing mouse myeloma cells. *Science* **182,** 164–166.

Bentley, D. L. (2005). Rules of engagement: Co-transcriptional recruitment of pre-mRNA processing factors. *Curr. Opin. Cell Biol.* **17,** 251–256.

Besmer, E., Market, E., and Papavasiliou, F. N. (2006). The transcription elongation complex directs activation-induced cytidine deaminase-mediated DNA deamination. *Mol. Cell. Biol.* **26,** 4378–4385.

Betz, A. G., Milstein, C., Gonzalez-Fernandez, A., Pannell, R., Larson, T., and Neuberger, M. S. (1994). Elements regulating somatic hypermutation of an immunoglobulin kappa gene: Critical role for the intron enhancer/matrix attachment region. *Cell* **77,** 239–248.

Bottaro, A., Lansford, R., Xu, L., Zhang, J., Rothman, P., and Alt, F. W. (1994). S region transcription *per se* promotes basal IgE class switch recombination but additional factors regulate the efficiency of the process. *EMBO J.* **13,** 665–674.

Chaudhuri, J., Tian, M., Khuong, C., Chua, K., Pinaud, E., and Alt, F. W. (2003). Transcription-targeted DNA deamination by the AID antibody diversification enzyme. *Nature* **422,** 726–730.

Conlon, T. M., and Meyer, K. B. (2006). The chicken Ig light chain 3′-enhancer is essential for gene expression and regulates gene conversion via the transcription factor E2A. *Eur. J. Immunol.* **36,** 139–148.

Di Noia, J., and Neuberger, M. S. (2002). Altering the pathway of immunoglobulin hypermutation by inhibiting uracil-DNA glycosylase. *Nature* **419,** 43–48.

Di Noia, J. M., and Neuberger, M. S. (2004). Immunoglobulin gene conversion in chicken DT40 cells largely proceeds through an abasic site intermediate generated by excision of the uracil produced by AID-mediated deoxycytidine deamination. *Eur. J. Immunol.* **34,** 504–508.

Di Noia, J. M., Rada, C., and Neuberger, M. S. (2006). SMUG1 is able to excise uracil from immunoglobulin genes: Insight into mutation versus repair. *EMBO J.* **25,** 585–595.

Dickerson, S. K., Market, E., Besmer, E., and Papavasiliou, F. N. (2003). AID mediates hypermutation by deaminating single stranded DNA. *J. Exp. Med.* **197,** 1291–1296.

Faili, A., Aoufouchi, S., Gueranger, Q., Zober, C., Leon, A., Bertocci, B., Weill, J. C., and Reynaud, C. A. (2002). AID-dependent somatic hypermutation occurs as a DNA single-strand event in the BL2 cell line. *Nat. Immunol.* **3,** 815–821.

Franco, S., Gostissa, M., Zha, S., Lombard, D. B., Murphy, M. M., Zarrin, A. A., Yan, C., Tepsuporn, S., Morales, J. C., Adams, M. M., Lou, Z., Bassing, C. H., *et al.* (2006). H2AX prevents DNA breaks from progressing to chromosome breaks and translocations. *Mol. Cell* **21,** 201–214.

Fukita, Y., Jacobs, H., and Rajewsky, K. (1998). Somatic hypermutation in the heavy chain locus correlates with transcription. *Immunity* **9,** 105–114.

Goldfarb, A. N., Flores, J. P., and Lewandowska, K. (1996). Involvement of the E2A basic helix-loop-helix protein in immunoglobulin heavy chain class switching. *Mol. Immunol.* **33,** 947–956.

Gordon, M. S., Kanegai, C. M., Doerr, J. R., and Wall, R. (2003). Somatic hypermutation of the B cell receptor genes B29 (Igbeta, CD79b) and mb1 (Igalpha, CD79a). *Proc. Natl. Acad. Sci. USA* **100,** 4126–4131.

Gourzi, P., Leonova, T., and Papavasiliou, F. N. (2006). A role for activation-induced cytidine deaminase in the host response against a transforming retrovirus. *Immunity* **24,** 779–786.

Harris, R. S., and Liddament, M. T. (2004). Retroviral restriction by APOBEC proteins. *Nat. Rev. Immunol.* **4,** 868–877.

Harris, R. S., Sale, J. E., Petersen-Mahrt, S. K., and Neuberger, M. S. (2002). AID is essential for immunoglobulin V gene conversion in a cultured B cell line. *Curr. Biol.* **12**, 435–438.

Harvey, C. A., and Downs, J. A. (2004). What functions do linker histones provide? *Mol. Microbiol.* **53**, 771–775.

Kee, B. L., Quong, M. W., and Murre, C. (2000). E2A proteins: Essential regulators at multiple stages of B-cell development. *Immunol. Rev.* **175**, 138–149.

Kleinstein, S. H., Louzoun, Y., and Shlomchik, M. J. (2003). Estimating hypermutation rates from clonal tree data. *J. Immunol.* **171**, 4639–4649.

Kuppers, R., and Dalla-Favera, R. (2001). Mechanisms of chromosomal translocations in B cell lymphomas. *Oncogene* **20**, 5580–5594.

Landowski, T. H., Qu, N., Buyuksal, I., Painter, J. S., and Dalton, W. S. (1997). Mutations in the Fas antigen in patients with multiple myeloma. *Blood* **90**, 4266–4270.

Larijani, M., Frieder, D., Sonbuchner, T. M., Bransteitter, R., Goodman, M. F., Bouhassira, E. E., Scharff, M. D., and Martin, A. (2005). Methylation protects cytidines from AID-mediated deamination. *Mol. Immunol.* **42**, 599–604.

Lebecque, S. G., and Gearhart, P. J. (1990). Boundaries of somatic mutation in rearranged immunoglobulin genes: 5′ boundary is near the promoter, and 3′ boundary is approximately 1 kb from V(D)J gene. *J. Exp. Med.* **172**, 1717–1727.

Li, Z., Luo, Z., and Scharff, M. D. (2004). Differential regulation of histone acetylation and generation of mutations in switch regions is associated with Ig class switching. *Proc. Natl. Acad. Sci. USA* **101**, 15428–15433.

Lomvardas, S., Barnea, G., Pisapia, D. J., Mendelsohn, M., Kirkland, J., and Axel, R. (2006). Interchromosomal interactions and olfactory receptor choice. *Cell* **126**, 403–413.

Longerich, S., Basu, U., Alt, F., and Storb, U. (2006). AID in somatic hypermutation and class switch recombination. *Curr. Opin. Immunol.* **18**, 164–174.

Martin, A., and Scharff, M. D. (2002). Somatic hypermutation of the AID transgene in B and non-B cells. *Proc. Natl. Acad. Sci. USA* **99**, 12304–12308.

McBride, K. M., Gazumyan, A., Woo, E. M., Barreto, V. M., Robbiani, D. F., Chait, B. T., and Nussenzweig, M. C. (2006). Regulation of hypermutation by activation-induced cytidine deaminase phosphorylation. *Proc. Natl. Acad. Sci. USA* **103**, 8798–8803.

McKean, D., Huppi, K., Bell, M., Staudt, L., Gerhard, W., and Weigert, M. (1984). Generation of antibody diversity in the immune response of BALB/c mice to influenza virus hemagglutinin. *Proc. Natl. Acad. Sci. USA* **81**, 3180–3184.

Michael, N., Shen, H. M., Longerich, S., Kim, N., Longacre, A., and Storb, U. (2003). The E box motif CAGGTG enhances somatic hypermutation without enhancing transcription. *Immunity* **19**, 235–242.

Morgan, H. D., Dean, W., Coker, H. A., Reik, W., and Petersen-Mahrt, S. K. (2004). Activation-induced cytidine deaminase deaminates 5-methylcytosine in DNA and is expressed in pluripotent tissues: Implications for epigenetic reprogramming. *J. Biol. Chem.* **279**, 52353–52360.

Muramatsu, M., Kinoshita, K., Fagarasan, S., Yamada, S., Shinkai, Y., and Honjo, T. (2000). Class switch recombination and hypermutation require activation-induced cytidine deaminase (AID), a potential RNA editing enzyme. *Cell* **102**, 553–563.

Muschen, M., Re, D., Jungnickel, B., Diehl, V., Rajewsky, K., and Kuppers, R. (2000). Somatic mutation of the CD95 gene in human B cells as a side-effect of the germinal center reaction. *J. Exp. Med.* **192**, 1833–1840.

Nambu, Y., Sugai, M., Gonda, H., Lee, C. G., Katakai, T., Agata, Y., Yokota, Y., and Shimizu, A. (2003). Transcription-coupled events associating with immunoglobulin switch region chromatin. *Science* **302**, 2137–2140.

Odegard, V. H., and Schatz, D. G. (2006). Targeting of somatic hypermutation. *Nat. Rev. Immunol.* **6**, 573–583.

Odegard, V. H., Kim, S. T., Anderson, S. M., Shlomchik, M. J., and Schatz, D. G. (2005). Histone modifications associated with somatic hypermutation. *Immunity* **23**, 101–110.

Okazaki, I. M., Kinoshita, K., Muramatsu, M., Yoshikawa, K., and Honjo, T. (2002). The AID enzyme induces class switch recombination in fibroblasts. *Nature* **416**, 340–345.

Papavasiliou, F. N., and Schatz, D. G. (2000). Cell-cycle-regulated DNA double-stranded breaks in somatic hypermutation of immunoglobulin genes. *Nature* **408**, 216–221.

Parsa, J. Y., Basit, W., Wang, C. L., Gommerman, J. L., Carlyle, J. R., and Martin, A. (2007). AID mutates a non-immunoglobulin transgene independent of chromosomal position. *Mol. Immunol.* **44**(4), 567–575.

Pasqualucci, L., Migliazza, A., Fracchiolla, N., William, C., Neri, A., Baldini, L., Chaganti, R. S., Klein, U., Kuppers, R., Rajewsky, K., and Dalla-Favera, R. (1998). BCL-6 mutations in normal germinal center B cells: Evidence of somatic hypermutation acting outside Ig loci. *Proc. Natl. Acad. Sci. USA* **95**, 11816–11821.

Pasqualucci, L., Neumeister, P., Goossens, T., Nanjangud, G., Chaganti, R. S., Kuppers, R., and Dalla-Favera, R. (2001). Hypermutation of multiple proto-oncogenes in B-cell diffuse large-cell lymphomas. *Nature* **412**, 341–346.

Peters, A., and Storb, U. (1996). Somatic hypermutation of immunoglobulin genes is linked to transcription initiation. *Immunity* **4**, 57–65.

Petersen-Mahrt, S. K., Harris, R. S., and Neuberger, M. S. (2002). AID mutates *E. coli* suggesting a DNA deamination mechanism for antibody diversification. *Nature* **418**, 99–103.

Pham, P., Bransteitter, R., Petruska, J., and Goodman, M. F. (2003). Processive AID-catalysed cytosine deamination on single-stranded DNA simulates somatic hypermutation. *Nature* **424**, 103–107.

Quong, M. W., Harris, D. P., Swain, S. L., and Murre, C. (1999). E2A activity is induced during B-cell activation to promote immunoglobulin class switch recombination. *EMBO J.* **18**, 6307–6318.

Rada, C., and Milstein, C. (2001). The intrinsic hypermutability of antibody heavy and light chain genes decays exponentially. *EMBO J.* **20**, 4570–4576.

Rada, C., Gonzalez-Fernandez, A., Jarvis, J. M., and Milstein, C. (1994). The 5' boundary of somatic hypermutation in a V kappa gene is in the leader intron. *Eur. J. Immunol.* **24**, 1453–1457.

Rada, C., Williams, G. T., Nilsen, H., Barnes, D. E., Lindahl, T., and Neuberger, M. S. (2002). Immunoglobulin isotype switching is inhibited and somatic hypermutation perturbed in UNG-deficient mice. *Curr. Biol.* **12**, 1748–1755.

Rada, C., Di Noia, J. M., and Neuberger, M. S. (2004). Mismatch recognition and uracil excision provide complementary paths to both Ig switching and the A/T-focused phase of somatic mutation. *Mol. Cell* **16**, 163–171.

Ramiro, A. R., Stavropoulos, P., Jankovic, M., and Nussenzweig, M. C. (2003). Transcription enhances AID-mediated cytidine deamination by exposing single-stranded DNA on the non-template strand. *Nat. Immunol.* **4**, 452–456.

Ramiro, A. R., Jankovic, M., Callen, E., Difilippantonio, S., Chen, H. T., McBride, K. M., Eisenreich, T. R., Chen, J., Dickins, R. A., Lowe, S. W., Nussenzweig, A., and Nussenzweig, M. C. (2006). Role of genomic instability and p53 in AID-induced c-myc-Igh translocations. *Nature* **440**, 105–109.

Raschke, E. E., Albert, T., and Eick, D. (1999). Transcriptional regulation of the Ig kappa gene by promoter-proximal pausing of RNA polymerase II. *J. Immunol.* **163**, 4375–4382.

Revy, P., Muto, T., Levy, Y., Geissmann, F., Plebani, A., Sanal, O., Catalan, N., Forveille, M., Dufourcq-Labelouse, R., Gennery, A., Tezcan, I., Ersoy, F., *et al.* (2000). Activation-induced cytidine deaminase (AID) deficiency causes the autosomal recessive form of the Hyper-IgM syndrome (HIGM2). *Cell* **102**, 565–575.

Ruckerl, F., and Bachl, J. (2005). Activation-induced cytidine deaminase fails to induce a mutator phenotype in the human pre-B cell line Nalm-6. *Eur. J. Immunol.* **35**, 290–298.

Ruckerl, F., Mailhammer, R., and Bachl, J. (2004). Dual reporter system to dissect cis- and trans-effects influencing the mutation rate in a hypermutating cell line. *Mol. Immunol.* **41**, 1135–1143.

Ruckerl, F., Busse, B., and Bachl, J. (2006). Episomal vectors to monitor and induce somatic hypermutation in human Burkitt-Lymphoma cell lines. *Mol. Immunol.* **43**(10), 1645–1652.

Sablitzky, F., Wildner, G., and Rajewsky, K. (1985). Somatic mutation and clonal expansion of B cells in an antigen-driven immune response. *EMBO J.* **4**, 345–350.

Sale, J. E., and Neuberger, M. S. (1998). TdT-accessible breaks are scattered over the immunoglobulin V domain in a constitutively hypermutating B cell line. *Immunity* **9**, 859–869.

Saribasak, H., Saribasak, N. N., Ipek, F. M., Ellwart, J. W., Arakawa, H., and Buerstedde, J. M. (2006). Uracil DNA glycosylase disruption blocks Ig gene conversion and induces transition mutations. *J. Immunol.* **176**, 365–371.

Sayegh, C. E., Quong, M. W., Agata, Y., and Murre, C. (2003). E-proteins directly regulate expression of activation-induced deaminase in mature B cells. *Nat. Immunol.* **4**, 586–593.

Schoetz, U., Cervelli, M., Wang, Y. D., Fiedler, P., and Buerstedde, J. M. (2006). E2A expression stimulates Ig hypermutation. *J. Immunol.* **177**, 395–400.

Schreck, S., Buettner, M., Kremmer, E., Bogdan, M., Herbst, H., and Niedobitek, G. (2006). Activation-induced cytidine deaminase (AID) is expressed in normal spermatogenesis but only infrequently in testicular germ cell tumours. *J. Pathol.* **210**(1), 26–31.

Schroeder, S. C., Schwer, B., Shuman, S., and Bentley, D. (2000). Dynamic association of capping enzymes with transcribing RNA polymerase II. *Genes Dev.* **14**, 2435–2440.

Shen, H. M., Peters, A., Baron, B., Zhu, X., and Storb, U. (1998). Mutation of BCL-6 gene in normal B cells by the process of somatic hypermutation of Ig genes. *Science* **280**, 1750–1752.

Shen, H. M., Michael, N., Kim, N., and Storb, U. (2000). The TATA binding protein, c-Myc and survivin genes are not somatically hypermutated, while Ig and BCL6 genes are hypermutated in human memory B cells. *Int. Immunol.* **12**, 1085–1093.

Shen, H. M., Peters, A., Kao, D., and Storb, U. (2001). The 3′ Igkappa enhancer contains RNA polymerase II promoters: Implications for endogenous and transgenic kappa gene expression. *Int. Immunol.* **13**, 665–674.

Shen, H. M., Ratnam, S., and Storb, U. (2005). Targeting of the activation-induced cytosine deaminase is strongly influenced by the sequence and structure of the targeted DNA. *Mol. Cell. Biol.* **25**, 10815–10821.

Sohail, A., Klapacz, J., Samaranayake, M., Ullah, A., and Bhagwat, A. S. (2003). Human activation-induced cytidine deaminase causes transcription-dependent, strand-biased C to U deaminations. *Nucleic Acids Res.* **31**, 2990–2994.

Spilianakis, C. G., Lalioti, M. D., Town, T., Lee, G. R., and Flavell, R. A. (2005). Interchromosomal associations between alternatively expressed loci. *Nature* **435**, 637–645.

Tumas-Brundage, K., and Manser, T. (1997). The transcriptional promoter regulates hypermutation of the antibody heavy chain locus. *J. Exp. Med.* **185**, 239–250.

Wang, C. L., Harper, R. A., and Wabl, M. (2004). Genome-wide somatic hypermutation. *Proc. Natl. Acad. Sci. USA* **101**, 7352–7356.

Wang, L., Whang, N., Wuerffel, R., and Kenter, A. L. (2006). AID-dependent histone acetylation is detected in immunoglobulin S regions. *J. Exp. Med.* **203**, 215–226.

Winter, D. B., Sattar, N., Mai, J. J., and Gearhart, P. J. (1997). Insertion of 2 kb of bacteriophage DNA between an immunoglobulin promoter and leader exon stops somatic hypermutation in a kappa transgene. *Mol. Immunol.* **34**, 359–366.

Woo, C. J., Martin, A., and Scharff, M. D. (2003). Induction of somatic hypermutation is associated with modifications in immunoglobulin variable region chromatin. *Immunity* **19**, 479–489.

Yang, S. Y., Fugmann, S. D., and Schatz, D. G. (2006). Control of gene conversion and somatic hypermutation by immunoglobulin promoter and enhancer sequences. *J. Exp. Med.* **203**(13), 2919–2928.

Yang, S. Y., Fugmann, S. D., Gramlich, H. S., and Schatz, D. G. AID-mediated sequence diversification is transiently targeted to newly integrated DNA substrates. (Submitted for publication.)

Yelamos, J., Klix, N., Goyenechea, B., Lozano, F., Chui, Y. L., Gonzalez Fernandez, A., Pannell, R., Neuberger, M. S., and Milstein, C. (1995). Targeting of non-Ig sequences in place of the V segment by somatic hypermutation. *Nature* **376**, 225–229.

Yoshikawa, K., Okazaki, I. M., Eto, T., Kinoshita, K., Muramatsu, M., Nagaoka, H., and Honjo, T. (2002). AID enzyme-induced hypermutation in an actively transcribed gene in fibroblasts. *Science* **296**, 2033–2036.

Zaidi, S. K., Young, D. W., Choi, J. Y., Pratap, J., Javed, A., Montecino, M., Stein, J. L., Van Wijnen, A. J., Lian, J. B., and Stein, G. S. (2005). The dynamic organization of gene-regulatory machinery in nuclear microenvironments. *EMBO Rep.* **6**, 128–133.

AID-Initiated Purposeful Mutations in Immunoglobulin Genes

Myron F. Goodman,[*,†] Matthew D. Scharff,[‡] and Floyd E. Romesberg[§]

[*]Department of Biological Sciences, University of Southern California, Los Angeles, California
[†]Department of Chemistry, University of Southern California, Los Angeles, California
[‡]Department of Cell Biology, Albert Einstein College of Medicine, Bronx, New York
[§]Department of Chemistry, The Scripps Research Institute, La Jolla, California

    Abstract 127
 1. Introduction 128
 2. Biochemical Basis of C Deamination by APOBEC Enzymes 132
 3. How and Why Might AID-Specific Mutations Be Targeted? 141
 4. Selection of AID-Induced Mutations During Ab Maturation 143
    References 149

Abstract

Exposure brings risk to all living organisms. Using a remarkably effective strategy, higher vertebrates mitigate risk by mounting a complex and sophisticated immune response to counter the potentially toxic invasion by a virtually limitless army of chemical and biological antagonists. Mutations are almost always deleterious, but in the case of antibody diversification there are mutations occurring at hugely elevated rates within the variable (V) and switch regions (SR) of the immunoglobulin (Ig) genes that are responsible for binding to and neutralizing foreign antigens throughout the body. These mutations are truly purposeful. This chapter is centered on activation-induced cytidine deaminase (AID). AID is required for initiating somatic hypermutation (SHM) in the V regions and class switch recombination (CSR) in the SR portions of Ig genes. By converting $C \rightarrow U$, while transcription takes place, AID instigates a cascade of mutational events involving error-prone DNA polymerases, base excision and mismatch repair enzymes, and recombination pathways. Together, these processes culminate in highly mutated antibody genes and the B cells expressing antibodies that have achieved optimal antigenic binding undergo positive selection in germinal centers. We will discuss the biological role of AID in this complex process, primarily in terms of its biochemical properties in relation to SHM in vivo. The chapter also discusses recent advances in experimental methods to characterize antibody dynamics as a function of SHM to help elucidate the role that the AID-induced mutations play in tailoring molecular recognition. The emerging experimental techniques help to address long-standing conundrums concerning evolution-imposed constraints on antibody structure and function.

1. Introduction

The immune response has evolved to protect us from pathogenic infectious agents and toxic foreign substances. Aspects of the innate immune response are present in nonvertebrates and play an important role in vertebrates while adaptive immunity arose with the advent of vertebrates. In mice and humans, the adaptive humoral response becomes functional with the differentiation of antibody (Ab)-forming B cells in the bone marrow that have rearranged their heavy chain variable (V), diversity (D) and joining (J) germ line genes, as well as their light chain V and J germ line genes, to encode the light and heavy chains of the IgM Ab that is expressed on the surface of the B cell (Fig. 1). A vast repertoire of Ab-binding sites is expressed through the combinatorial rearrangement of numerous different V(D)J regions, sequence variation during V(D)J joining, and the expression of different combinations of heavy and light chain V regions in each of the large numbers of B cells that arise in the bone marrow every day (Maizels, 2005).

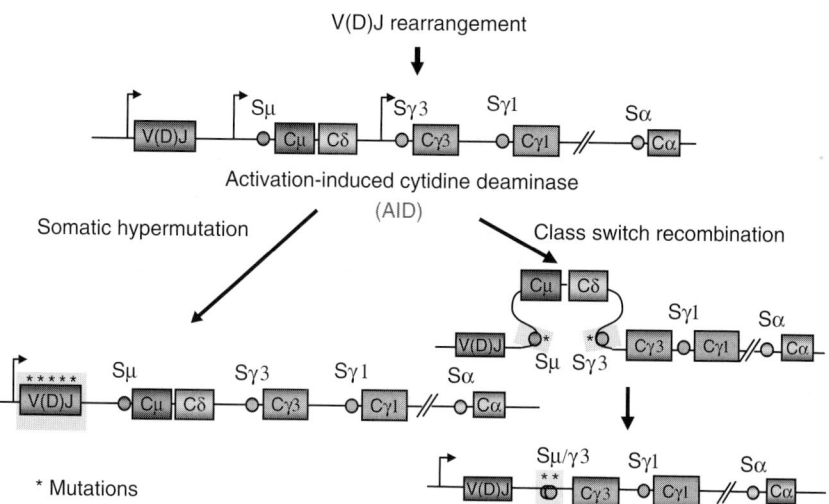

Figure 1 In the absence of antigen, pre-B cells in the bone marrow undergo V(D)J rearrangement and express IgM (V(D)J-Cμ) heavy chains on their surface. Following stimulation with antigen, the V(D)J region undergoes AID-induced mutations (*) to change the affinity and specificity of the Ab variable region (left diagram). If stimulated by specific lymphokine(s), the B cells make the donor Sμ and recipient Sγ3 SR accessible to AID-induced mutations (*) (right diagram). In this example, Sμ and Sγ SR recombine to produce a new, chimeric, Sμ/Sγ SR to bring the V(D)J region in close proximity with Cγ3 and encode an IgG3 heavy chain (right diagram). (**See Color Plate 5.**)

In spite of this initial diversity, most of these germ line-encoded IgM antibodies are of low affinity and do not leave the circulation to enter the tissues and the mucosal secretions. Furthermore, these low-affinity antibodies frequently do not neutralize pathogens and toxins and are not always effective in protecting us from the environment. When first encountered, infectious agents have to be dealt with by macrophages and complement, and other participants in the innate immune response. However, within a few days, higher affinity antibodies of IgG, IgA, and IgE isotypes that can inactivate invading organisms appear in the circulation and spread throughout the body and into the mucosal spaces (Rajewsky, 1996).

These affinity-matured and isotype-switched antibodies are generated when the B cells interact with antigens (Ags) through their surface immunoglobulin (Ig) and are stimulated to further differentiate into centroblasts in the germinal centers of secondary lymphoid organs like the spleen and lymph nodes. A critical feature of germinal center B cells is that they turn on the expression of large amounts of activation-induced cytidine deaminase (AID) (Muramatsu *et al.*, 2000). AID is a B-cell-specific molecule that plays a central role in adaptive immunity because it initiates the process of somatic hypermutation (SHM) of V regions to produce antibodies that have higher affinity and changes in fine specificity (Longo and Lipsky, 2006; Rajewsky, 1996; Fig. 1). At approximately the same time AID initiates class switch recombination (CSR) to allow those modified antigen-binding sites to be expressed with all possible constant (C) regions and carry out a variety of combinations of effector functions throughout the body (Fig. 1). Patients and mice that are unable to express AID have a hyper-IgM syndrome and are very susceptible to infections (Muramatsu *et al.*, 2000; Revy *et al.*, 2000). Thus, AID is the critical molecule in the initiation of the generation of Ab diversity.

The overexpression of AID in *Escherichia coli* (Petersen-Mahrt *et al.*, 2002) and cultured human cells (Martin *et al.*, 2002; Yoshikawa *et al.*, 2002) caused increased C → T mutations, which strongly suggested that AID is targeting DNA. Data obtained with partially purified AID provided direct biochemical evidence that AID deaminates C → U on single-stranded DNA (ssDNA) (Bransteitter *et al.*, 2003; Chaudhuri *et al.*, 2003; Dickerson *et al.*, 2003; Sohail *et al.*, 2003). Deamination was not observed on double-stranded DNA (dsDNA), RNA, or RNA–DNA hybrid molecules (Bransteitter *et al.*, 2003; Chaudhuri *et al.*, 2003). However, there is an alternative point of view regarding whether AID acts directly on ssDNA in implementing SHM (Honjo *et al.*, 2004).

AID-induced SHMs accumulate at a rate of $\sim 1 \times 10^{-3}$ mutations per base per generation (McKean *et al.*, 1984; Rajewsky, 1996) and *in vivo* it is preferentially targeted to WRCH (W = A/T, R = A/G, H = A/C/T) motifs and the complementary DGYW (D = A/G/T, Y = C/T) motifs (Rogozin and Diaz, 2004). Codon usage leads to an enrichment for these motifs in the complementarity determining regions (CDRs) that encode the antigen-binding sites of the heavy and light chain V regions (Wagner *et al.*, 1995). This suggests that the germ line Ig genes have coevolved with AID to focus its action on the antigen-binding sites and to protect the other parts of the Ab protein from mutations that might block its assembly, secretion, or effector functions. In the V region, AID-induced mutations are found in approximately equal abundance on both the transcribed and untranscribed strand, begin ~100- to 200-bp downstream from the site of initiation of transcription, are most frequent in the coding exon of the V region and end ~1.5- to 2-kb downstream of the promoter sparing the intronic enhancer and C region from mutation (Rada and Milstein, 2001). In the V region, once AID has deaminated C → U, the G:U that has been generated can be replicated to generate C → T or G → A transition mutations, removed by the UNG uracil-DNA glycosylase to create an abasic site that can then be bypassed by error-prone polymerases (Di Noia and Neuberger, 2002), perhaps with the help of monoubiquitinated PCNA (Bachl *et al.*, 2006), or processed by the MRE11 complex (Larson *et al.*, 2005). Alternatively, the G:U can be targeted by mismatch repair (MMR) to initiate an error-prone polymerase-mediated mutation process that introduces A:T and perhaps G:C mutations that are proximal to but not located within hot spots (Li *et al.*, 2004c). Thus, there are many alternative pathways and enzymes involved in SHM, but the details of how these different pathways are recruited and regulated are largely unknown.

CSR is also triggered by and requires AID, but the exact role of AID and of the other enzymes involved is even less well understood than it is for SHM. It is clear that there are highly reiterated sequences 5' to the μ, γ, ε, and α heavy chain constant region genes that are downstream from the μ constant region and that these switch regions (SRs) are rich in hot spots that are targeted by AID for mutation (Chaudhuri and Alt, 2004; Fig. 1). The μ SR serves as the donor and the γ, ε, and α SRs serve as the recipients for the recombinational event that fuses the V region with one or another of the downstream constant region genes. CSR allows the B cell to switch from making an IgM to an IgG, IgE, or IgA Ab. The choice of which SRs serve as recipient for CSR is determined by which cytokines are released by the helper T cells that interact with the IgM-producing B cell (Stavnezer, 1996). Furthermore, there is considerable evidence that once AID deaminates C → U in both the donor and recipient SRs, the resulting G:U recruits all of the same enzymes as are recruited during SHM and that ssDNA breaks are created through the action of UNG, BER, MMR, and perhaps as yet unidentified endonucleases and other enzymes (Chaudhuri and Alt, 2004). One proposal is that staggered double-stranded breaks are generated by AID and base excision and MMR enzymes are recruited to the G:U or G:abasic site that is created and that these double-stranded breaks then recruit the enzymes that complete the process of CSR by nonhomologous end joining (Chen et al., 2001; Rush et al., 2004; Schrader et al., 2005).

It is also important to note that the mistargeting of AID-induced SHM to proto-oncogenes such as Bcl6 and *c-myc*, and perhaps many others, sometimes results in point mutations that lead to the uncontrolled overexpression of these genes and the malignant transformation of B cells (Gaidano et al., 2003; Kuppers and Dalla-Favera, 2001). In addition, the dsDNA breaks that occur in the Ig gene during CSR lead to the chromosomal translocations that place the same oncogenes under the regulation of Ig gene enhancers and promoters and also contribute to B-cell lymphomagenesis (Kuppers and Dalla-Favera, 2001; Ramiro et al., 2006). Together these events are thought to be responsible for 85% of the B-cell lymphomas, which are one of the most common cancers in young people. In order to understand how Ab diversity is generated and how the genomic instability that is a critical part of SHM and CSR is sometimes mistargeted, it is important to understand exactly how AID is normally targeted to the V and SRs and not to other parts of the Ig genes or to other genes in the germinal center B cells.

It is axiomatic that the overwhelming number of mutations are either neutral or deleterious. But there are enzymes that are designed mutators whose principal role is to provide the cell with sufficient flexibility to adapt rapidly in stressful environments and also to evolve on millennia time frames. In this chapter, we will first describe the biochemical characteristics of one of those mutagenic enzymes, AID, and examine the degree to which the properties of the enzyme itself contribute to its highly mutagenic effect and its preferential targeting of hot spots in the heavy and light chain V region and SRs. We will then review the evidence that additional factors that are not inherent in biochemical properties of AID also contribute to the restriction of the mutagenic activity of AID to Ig genes. We also examine how the involvement of AID enables complex organisms to make protective antibodies. Finally, we review recent biophysical techniques that are capable of directly characterizing changes in protein structure and dynamics as a function of evolution, as it is these changes that are ultimately responsible for the functional manifestation of AID-induced mutations. By including recent advances in immunology, biochemistry, and biophysics, we hope to provide a more comprehensive and interdisciplinary view of the mechanisms of, and the selection pressures shaping, Ab diversification.

2. Biochemical Basis of C Deamination by APOBEC Enzymes

There are 12 members of the APOBEC family of nucleic acid-dependent C deaminases. APOBEC1, the first to be discovered, has the unusual highly selective property of deaminating just a single C residue on mRNA (Davidson and Shelness, 2000). The remaining APOBEC enzymes are either known to deaminate C at multiple sites on ssDNA or have no known substrate. We have examined the biochemical basis of C deamination for AID and Apo3G, and we will describe current approaches to delineate their biochemical properties and mechanisms.

2.1. AID Targets C Motifs on ssDNA

In 1999, AID was found to be required for SHM and CSR (Muramatsu et al., 2000), but it was not until 2003 that the partially purified enzyme was shown to act on ssDNA (Bransteitter et al., 2003; Chaudhuri et al., 2003; Dickerson et al., 2003; Sohail et al., 2003). The initial problem was that attempts to purify AID did not provide active enzyme (Muramatsu et al., 1999). This was overcome when we discovered that the activity of AID purified from insect cells had been masked owing to the presence of an avidly bound ssRNA inhibitor (Bransteitter et al., 2003). AID has biochemical properties that recapitulate several basic properties of V-gene C $\to$ T mutations *in vivo* (Pham et al., 2003). Perhaps the most important of these is its ability to select out specific mutational hot spots by favoring deamination of canonical WRC motifs (W = A/T, R = A/G) while suppressing deamination of SYC (S = G/C, Y = T/C). The deamination specificity of AID *in vitro* was determined using a *lacZ* reporter gene located in an ssDNA-gapped region of bacteriophage M13 dsDNA. Following incubation with AID, the DNA was transfected into uracil-glycosylase deficient *E. coli*. AID-catalyzed deaminations generate C $\to$ T mutations in the *lacZ* reporter gene, leading to the production of clear or light blue mutant M13 phage plaques, or nonmutated wild-type dark blue plaques. The C $\to$ T mutations occur precisely at the C $\to$ U deamination sites. The DNA sequence analysis revealed that under conditions for which there was a very low frequency of mutant plaques ($\sim$2 to 5%), roughly half of the mutant DNA clones had between 1 and 20 mutations and the other half had between 21 and 80 mutations (Pham et al., 2003). Since a large majority of DNA molecules contain no mutations, the observation that multiple mutations occur on a single DNA molecule strongly suggests that AID is acting processively on ssDNA in this *in vitro* system.

The distribution of mutations in sparsely deaminated clones showed just a few mutant sites, typically but not always in WRC hot spot motifs, separated by sizable regions containing nonmutated hot spot motifs. In the much more densely deaminated clones, one observes mutational clusters often containing 3–5 deaminated C residues within about a 10-base region with deaminations occurring in WRC motifs as well as neighboring cold spot SYC and all other motifs. The upshot of the clonal analysis is that AID appears to bind randomly to ssDNA and is able to deaminate a large number of C residues while bound to the same DNA substrate. Since only ~25% of C residues mutated to T in lacZ result in a lacZ mutant phenotype, it was essential to sequence DNA clones isolated from "nonmutated" blue plaques to ensure that silent C sites were not mutated. Data showing that there were in fact no lacZ mutations occurring in more than 50 DNA clones isolated from wild-type lacZ (dark blue) plaques strongly support a processive scanning mechanism (Pham *et al.*, 2003).

But what exactly is meant by the term "processive" in the context of the behavior of AID? The familiar definition of processivity was coined for DNA polymerase as a measure of the number of nucleotides incorporated after the enzymes binds to a primer/template DNA substrate prior to its dissociation. In the case of DNA polymerase, once released from DNA, the enzyme reequilibrates in the bulk solution and subsequently binds to any available primer/template DNA. In contrast, APOBEC enzymes which do not have to act on each nucleotide as they move along the DNA may have a number of microscopic dissociations from ssDNA, but are much more likely to reassociate with and continue to deaminate the *same* DNA substrate (Chelico *et al.*, 2006; Pham *et al.*, 2003). The property of preferential association with a single substrate accounts for the processive action of AID; a similar processive mechanism has been proposed for restriction nucleases (Halford and Marko, 2004).

A second important distinction between AID and DNA polymerase is that while each template base is a candidate for copying by polymerase, APOBEC C deaminases only attack C residues. Individual ssDNA molecules attacked by AID exhibit significantly different patterns both for the number and distribution of deaminations (Bransteitter *et al.*, 2004; Pham *et al.*, 2003). An examination of individual DNA clones shows the presence of densely clustered mutations separated by lightly mutated regions (Bransteitter *et al.*, 2004; Pham *et al.*, 2003). The wide variability in the locations and number of mutations for different clones suggests that AID initially binds at a random position on ssDNA and deaminates C residues processively over a short (~10 base) region but then translocates randomly to a different region on the same DNA substrate. Further support for a random binding mechanism is that AID exhibits a similar apparent equilibrium-binding constant to ssDNA substrates containing multiple WRC hot spot or SYC cold spot motifs, no C residues, or only product U residues (R. Bransteitter, P. Pham, and M. F. Goodman, unpublished data).

Although AID favors deamination of WRC hot spot motifs by a ratio of about six to one over SYC cold spot motifs (Pham et al., 2003), there are many instances when non-hot spot C residues are attacked while proximal hot spot Cs are not. This observation reveals an essential stochastic aspect of AID that is consistent with V-gene mutational patterns *in vivo*. A "mutability index" characterizing SHM is defined as the frequency of mutations found to occur in a specific V-gene sequence motif compared to mutation frequency predicted to occur with no sequence bias (Shapiro et al., 2002). We have shown that the average mutability index for both hot WRC and cold SYC motifs generated by AID acting on ssDNA *in vitro* is virtually indistinguishable from SHM *in vivo* (Pham et al., 2003; Table 2), which validates the importance of studying AID in a variety of model biochemical systems. The fact that V-gene mutations are relatively few and far between may imply that most of the deaminated Cs are repaired. Even so, SHM mutations in a 3' intronic region of VDJ from mice (Rada et al., 2004) reveal a clustered deamination pattern reminiscent of the T7-transcriptional deamination pattern (Pham et al., 2005), suggesting that the biological consequences of AID might be reflective of its biochemical properties *in vitro*.

A model for AID that perhaps best reflects its behavior pictures the enzyme binding randomly to ssDNA and then scanning along the DNA by jumping and sliding in either direction to catalyze multiple deaminations, preferentially, although not exclusively in WRC motifs. A sketch showing how AID might act depicts the enzyme as a multimer, most likely a dimer (Fig. 2). If each monomer, constrained to operate as part of a dimer, can in principal bind to different regions on ssDNA independently of whether the other monomer is bound, then independent sliding motions of each of them over distances ~10 nt can give rise to clustered deamination patterns with regions containing few or no deaminations in between clusters, as has been observed *in vitro* when AID acts on naked ssDNA (Pham et al., 2003) or when supercoiled circular dsDNA is transcribed by T7 RNA polymerase (Bransteitter et al., 2004). On the basis of data from Honjo (Wang et al., 2006a), AID appears to be active as a dimer. Mutations that are predicted to interfere with multimer formation strongly reduce AID activity (Procknow et al., 2007; Wang et al., 2006a).

The presence of an unusually high concentration of basic amino acids located near the N-terminal domain of AID, resulting in a localized +11 charge, is likely to result in a strong interaction with the negatively charged ssDNA phosphate backbone (Bransteitter et al., 2004). The replacement of two basic amino acids by acidic residues to reduce the N-terminal charge to +7 (R35E/R36D) causes a significant decline in AID processivity revealed by the *in vitro* system, with far fewer C deaminations observed on individual ssDNA

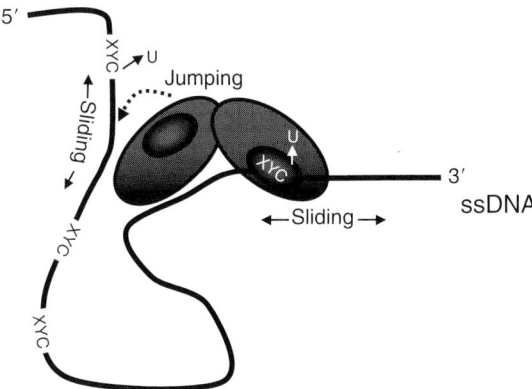

Figure 2 Jumping and sliding model for processive C → U deaminations catalyzed by Apo3G or AID. Apo3G or AID is shown as a dimer, with one of the monomers binding prior to the other. Binding occurs randomly, and sliding occurs in either direction along the ssDNA substrate. In the case of Apo3G, deamination occurs only when either monomer confronts a target 5′CCC (i.e., X = C, Y = C) while sliding 3′ → 5′. Structural constraints might favor binding of other monomer toward the 5′ end of the substrate, with either sliding or jumping constraints strongly favoring deamination in a 3′ → 5′, in the absence of an external energy source, for example ATP or GTP hydrolysis. Once bound, the other monomer also moves bidirectionally and deaminates C only when sliding 3′ → 5′. Asymmetric catalysis and jumping could account for the strong 3′ → 5′ deamination polarity of Apo3G, shown in Fig. 3. AID binds randomly to ssDNA and performs processive deamination of C → U on ssDNA, but, unlike Apo3G, deamination is unbiased, occurring equally in 5′ and 3′ directions, with preferential targeting in WRC motifs (W = A/T, R = A/G). (**See Color Plate 6.**)

molecules accompanied by a significant reduction in clustered mutations (Bransteitter *et al.*, 2004). Although mutations in these specific amino acid residues have not been associated with human disease, it is important to note that two mutations in the N-terminal domain, K10R and R24W, have been linked to a Hyper-IgM2 syndrome (Revy *et al.*, 2000). Although patients with this syndrome usually have normal or elevated serum IgM levels, they do not appear to have IgG, IgA, and IgE nor do they have V-gene mutations (Revy *et al.*, 2000).

The likely importance of N-region positive charge in modulating the properties of AID raises the key issue of the role of phosphorylation in Ab diversification. It is incontrovertible that AID isolated from B-cell nuclei is phosphorylated, for example, at Ser38, and possibly at other residues. Yet only a small fraction (∼10%) of nuclear AID appears to be phosphorylated at S38 (Basu *et al.*, 2005; McBride *et al.*, 2006; Pasqualucci *et al.*, 2006). One report suggests that although AID purified from human cells can attack ssDNA in the absence of phosphorylation, it cannot deaminate linear dsDNA transcribed by T7 RNA polymerase (Chaudhuri et al., 2004). It was reported that human single-stranded binding protein (RPA) was also required for transcription-dependent deamination by B-cell-phosphorylated AID (Chaudhuri et al., 2004). We are currently investigating the effect of phosphorylation on partially purified GST-tagged human AID expressed in baculovirus-infected cells. Our preliminary data substantiate the importance of phosphorylation of AID vis-a-vis its biochemical activity. We observe, for example, that the recombinant AID from insect cells is phosphorylated at at least two residues, Ser38 and Ser43. The specific activity of AID is reduced significantly by replacing these amino acids with Ala, and it is increased by replacement of Ser38 and Ser43 with phosphorylation-mimic Asp residues (S. Allen et al., unpublished data). However, we have not as yet been able to identify an essential role for phosphorylation or for RPA in T7 RNA polymerase transcription-dependent deamination. A more extensive biochemical analysis will likely be necessary to simulate transcription-dependent AID-catalyzed deamination and to elucidate the roles of accessory protein factors, *cis*-transcriptional elements, and AID phosphorylation.

We have measured the activity of AID on model transcription bubbles (Bransteitter et al., 2003) and on dsDNA undergoing active transcription (Bransteitter et al., 2004; Pham et al., 2003). AID is able to deaminate C in bubbles with as few as three displaced nucleotides, but appears to be most active with a displaced strand of nine nucleotides (Bransteitter et al., 2003). We have used two types of dsDNA substrates containing a T7 promoter to measure transcription-dependent C deamination, one composed of covalently closed supercoiled M13 DNA containing a lacZ reporter sequence (Pham et al., 2003), and one which is linear containing a single WRC target motif (S. Allen et al., unpublished data). The lacZ mutational spectra show a decided preference for deaminations in WRC motifs. Sequence data from individual DNA clones reveal a clustered mutational pattern (Bransteitter et al., 2004) reminiscent of the action of AID on nontranscribed ssDNA (Pham et al., 2003). An added element specific to the transcription assay is the observation that the mutations exhibit a polar gradient beginning proximal to the T7 promoter, gradually diminishing for about 500 nt further downstream from the promoter. The data suggest that AID might move with the transcription bubble, perhaps by jumping and sliding in accordance with our proposed model (Fig. 2). We speculate that the reduction in mutations with distance from the end of the promoter might be caused by a peeled-off ssRNA transcript binding to AID—recall that AID is strongly inhibited when bound to ssRNA (Bransteitter et al., 2003). In neither the M13 nor the linear dsDNA assay do we observe an absolute requirement either for phosphorylation or for RPA.

We have no explanation for why our T7 transcription-based assay with linear dsDNA differs from a similar assay which requires phosphorylated AID + RPA (Chaudhuri et al., 2004). Since human AID expressed in insect cells is phosphorylated at S38 as observed for AID from human B cells, perhaps there are more subtle features of B-cell AID or other factors in B-cell extracts that can account for the differences. The T7 transcription assays all show a strong preference (about 15:1) for deamination on the nontranscribed strand. These results are in accordance with AID's ability to bind to and catalyze C deamination on ssDNA; whereas AID cannot bind to nor deaminate dsDNA or RNA–DNA hybrids (Bransteitter et al., 2003). Presumably, low levels of deamination occurring on the transcribed strand result from transient melting of the RNA–DNA hybrid. Yet V-gene mutations occur roughly equally on both nontranscribed and transcribed DNA strands *in vivo*.

Several interesting questions and possibilities are raised by the large numbers of mutations that occur on the transcribed strand *in vivo*. Initially it was suggested that sites of AID-catalyzed C deamination were processed in parallel in either of three ways (Di Noia and Neuberger, 2002; Poltoratsky et al., 2000): replication of U giving rise to C → T mutations at the deamination site, processing of a U:G mismatch by MMR enzymes, and conversion of U to an abasic moiety by UNG which could be processed by a BER pathway. The latter two repair pathways would expose the transcribed strand to copying by error-prone DNA polymerases thus facilitating mutations at A and T sites, perhaps in accord with the specificity of pol η (Rogozin et al., 2001) inaccurately copying a secondary WA hot spot motif, or perhaps to further attack by AID. Although data from mice deficient in MMR or BER provide definitive support for this model (Li et al., 2004b; Martomo et al., 2004; Rada et al., 2004), the question still remains "is the transcribed strand accessible to AID during transcription"? The short answer in our opinion is "probably no," or at least not to any major extent. Yet there are data that suggest the opposite could be true. It has been suggested that unwinding of supercoiled regions at the end of a transcription bubble might make both strands accessible to AID (Shen and Storb, 2004). An experiment using an *E. coli* transcription system finds mutations occurring in equal numbers on both strands (Bessmer et al., 2006). Although these authors proposed that the *E. coli* system was considerably more eukaryotic-like than the T7 system, it is also the case that the T7 promoter is strictly unidirectional, whereas bidirectional transcription might be occurring in *E. coli*. A potential difficulty using *E. coli* transcription is that there are several promoters having opposite orientations on the same plasmid substrate, which is not the case for T7, which just has a single T7 promoter on the plasmid substrate. Data were not presented to rule out this possibility. Much more to the point is a study mapping transcription in B cells, which showed that

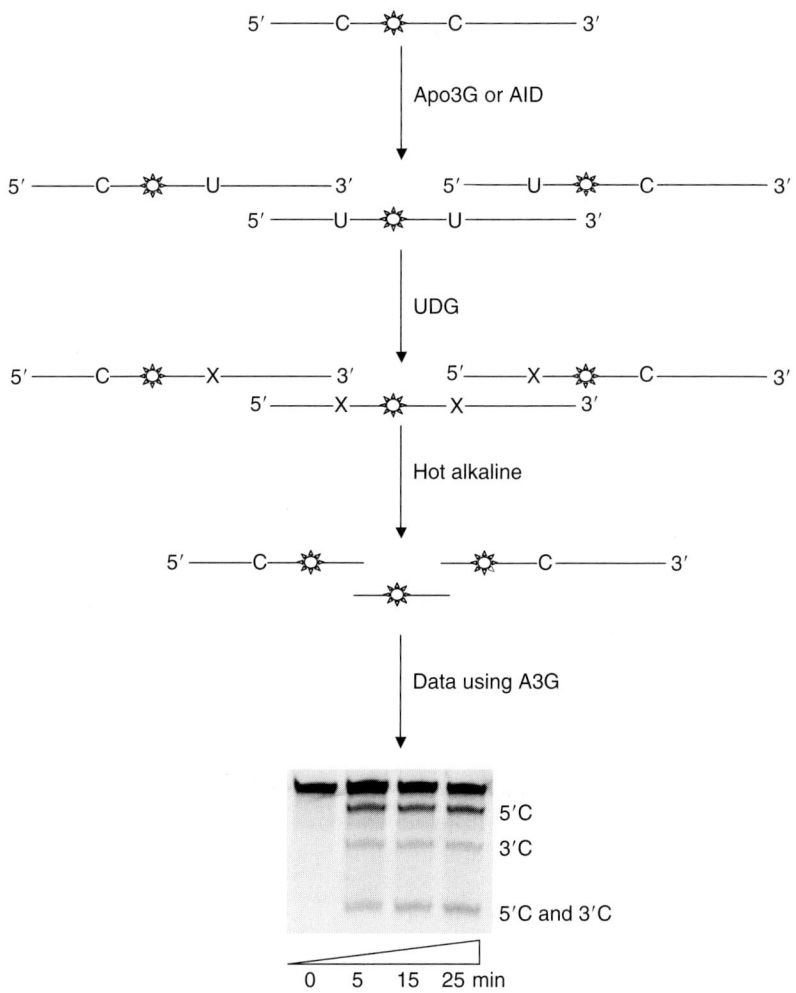

Figure 3 Analysis for Apo3G and AID processive C → U deaminations on ssDNA. An ssDNA substrate containing two C target motifs and either a fluorescent molecule or ^{32}P located in between the two motifs is incubated with Apo3G or AID, leading to three alternative outcomes, a single C → U conversion in the target motif located either nearer the 3' end or nearer the 5' end, or double C → U conversions occurring in both 3' and 5' target motifs. Incubation with uracil glycosylase (UDG) will convert U to an abasic moiety (X), and subsequent exposure to hot alkaline conditions will cause a break in the DNA strand at X, resulting is DNA strands having different lengths. Strands arising from 5' C, 3' C or 5' C, and 3' C deamination events are resolved by gel electrophoresis. Enzyme, ssDNA substrate concentrations, and incubation times are adjusted to ensure that C → U deaminations result from the action of no more than one Apo3G or AID encounter with an ssDNA substrate, which we refer to as single-hit conditions (Chelico *et al.*, 2006). Data are shown for Apo3G, where one observes favored deamination at 5' over 3'-target motifs,

transcription is occurring bidirectionally (D. Ronai and M. Scharff *et al.*, unpublished data). If this observation proves to be correct *in vivo*, AID could deaminate both DNA strands in B cells by attacking the nontranscribed strands of transcription bubbles moving in opposite directions.

Whether *E. coli* transcription is more eukaryotic-like than T7 transcription, an *in vitro* mammalian transcription model system will be required not only to address nontranscribed versus transcribed strand C deamination and the reasons for the lack of mutations in the first 100–200 bases, but more importantly to begin investigating how AID is targeted to V-gene, but not C-gene transcription bubbles. And, more generally, how AID and other APOBEC C deaminases are prevented from acting in an inopportune manner at the wrong place or at the wrong time (Pham *et al.*, 2005). Clearly a variety of *cis*- and *trans*-acting transcriptional elements must be involved such as enhancer and MAR elements. There could well be a combination of positive and negative regulatory factors that determine how, when, and where AID acts during transcription. One idea is that AID might be recruited to a specific region undergoing transcription by a transcription factor while perhaps interacting with RPA (Chaudhuri *et al.*, 2004). Alternatively, it is possible that AID access is negatively regulated by factors that prevent AID from binding to ssDNA during transcription, as deduced from data in Ronai *et al.* (2005) or, a combination of negative and positive acting factors might be required to govern the access of AID to ssDNA exposed during transcription.

2.2. APOBEC-Targeting Mechanisms Involve Jumping and Sliding Along ssDNA

Random binding to ssDNA and bidirectional processive movement of AID was deduced, as described above, from the distribution of C deamination clusters on individual DNA clones (Bransteitter *et al.*, 2004; Pham *et al.*, 2003). To obtain a more precise picture describing the dynamics of scanning for any APOBEC enzyme, we have designed an assay to measure correlated multiple C deaminations occurring on individual ssDNA molecules that interact at most once with an APOBEC enzyme (Chelico *et al.*, 2006). In its simplest form, the assay monitors deamination of two target C residues located on an ssDNA substrate, separated by an arbitrary number of nucleotides, containing either a ^{32}P or fluorescent (fluorescein) tag located between the two motifs (Fig. 3). There are three possible outcomes for an ssDNA substrate acted on by an

---

along with processive coordinated double deaminations at 5′ C and 3′ C occurring during a single encounter of Apo3G with an ssDNA substrate.

APOBEC C deaminase: a single conversion of C → U in either the 3′-motif or 5′-motif, or double C → U conversions occurring in both 3′- and 5′-motifs on the *same* DNA molecule. Treatment with UNG to convert U to an abasic site followed by strand breakage at the abasic moiety results in different length fluorescent or ^{32}P-tagged fragments that are clearly resolved by PAGE (Fig. 3). An APOBEC enzyme acts processively if it catalyzes C deaminations in both motifs. Practically speaking, to ensure that double deaminations are in fact catalyzed by the action of at most one APOBEC molecule, enzyme/substrate ratios and incubation times are chosen so that no more than about 10% of the substrates are deaminated. A thorough description of the assay is given in Chelico *et al.* (2006).

The analysis reveals a remarkable scanning mechanism for Apo3G. Apo3G catalyzes coordinated double deaminations caused by the action of a single enzyme at 3′- and 5′-target motifs sevenfold more frequently than predicted by the product of independent deaminations at 3′- and 5′-sites catalyzed by two different Apo3G molecules on the same ssDNA substrate (Chelico *et al.*, 2006). Apo3G acts processively over at least 100 nt, but what's "remarkable" is that although the enzyme appears to bind randomly to ssDNA, deamination proceeds predominantly 3′ → 5′, as seen by the presence of much more deamination at the 5′- compared to 3′-target motif. In other words, the band intensities corresponding to single deaminations are far more intense for deamination of the 5′-target (Fig. 3). However, there is no apparent energy source present to impart directionality—notably, the strong asymmetry favoring 5′- over 3′-C deamination occurs to the same extent either in the absence or presence of nucleotides, for example ATP or GTP. To account for the differential pattern of deamination, we have proposed that Apo3G attacks its preferred CCC target motif with a strong 3′ to 5′ polarity, that is Apo3G attacks from the 3′-side. In the absence of a source of energy to impart directional motion, the enzyme can move along the ssDNA in either direction, but catalysis is restricted to occur from the 3′ to 5′ direction. Apo3G cannot bind to dsDNA (Chelico *et al.*, 2006). By annealing an ssDNA oligonucleotide in between the two target C motifs to create a partially dsDNA region on the ssDNA substrate along which Apo3G cannot slide, we have shown that in addition to sliding along ssDNA, the enzyme can also jump over the dsDNA block (Chelico *et al.*, 2006).

A sketch depicting a sliding and jumping action of Apo3G is shown in Fig. 2. Apo3G is believed to operate as a multimer, possibly as a dimer (Chelico *et al.*, 2006). We have speculated that an asymmetric head to tail arrangement of monomer subunits could in principle provide for the type of asymmetric 3′ to 5′ attack (Chelico *et al.*, 2006). Using the same assay, we observe that AID slides and jumps along ssDNA, thus acting in a manner similar to Apo3G. However, AID behaves very differently from Apo3G in that it deaminates 5′- and 3′-target motifs equally well (Pham *et al.*, 2007). One can imagine a symmetric head-to-head arrangement of monomers for AID. Imagination aside, it is essential to determine just what the biochemically and, of course, biologically active forms are for Apo3G and AID. A study using an Apo3G mutant incapable of forming dimers finds that the monomer is catalytically active both *in vitro* and *in vivo* (Opi *et al.*, 2006). Although, it would be interesting to see if the mutant is able to catalyze processive deaminations, what would be unquestionably most beneficial at this time would be to have a crystal structure for AID and Apo3G, even better, a cocrystal with ssDNA.

Although a precise structural explanation for the scanning awaits high-resolution crystal structures for the APOBEC nucleic acid deaminases, the scanning behavior of Apo3G and AID appears to simulate their most salient *in vivo* properties. For example, it is known that the HIV-1 AIDS virus contains a strong mutational polarity with C → U deaminations concentrated toward the 5′-region of the virus minus strand (Yu *et al.*, 2004). The intrinsic ability of Apo3G to carry out a 3′ to 5′ attack on proviral cDNA *in vitro* could account for the distribution of viral mutations skewed heavily toward the 3′-DNA end of the plus strand. A finding that there's actually a twin gradient emanating from two priming positions for second-strand DNA to DNA synthesis (Suspene *et al.*, 2006), makes matters somewhat more complicated, but the intrinsic 3′ → 5′ attack by Apo3G involving sliding *and* jumping might account (Chelico *et al.*, 2006), at least in part, for both mutational gradients on different parts of the cDNA. A strict directionality might also be imposed on AID by the requirement that deamination takes place while tracking along with a moving transcription bubble translocating 5′ to 3′ along V-gene DNA.

3. How and Why Might AID-Specific Mutations Be Targeted?

The properties of AID that have been revealed by the biochemical studies described above suggest that it is targeted to specific motifs within highly transcribed genes. The sparing of the first 100–200 bp and decrease in SHM 1.5-kb downstream from the transcription start site may ultimately be attributable to the inherent properties of the enzyme as it interacts with DNA and the transcription apparatus. However, the inherent biochemical properties of AID probably are less likely to explain how its mutagenic action is preferentially targeted to Ig heavy and light chains and why it is sometimes mistargeted to other highly transcribed genes in centroblast B cells. It is likely that associated proteins contribute to the targeting to the Ig genes and to the apparent differential targeting to V and SRs. This is supported by the finding that mutations in the C-terminal end of AID lead to an inability of the enzyme to mediate CSR, while mutations in the N-terminal portion lead to the loss of ability to mediate V region mutation while CSR continues (Barreto et al., 2003; Shinkura et al., 2004). Further support for the differential targeting to V and SRs occurs comes from the observation that when AID is induced in naive mouse B cells, those cells carry out what appears to be normal CSR and undergo high rates of mutation in the SRs including the regions 5′ to the μ SR, but no mutations occur in the V regions of those same cells (Nagaoka et al., 2002; Reina-San-Martin et al., 2003). AID has been reported to associate with RNAP II (Nambu et al., 2003), but the detailed relationship between AID-induced mutations and the transcription have yet to be elucidated. It has been suggested that there may be a mutasome that includes AID and some or many of the other proteins that participate in SHM and CSR, but such complexes have yet to be identified (Reynaud et al., 2003).

In addition to the role of associated proteins, there are probably other mechanisms that are responsible for the selective targeting of AID to the V and SRs of the Ig genes and the protection of other highly transcribed genes in centroblast B cells. Some of the studies suggesting such mechanisms have been reviewed in detail (Odegard and Schatz, 2006). Briefly, various combinations of cytokines target AID to the different SR that are 5′ to the α, ε, and each of four IgG constant regions. This selective targeting could be facilitated by increased accessibility that is associated with changes in acetylation and methylation of chromatin (Li et al., 2004a; Nambu et al., 2003; Wang et al., 2006b). These changes in chromatin structure are also associated with the onset of transcription in these regions, so it is unclear whether specific patterns of chromatin modifications are required for the correct targeting of AID to particular SRs (Li et al., 2004a; Wang et al., 2006b). However, the different patterns of histone modifications suggest that chromatin structure may play a greater role than just providing accessibility for RNAP II. Studies in tissue culture cells undergoing SHM show that the protection of the first 100–200 bps and of the C region is lost when there is global hyperacetylation of histones, suggesting that chromatin structure may play some specific role (Woo et al., 2003). Differences in the acetylation of the histones associated with V and C are also observed *in vivo* in mice but precede the induction of AID, so it is still unclear if targeting requires changes in chromatin structure (Odegard and Schatz, 2006; Odegard et al., 2005).

There are similar uncertainties about the requirement for and the role of *cis*-acting sequences in the targeting of AID to the V region. The observations that when AID is overexpressed both in cultured cells and *in vivo* it can target non-Ig genes (Gaidano et al., 2003; Gordon et al., 2003; Okazaki et al., 2003; Wang et al., 2004), including itself (Martin and Scharff, 2002), suggest that particular *cis*-acting DNA motifs are not required. Although there is evidence of a need for enhancers and promoters in ectopically located Ig genes in cultured cells and *in vivo* (Jolly *et al.*, 1996; Tumas-Brundage *et al.*, 1996), the deletion of some of these elements in the endogenous genes does not always confirm these findings (Odegard and Schatz, 2006; Tumas-Brundage *et al.*, 1996). However, the specific deletion or manipulation of some of these elements in cultured cells suggests that the targeting of AID to the V region may be complex and that are a mixture of negative and positive controls (Ronai *et al.*, 2005). The potential role of enhancers and promoters is particularly difficult to dissect because transcription is required for AID-induced mutations so any change in the putative *cis*-acting sequences that results in a decrease in transcription will also cause a decrease in SHM. It is also possible that there are particular DNA structures, such as G-quartets in SRs, that serve as a niche for the targeting of AID (Maizels, 2005).

It will probably be necessary to reconstruct the processes of SHM and CSR *in vitro* to determine the role of chromatin modifications, *cis*-acting sequences, and specific DNA structures in creating and fixing the large numbers of mutation that are required for both SHM and CSR.

4. Selection of AID-Induced Mutations During Ab Maturation

Why might AID hot spots have been selected for during evolution? To frame this question in an appropriate context, it is critical to consider the various selection pressures under which antibodies evolve. It is obvious that no mutations are tolerated which prevent assembly or appropriate folding of the Ab (Horne *et al.*, 1982; Kranz and Voss, 1981; Wiens *et al.*, 1998). Thus, germ line gene sequences may have been selected that are prone not to mutate residues that form parts of the interchain interface or structural motifs within the framework (FR) regions.

However, more subtle selection pressures may have helped select for AID hot spot sequences. One of the earliest understood challenges to the immune system was "horror autotoxicus" (Silverstein, 2001). How are Ab molecules generated with the bewildering array of specificities required to recognize a virtually infinite set of foreign epitopes, without producing Ab that bind any self molecules (Landsteiner, 1936). This problem is at least partially solved if evolution has selected for germ line antibodies that are polyspecific, thus, greatly expanding the range of foreign molecules that are recognized with sufficient affinity to initiate SHM. But this immediately leads to another problem, if these antibodies remain polyspecific, they are also likely to bind self molecules and cause autoimmunity. How might the control of AID-dependent mutations help select against the evolution of self-reactive antibodies

One way that AID-dependent mutations might simultaneously optimize affinity and specificity is by manipulating protein flexibility. Flexible germ line combining sites that adopt different conformations would be able to recognize a broad range of Ags with an induced-fit-like mechanism (Berzofsky, 1985; Bosshard, 2001; Foote and Milstein, 1994; Ma et al., 2002; Sundberg and Mariuzza, 2003). Although these flexible antibodies would also be expected to bind self-molecules (Comtesse et al., 2000), they are only present in low concentrations (Souroujon et al., 1988). A rapid change in the concentration or presentation of a foreign molecule may then induce SHM (Baumgarth, 2000; Jegerlehner et al., 2002). If mutations are introduced that rigidify the protein in a conformation suitable for target recognition, they may be selected as they will decrease the entropic cost of binding and increase affinity (Comtesse et al., 2000; Guigou et al., 1991; Hodgkin, 1998; James et al., 2003; Joyce, 1997; Mason, 1998; Patten et al., 1996; Souroujon et al., 1988; Wedemayer et al., 1997). The mature antibodies may then be produced in the large quantities required to fight an infection because they are now highly specific, recognizing only their target with a lock-and-key-like mechanism (Pauling, 1946; Sundberg and Mariuzza, 2003).

By comparing Ab structures with and without bound small molecule Ags, researchers began in the 1990s to characterize Ab–Ag recognition in terms of induced-fit and lock-and-key. The first reported studies by Wilson of an antipeptide antibody (Stanfield et al., 1990) and by Poljak and Milstein of an anti-2-phenyloxazone Ab (Alzari et al., 1990) in 1990 found that Ag binding did not induce a significant change in protein structure. However, significant changes in Ab structure on Ag binding were observed in several subsequent studies, most notably with an anti-DNA Ab (Herron et al., 1991), an antiprogesterone Ab (Arevalo et al., 1993), and another antipeptide Ab (Rini et al., 1992).

The structural consequences of SHM have been elegantly examined by the groups of Ray Stevens and Peter Schultz. They approached the problem by characterizing the protein rearrangements induced by Ag binding in both germ line and mature Ab (Hsieh-Wilson et al., 1996; Mundorff et al., 2000; Patten et al., 1996; Wedemayer et al., 1997; Yin et al., 2001). These studies unambiguously illustrated two important aspects of SHM: first, many of the selected mutations are distal from the combining site and second, at least some of them appear to preorganize the combining site for Ag recognition. Two examples are especially illuminating. During the affinity maturation of Ab 48G7, which binds a p-nitrophenyl phosphonate analogue (Jacobs, 1990), nine mutations were introduced, none of which directly contact the Ag (Patten et al., 1996). Comparison of the Ag-free and Ag-bound combining sites of mutated, affinity-matured Ab 48G7 shows that there are no significant changes on Ag binding. However, significant structural changes are observed on Ag binding to the germ line Ab (Wedemayer et al., 1997). Thus, it was suggested that several of the somatic mutations, especially heavy chain mutations N^H56D and G^H55V, preorganize the combining site appropriately to bind Ag. Ab 28B4 provides a second example. 28B4 evolved to bind an aminophosphonic acid analogue (Hsieh *et al.*, 1994) via nine mutations. Again, germ line and affinity-matured Ab structures, both with and without bound Ag, were determined (Hsieh-Wilson *et al.*, 1996; Yin *et al.*, 2001). While in this case the differences were smaller, heavy chain CDR3 and light chain CDR1 of the germ line Ab displayed conformational changes on Ag binding that were not apparent in the mature receptor. It was suggested that the $D^H 95W$ mutation in the heavy chain is important for preorganizing the CDR3 loop.

The structural studies described above identify regions of the Ab that undergo Ag-induced changes in structure. However, in other cases the observed structural changes are small in the germ line as well as the mature Ab (Romesberg *et al.*, 1998). Even when large structural changes are apparent, it is not clear if they reflect interconversion between two well-ordered and rigid conformations, or if they actually reflect the ability of the combining site to adopt a wide range of structures, that is flexibility. To more rigorously test the hypothesis that SHM optimizes Ab flexibility and conformational heterogeneity, a combination of structural and dynamic approaches is required.

Protein dynamics have been described as conformational disorder according to Frauenfelder's model of a hierarchical energy landscape wherein proteins exist in a limited number of conformations, each consisting of a large number of conformational substates (Frauenfelder and Leeson, 1998; Frauenfelder and McMahon, 2000; Frauenfelder *et al.*, 1988, 1991; Kitao *et al.*, 1998). Fluctuations between different conformational substates result in diffusive motion on the picosecond to nanosecond timescale, while large-scale conformational changes result from a superposition of diffusive motions, and accordingly they occur on a slower timescale (Frauenfelder *et al.*, 1988; Parak, 2003; Zaccai, 2000). While NMR is a promising technique to measure Ab dynamics, potentially as a function of SHM, it has not yet been applied to this problem.

One optical technique that has been applied to the problem is 3-photon echo peak shift spectroscopy (3PEPS). The 3PEPS experiment is similar to the well-known NMR spin echo experiment, but requires three pulses of light resonant with the absorption of the bound chromophore. Briefly, in these experiments a force is applied to the chromophore's environment by absorption-induced changes in the chromophore's dipole moment, and the time scale and energy of the protein's response to this force are characterized by following coherence decay with second and third pulses of femtosecond light. Additionally, in a homogeneous environment (i.e., a single well-ordered Ab combining site), the 3PEPS signal decays to zero; however, in a heterogeneous environment, the 3PEPS signal decays asymptotically to a nonzero value. This feature is particularly interesting as it renders 3PEPS the only technique that can detect conformational heterogeneity under biological conditions (i.e., above cryogenic temperatures) (Fleming and Cho, 1996; Homoelle and Beck, 1997; Homoelle et al., 1998; Nagasawa et al., 1997, 2003). The 3PEPS technique was developed to study solvation dynamics, but is easily adopted to study Ab evolution with the use of antichromophoric antibodies.

To examine how protein dynamics may be manipulated by SHM, the well-characterized antifluorescein Ab, 4-4-20, for which there is also a published crystal structure, was employed. The germ line precursor of 4-4-20 was evolved to bind fluorescein via two light chain mutations and 10 heavy chain mutations (Jimenez et al., 2004). While the light chain mutations are proximal to the bound fluorescein, the heavy chain mutations group into two clusters, one >10 Å from the binding site and other >20 Å. Each mutation was individually examined in the context of both a germ line or mature Ab, and the effect on fluorescein affinity measured by surface plasmon resonance (Zimmermann et al., 2006). Remarkably, the greatest impact on affinity was due to a Cys to Arg mutation at position 38 of the heavy chain, located more than 20 Å removed from the binding site. In addition, because affinities must increase during affinity maturation, it was possible to conclude that the maturation of the heavy chain preceded the evolution of the light chain (Zimmermann et al., 2006).

The germ line Ab, a potential intermediate (with an evolved heavy chain and a germ line light chain), and the mature Ab were recombinantly expressed and characterized using 3PEPS (Fig. 4). The 3PEPS time domain data was Fourier transformed into a spectral density, where the amplitude of the protein motions induced by fluorecein excitation is plotted versus their frequency (Fig. 4B and C). It is immediately apparent that SHM systematically reduced the amplitude of low-frequency motion resulting in a fully mature Ab that displays only high-frequency motion. Remarkably, analysis of the spectral densities demonstrate that during maturation the average force constant of the protein motions displaced by fluorescein excitation was increased by 400-fold (Zimmermann et al., 2006). Even more remarkably, the 3PEPS terminal peak shift, a quantitative measure of heterogeneity, was systematically reduced during maturation (Fig. 4).

A physical basis for SHM-induced rigidification is apparent from a comparison of the structure of the mature Ab (Whitlow et al., 1995) with the computational model of the germ line. The heavy chain mutations appear to play a central role despite the fact that none involve residues that directly contact Ag. Instead, these mutations appear to rigidify the protein by introducing two clusters of mutually dependent interactions that act to cross-link β-strands and CDR loops of the combining site, localizing it to a conformation most appropriate for Ag binding (Fig. 4). Further deconvolution of the structural

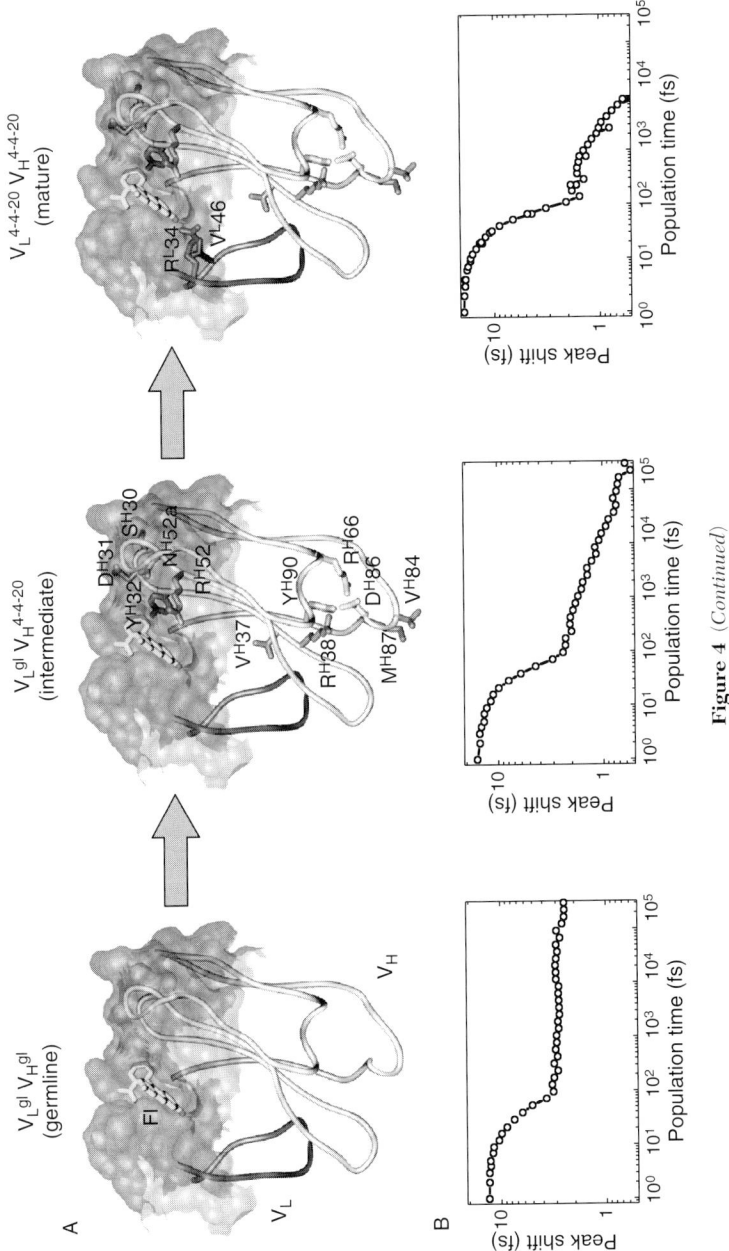

Figure 4 (*Continued*)

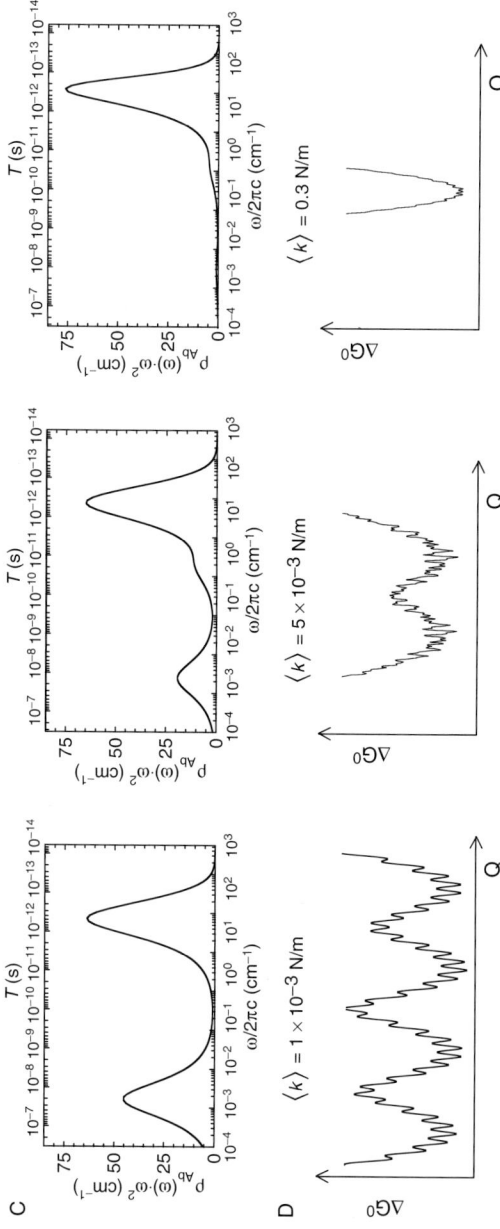

Figure 4 Evolution of Ab 4-4-20 structure and dynamics. (A) Ab structure with mutations introduced during SHM shown in orange (see text). Also shown in light blue are the residues that form the hydrogen bond network within the mature Ab that might help to rigidify the combining site. For clarity, only part of the light chain is shown. (B) Experimental 3PEPS decays. (C) Spectral densities that result from Fourier transform of the experimental 3PEPS time domain decays (see text). (D) Schematic representation of the Ab energy landscape as a function of SHM. The 3PEPS decays and terminal peak shifts suggest that SHM changed the Ab from a flexible precursor that samples many different potential energy minima, corresponding to different combining site conformations, to a more rigid receptor that is localized to a single, well-ordered conformation. Also shown is the average force constant of the induced combining site motions as determined from 3PEPS experiments (Zimmermann et al., 2006). (**See Color Plate 7.**)

and dynamic changes associated with the evolution of Ab 4-4-20 should be provided by structural analysis of the germ line progenitor.

While still at a very early stage in our understanding, the characterization of protein structure and dynamics as a function of SHM suggests that during evolution AID-dependent mutations are selected that convert flexible and polyspecific Ab into rigid and highly specific Ab. Further testing this model will require the use of other techniques, such as NMR-based approaches that are capable of characterizing dynamics as a function of maturation in both the free and Ag-bound Ab as well as additional structural studies. Nonetheless, the structural and dynamic data discussed suggest that evolution may have selected for AID-induced mutational hot spots in order to focus the mutations to sites within the combining site and to those elsewhere that tailor protein dynamics for molecular recognition. Thus, AID and the other proteins involved in SHM may have coevolved along with the Ig gene sequences to ensure elsewhere that mutations that evolve molecular recognition are quickly introduced. Further characterizing both the mechanisms of AID activity and how the selected mutations facilitate molecular recognition should test and refine the proposed models and also help to clarify the role of purposeful mutations in Ab evolution.

Acknowledgments

This work was supported by NIH grants R37GM21422 and RO1ES013192 (M.F.G.), RO1CA72649 and R01CA102705 (M.D.S), and the Skaggs Institute for Chemical Biology (F.E.R.).

References

Alzari, P. M., Spinelli, S., Mariuzza, R. A., Boulot, G., Poljak, R. J., Jarvis, J. M., and Milstein, C. (1990). Three-dimensional structure determination of an anti-2-phenyloxazolone antibody: The role of somatic mutation and heavy/light chain pairing in the maturation of an immune response. *EMBO J.* **9,** 3807–3814.

Arevalo, J. H., Stura, E. A., Taussig, M. J., and Wilson, I. A. (1993). Three-dimensional structure of an anti-steroid Fab' and progesterone-Fab' complex. *J. Mol. Biol.* **231,** 103–118.

Bachl, J., Ertongur, I., and Jungnickel, B. (2006). Involvement of Rad18 in somatic hypermutation. *Proc. Natl. Acad. Sci. USA* **103,** 12081–12086.

Barreto, V., Reina-San-Martin, B., Ramiro, A. R., McBride, K. M., and Nussenzweig, M. C. (2003). C-terminal deletion of AID uncouples class switch recombination from somatic hypermutation and gene conversion. *Mol. Cell* **12,** 501–508.

Basu, U., Chaudhuri, J., Alpert, C., Dutt, S., Ranganath, S., Li, G., Schrum, J. P., Manis, J. P., and Alt, F. W. (2005). The AID antibody diversification enzyme is regulated by protein kinase A phosphorylation. *Nature* **438,** 508–511.

Baumgarth, N. (2000). A two-phase model of B-cell activation. *Immunol. Rev.* **176,** 171–180.

Berzofsky, J. A. (1985). Intrinsic and extrinsic factors in protein antigenic structure. *Science* **229**, 932–940.

Bessmer, E., Market, E., and Papavasiliou, F. N. (2006). The transcription elongation complex directs activation-induced cytidine deaminase-mediated DNA deamination. *Mol. Cell. Biol.* **26**, 4378–4385.

Bosshard, H. R. (2001). Molecular recognition by induced fit: How fit is the concept. *News Physiol. Sci.* **16**, 171–173.

Bransteitter, R., Pham, P., Scharff, M. D., and Goodman, M. F. (2003). Activation-induced cytidine deaminase deaminates deoxycytidine on single-stranded DNA but requires the action of RNase. *Proc. Natl. Acad. Sci. USA* **100**, 4102–4107.

Bransteitter, R., Pham, P., Calabrese, P., and Goodman, M. F. (2004). Biochemical analysis of hyper-mutational targeting by wild type and mutant AID. *J. Biol. Chem.* **279**, 51612–51621.

Chaudhuri, J., and Alt, F. W. (2004). Class-switch recombination: Interplay of transcription, DNA deamination and DNA repair. *Nat. Rev. Immunol.* **4**, 541–552.

Chaudhuri, J., Tian, M., Khuong, C., Chua, K., Pinaud, E., and Alt, F. W. (2003). Transcription-targeted DNA deamination by the AID antibody diversification enzyme. *Nature* **422**, 726–730.

Chaudhuri, J., Khuong, C., and Alt, F. W. (2004). Replication protein A interacts with AID to promote deamination of somatic hypermutation targets. *Nature* **430**, 992–998.

Chelico, L., Pham, P., Calabrese, P., and Goodman, M. F. (2006). APOBEC3G DNA deaminase acts processively $3' \rightarrow 5'$ on single-stranded DNA. *Nat. Struct. Mol. Biol.* **13**, 392–399.

Chen, X., Kinoshita, K., and Honjo, T. (2001). Variable deletion and duplication at recombination junction ends: Implication for staggered double-strand cleavage in class-switch recombination. *Proc. Natl. Acad. Sci. USA* **98**, 13860–13865.

Comtesse, N., Heckel, D., Maldener, E., Glass, B., and Meese, E. (2000). Probing the human natural autoantibody repertoire using an immunoscreening approach. *Clin. Exp. Immunol.* **121**, 430–436.

Davidson, N. O., and Shelness, G. S. (2000). APOLIPOPROTEIN B: mRNA editing, lipoprotein assembly, and presecretory degradation. *Annu. Rev. Nutr.* **20**, 169–193.

Di Noia, J., and Neuberger, M. S. (2002). Altering the pathway of immunoglobulin hypermutation by inhibiting uracil-DNA glycosylase. *Nature* **419**, 43–48.

Dickerson, S. K., Market, E., Besmer, E., and Papavasiliou, F. N. (2003). AID mediates hypermutation by deaminating single stranded DNA. *J. Exp. Med.* **197**, 1291–1296.

Fleming, G. R., and Cho, M. (1996). Chromophore-solvent dynamics. *Annu. Rev. Phys. Chem.* **47**, 109–134.

Foote, J., and Milstein, C. (1994). Conformational isomerism and the diversity of antibodies. *Proc. Natl. Acad. Sci. USA* **91**, 10370–10374.

Frauenfelder, H., and Leeson, D. T. (1998). The energy landscape in non-biological and biological molecules. *Nat. Struct. Biol.* **5**, 757–759.

Frauenfelder, H., and McMahon, B. H. (2000). Energy landscape and fluctuations in proteins. *Annalen der Physik* **9**, 655–667.

Frauenfelder, H., Parak, F., and Young, R. (1988). Conformational substates in proteins. *Annu. Rev. Biophys. Biophys. Chem.* **17**, 451–479.

Frauenfelder, H., Sligar, S. G., and Wolynes, P. G. (1991). The energy landscapes and motions of proteins. *Science* **254**, 1598–1603.

Gaidano, G., Pasqualucci, L., Capello, D., Berra, E., Deambrogi, C., Rossi, D., Maria Larocca, L., Gloghini, A., Carbone, A., and Dalla-Favera, R. (2003). Aberrant somatic hypermutation in multiple subtypes of AIDS-associated non-Hodgkin lymphoma. *Blood* **102**, 1833–1841.

Gordon, M. S., Kanegai, C. M., Doerr, J. R., and Wall, R. (2003). Somatic hypermutation of the B cell receptor genes B29 (Igbeta, CD79b) and mb1 (Igalpha, CD79a). *Proc. Natl. Acad. Sci. USA* **100**, 4126–4131.

Guigou, V., Guilbert, B., Moinier, D., Tonnelle, C., Boubli, L., Avrameas, S., Fougereau, M., and Fumoux, F. (1991). Ig repertoire of human polyspecific antibodies and B-cell ontogeny. *J. Immunol.* **146**, 1368–1374.

Halford, S. E., and Marko, J. F. (2004). How do site specific DNA-binding proteins find their targets. *Nucleic Acids Res.* **32**, 3040–3052.

Herron, J. N., He, X.-M., Ballard, D. W., Blier, P. R., Pace, P. E., Bothwell, A. L., Voss, E. W., Jr., and Edmundson, A. B. (1991). An autoantibody to single-stranded DNA: Comparison of the three-dimensional structures of the unliganded Fab and a deoxynucleotide-Fab complex. *Proteins* **11**, 159–175.

Hodgkin, P. D. (1998). Role of cross-reactivity in the development of antibody responses. *Immunologist* **6**, 223–226.

Homoelle, B. J., and Beck, W. F. (1997). Solvent accessibility of the phycocyanobilin chromophore in the α subunit of c-phycocyanin: Implications for a molecular mechanism for inertial protein-matrix solvation dynamics. *Biochemistry* **36**, 12970–12975.

Homoelle, B. J., Edington, M. D., Diffey, W. M., and Beck, W. F. (1998). Stimulated photon-echo and transient-grating studies of protein-matrix solvation dynamics and interexciton-state radiationless decay in α phycocyanin and allophycocyanin. *J. Phys. Chem. B* **102**, 3044–3052.

Honjo, T., Muramatsu, M., and Fagarasan, S. (2004). AID: How does it aid antibody diversity. *Immunity* **20**, 659–668.

Horne, C., Klein, M., Polidoulis, I., and Dorrington, K. J. (1982). Noncovalent association of heavy and light chains of human immunoglobulins. III. Specific interactions between VH and VL. *J. Immunol.* **129**, 660–664.

Hsieh, L. C., Stephans, J. C., and Schultz, P. G. (1994). An efficient antibody-catalyzed oxygenation reaction. *J. Am. Chem. Soc.* **116**, 2167–2168.

Hsieh-Wilson, L., Schultz, P. G., and Stevens, R. C. (1996). Insight into antibody catalysis: Structure of an oxygenation catalyst at 1.9-Å resolution. *Proc. Natl. Acad. Sci. USA* **93**, 5363–5367.

Jacobs, J. W. (1990). "Department of Chemistry." University of California Berkeley, Berkeley, California.

James, L. C., Roversi, P., and Tawfik, D. S. (2003). Antibody multispecificity mediated by conformational diversity. *Science* **299**, 1362–1367.

Jegerlehner, A., Storni, T., Lipowsky, G., Schmid, M., Pumpens, P., and Bachmann, M. F. (2002). Regulation of IgG antibody responses by epitope density and CD21-mediated costimulation. *Eur. J. Immunol.* **32**, 3305–3314.

Jimenez, R., Salazar, G., Yin, J., Joo, T., and Romesberg, F. E. (2004). Protein dynamics and the immunological evolution of molecular recognition. *Proc. Natl. Acad. Sci. USA* **101**, 3803–3808.

Jolly, C. J., Wagner, S. D., Rada, C., Klix, N., Milstein, C., and Neuberger, M. S. (1996). The targeting of somatic hypermutation. *Semin. Immunol.* **8**, 159–168.

Joyce, G. F. (1997). Evolutionary chemistry: Getting there from here. *Science* **276**, 1658–1659.

Kitao, A., Hayward, S., and Go, N. (1998). Energy landscape of a native protein: Jumping-among-minima model. *Proteins* **33**, 496–517.

Kranz, D. M., and Voss, E. W., Jr. (1981). Restricted reassociation of heavy and light chains from hapten-specific monoclonal antibodies. *Proc. Natl. Acad. Sci. USA* **78**, 5807–5811.

Kuppers, R., and Dalla-Favera, R. (2001). Mechanisms of chromosomal translocations in B cell lymphomas. *Oncogene* **20**, 5580–5594.

Landsteiner, K. (1936). "The Specificity of Serological Reactions," Dover, New York.

Larson, E. D., Cummings, W. J., Bednarski, D. W., and Maizels, N. (2005). MRE11/RAD50 cleaves DNA in the AID/UNG-dependent pathway of immunoglobulin gene diversification. *Mol. Cell* **20**, 367–375.

Li, Z., Luo, Z., and Scharff, M. D. (2004a). Differential regulation of histone acetylation and generation of mutations in switch regions is associated with Ig class switching. *Proc. Natl. Acad. Sci. USA* **101**, 15428–15433.

Li, Z., Scherer, S. J., Ronai, D., Iglesias-Ussel, M. D., Peled, J. U., Bardwell, P. D., Zhuang, M., Lee, K., Martin, A., Edelmann, W., and Scharff, M. D. (2004b). Examination of Msh6- and Msh3-deficient mice in class switching reveals overlapping and distinct roles of mutS homologues in antibody diversification. *J. Exp. Med.* **200**, 47–59.

Li, Z., Woo, C. J., Iglesias-Ussel, M. D., Ronai, D., and Scharff, M. D. (2004c). The generation of antibody diversity through somatic hypermutation and class switch recombination. *Genes Dev.* **18**, 1–11.

Longo, N. S., and Lipsky, P. E. (2006). Why do B cells mutate their immunoglobulin receptors. *Trends Immunol.* **27**, 374–380.

Ma, B., Shatsky, M., Wolfson, H. J., and Nussinov, R. (2002). Multiple diverse ligands binding at a single protein site: A matter of pre-existing populations. *Protein Sci.* **11**, 184–197.

Maizels, N. (2005). Immunoglobulin gene diversification. *Annu. Rev. Genet.* **39**, 23–46.

Martin, A., and Scharff, M. D. (2002). Somatic hypermutation of the AID transgene in B and non-B cells. *Proc. Natl. Acad. Sci. USA* **99**, 12304–12308.

Martin, A., Bardwell, P. D., Woo, C. J., Fan, M., Shulman, M. J., and Scharff, M. D. (2002). Activation-induced cytidine deaminase turns on somatic hypermutation in hybridomas. *Nature* **415**, 802–806.

Martomo, S. A., Yang, W. W., and Gearhart, P. J. (2004). A role for Msh6 but not Msh3 in somatic hypermutation and class switch recombination. *J. Exp. Med.* **200**, 61–68.

Mason, D. (1998). A very high level of crossreactivity is an essential feature of the T-cell receptor. *Immunol. Today* **19**, 395–404.

McBride, K. M., Gazumyan, A., Woo, E. M., Barreto, V. M., Robbiani, D. F., Chait, B. T., and Nussenzweig, M. C. (2006). Regulation of hypermutation by activation-induced cytidine deaminase phosphorylation. *Proc. Natl. Acad. Sci. USA* **103**, 8798–8803.

McKean, D., Huppi, K., Bell, M., Staudt, L., Gerhard, W., and Weigert, M. (1984). Generation of antibody diversity in the immune response of BALB/c mice to influenza virus hemagglutinin. *Proc. Natl. Acad. Sci. USA* **81**, 3180–3184.

Mundorff, E. C., Hanson, M. A., Varvak, A., Ulrich, H., Schultz, P. G., and Stevens, R. C. (2000). Conformational effects in biological catalysis: An antibody catalyzed oxy-cope rearrangement. *Biochemistry* **39**, 627–632.

Muramatsu, M., Sankaranand, V. S., Anant, S., Sugai, M., Kinoshita, K., Davidson, N. O., and Honjo, T. (1999). Specific expression of activation-induced cytidine deaminase (AID), a novel member of the RNA-editing deaminase family in germinal center B cells. *J. Biol. Chem.* **274**, 18470–18476.

Muramatsu, M., Kinoshita, K., Fagarasan, S., Yamada, S., Shinkai, Y., and Honjo, T. (2000). Class switch recombination and hypermutation require activation-induced cytidine deaminase (AID), a potential RNA editing enzyme. *Cell* **102**, 553–563.

Nagaoka, H., Muramatsu, M., Yamamura, N., Kinoshita, K., and Honjo, T. (2002). Activation-induced deaminase (AID)-directed hypermutation in the immunoglobulin Smu region: Implication of AID involvement in a common step of class switch recombination and somatic hypermutation. *J. Exp. Med.* **195**, 529–534.

Nagasawa, Y., Passino, S. A., Joo, T., and Fleming, G. R. (1997). Temperature dependence of optical dephasing in an organic polymer glass (PMMA) from 300 K to 30 K. *J. Chem. Phys.* **106,** 4840–4852.

Nagasawa, Y., Seike, K., Muromoto, T., and Okada, T. (2003). Two-dimensional analysis of integrated three-pulse photon echo signals of Nile blue doped in PMMA. *J. Phys. Chem. A* **107,** 2431–2441.

Nambu, Y., Sugai, M., Gonda, H., Lee, C. G., Katakai, T., Agata, Y., Yokota, Y., and Shimizu, A. (2003). Transcription-coupled events associating with immunoglobulin switch region chromatin. *Science* **302,** 2137–2140.

Odegard, V. H., and Schatz, D. G. (2006). Targeting of somatic hypermutation. *Nat. Rev. Immunol.* **6,** 573–583.

Odegard, V. H., Kim, S. T., Anderson, S. M., Shlomchik, M. J., and Schatz, D. G. (2005). Histone modifications associated with somatic hypermutation. *Immunity* **23,** 101–110.

Okazaki, I. M., Hiai, H., Kakazu, N., Yamada, S., Muramatsu, M., Kinoshita, K., and Honjo, T. (2003). Constitutive expression of AID leads to tumorigenesis. *J. Exp. Med.* **197,** 1173–1181.

Opi, S., Takeuchi, H., Kao, S., Khan, M. A., Miyagi, E., Goila-Gaur, R., Iwatani, Y., Levin, J. G., and Strebel, K. (2006). Monomeric APOBEC3G is catalytically active and has antiviral activity. *J. Virol.* **80,** 4673–4682.

Parak, F. (2003). Physical aspects of protein dynamics. *Rep. Prog. Phys.* **66,** 103–129.

Pasqualucci, L., Kitaura, Y., Gu, H., and Dalla-Favera, R. (2006). PKA-mediated phosphorylation regulates the function of activation-induced deaminase (AID) in B cells. *Proc. Natl. Acad. Sci. USA* **103,** 395–400.

Patten, P. A., Gray, N. S., Yang, P. L., Marks, C. B., Wedemayer, G. J., Boniface, J. J., Stevens, R. C., and Schultz, P. G. (1996). The immunological evolution of catalysis. *Science* **271,** 1086–1091.

Pauling, L. (1946). Molecular architecture and biological reactions. *Chem. Eng. News* **24,** 1375–1377.

Petersen-Mahrt, S. K., Harris, R. S., and Neuberger, M. S. (2002). AID mutates *E. coli* suggesting a DNA deamination mechanism for antibody diversification. *Nature* **418,** 99–103.

Pham, P., Bransteitter, R., Petruska, J., and Goodman, M. F. (2003). Processive AID-catalysed cytosine deamination on single-stranded DNA simulates somatic hypermutation. *Nature* **424,** 103–107.

Pham, P., Bransteitter, R., and Goodman, M. F. (2005). Reward versus risk: DNA cytidine deaminases triggering immunity and disease. *Biochemistry* **44,** 2703–2715.

Pham, P., Chelico, L., and Goodman, M. F. (2007). DNA deaminases AID and APOBEC3G act processively on single-stranded DNA. *DNA Repair* (in press).

Poltoratsky, V., Goodman, M. F., and Scharff, M. D. (2000). Error prone candidates vie for somatic mutation. *J. Exp. Med.* **192,** F27–F30.

Procknow, C., Bronsteitter, R., Klien, M. G., Goodman, M. F., and Chen, X. S. (2007). The APOBEC-2 crystal structure and functional implications for the deaminase AID. *Nature* **445,** 447–451.

Rada, C., and Milstein, C. (2001). The intrinsic hypermutability of antibody heavy and light chain genes decays exponentially. *EMBO J.* **20,** 4570–4576.

Rada, C., Di Noia, J. M., and Neuberger, M. S. (2004). Mismatch recognition and uracil excision provide complementary paths to both Ig switching and the A/T-focused phase of somatic mutation. *Mol. Cell* **16,** 163–171.

Rajewsky, K. (1996). Clonal selection and learning in the antibody system. *Nature* **381,** 751–758.

Ramiro, A. R., Nussenzweig, M. C., and Nussenzweig, A. (2006). Switching on chromosomal translocations. *Cancer Res.* **66,** 7837–7839.

Reina-San-Martin, B., Difilippantonio, S., Hanitsch, L., Masilamani, R. F., Nussenzweig, A., and Nussenzweig, M. C. (2003). H2AX is required for recombination between immunoglobulin switch regions but not for intra-switch region recombination or somatic hypermutation. *J. Exp. Med.* **197,** 1767–1778.

Revy, P., Muto, T., Levy, Y., Geissmann, F., Plebani, A., Sanal, O., Catalan, N., Forveille, M., Dufourcq-Labelouse, R., Gennery, A., Tezcan, I., Ersoy, F., *et al.* (2000). Activation-induced cytidine deaminase (AID) deficiency causes the autosomal recessive form of the Hyper-IgM syndrome (HIGM2). *Cell* **102,** 565–575.

Reynaud, C. A., Aoufouchi, S., Faili, A., and Weill, J. C. (2003). What role for AID: Mutator, or assembler of the immunoglobulin mutasome. *Nat. Immunol.* **4,** 631–638.

Rini, J. M., Schulze-Gahmen, U., and Wilson, I. A. (1992). Structural evidence for induced fit as a mechanism for antibody-antigen recognition. *Science* **255,** 959–965.

Rogozin, I. B., and Diaz, M. (2004). Cutting edge: DGYW/WRCH is a better predictor of mutability at G:C bases in Ig hypermutation than the widely accepted RGYW/WRCY motif and probably reflects a two-step activation-induced cytidine deaminase-triggered process. *J. Immunol.* **172,** 3382–3384.

Rogozin, I. B., Pavlov, Y. I., Bebenek, K., Matsuda, T., and Kunkel, T. A. (2001). Somatic mutation hotspots correlate with DNA polymerase eta error spectrum. *Nat. Immunol.* **2,** 530–536.

Romesberg, F. E., Spiller, B., Schultz, P. G., and Stevens, R. C. (1998). Immunological origins of binding and catalysis in a Diels-Alderase antibody. *Science* **279,** 1929–1933.

Ronai, D., Iglesias-Ussel, M. D., Fan, M., Shulman, M. J., and Scharff, M. D. (2005). Complex regulation of somatic hypermutation by cis-acting sequences in the endogenous IgH gene in hybridoma cells. *Proc. Natl. Acad. Sci. USA* **102,** 11829–11834.

Rush, J. S., Fugmann, S. D., and Schatz, D. G. (2004). Staggered AID-dependent DNA double strand breaks are the predominant DNA lesions targeted to S mu in Ig class switch recombination. *Int. Immunol.* **16,** 549–557.

Schrader, C. E., Linehan, E. K., Mochegova, S. N., Woodland, R. T., and Stavnezer, J. (2005). Inducible DNA breaks in Ig S regions are dependent on AID and UNG. *J. Exp. Med.* **202,** 561–568.

Shapiro, G. S., Aviszus, K., Murphy, J., and Wysocki, L. J. (2002). Evolution of Ig DNA Sequence to target specific base positions within codons for somatic hypermutation. *J. Immunol.* **168,** 2302–2306.

Shen, H. M., and Storb, U. (2004). Activation-induced cytidine deaminase (AID) can target both DNA strands when the DNA is supercoiled. *Proc. Natl. Acad. Sci. USA* **101,** 12997–13002.

Shinkura, R., Ito, S., Begum, N. A., Nagaoka, H., Muramatsu, M., Kinoshita, K., Sakakibara, Y., Hijikata, H., and Honjo, T. (2004). Separate domains of AID are required for somatic hypermutation and class-switch recombination. *Nat. Immunol.* **5,** 707–712.

Silverstein, A. M. (2001). Autoimmunity versus horror autotoxicus: The struggle for recognition. *Nat. Immunol.* **2,** 279–281.

Sohail, A., Klapacz, J., Samaranayake, M., Ullah, A., and Bhagwat, A. S. (2003). Human activation-induced cytidine deaminase causes transcription-dependent, strand-biased C to U deaminations. *Nucleic Acids Res.* **31,** 2990–2994.

Souroujon, M., White-Scharf, M. E., Andre-Schwartz, J., Gefter, M. L., and Schwartz, R. S. (1988). Preferential autoantibody reactiviy of the preimmune B-cell repertoire in normal mice. *J. Immunol.* **140,** 4173–4179.

Stanfield, R. L., Fieser, T. M., Lerner, R. A., and Wilson, I. A. (1990). Crystal structures of an antibody to a peptide and its complex with peptide antigen at 2.8 Å. *Science* **248,** 712–719.

Stavnezer, J. (1996). Antibody class switching. *Adv. Immunol.* **61,** 79–146.

Sundberg, E. J., and Mariuzza, R. A. (2003). Molecular recognition in antibody-antigen complexes. *Adv. Protein Chem.* **61,** 119–160.

Suspene, R., Rusniok, C., Vartanian, J. P., and Wain-Hobson, S. (2006). Twin gradients in APOBEC3 edited HIV-1 DNA reflect the dynamics of lentiviral replication. *Nucleic Acids Res.* **34,** 4677–4684.

Tumas-Brundage, K., Vora, K. A., Giusti, A. M., and Manser, T. (1996). Characterization of the cis-acting elements required for somatic hypermutation of murine antibody V genes using conventional transgenic and transgene homologous recombination approaches. *Semin. Immunol.* **8,** 141–150.

Wagner, S. D., Milstein, C., and Neuberger, M. S. (1995). Codon bias targets mutation. *Nature* **376,** 732.

Wang, C. L., Harper, R. A., and Wabl, M. (2004). Genome-wide somatic hypermutation. *Proc. Natl. Acad. Sci. USA* **101,** 7352–7356.

Wang, J., Shinkura, R., Muramatsu, M., Nagaoka, H., Kinoshita, K., and Honjo, T. (2006a). Identification of a specific domain required for dimerization of activation-induced cytidine deaminase. *J. Biol. Chem.* **281,** 19115–19123.

Wang, L., Whang, N., Wuerffel, R., and Kenter, A. L. (2006b). AID-dependent histone acetylation is detected in immunoglobulin S regions. *J. Exp. Med.* **203,** 215–226.

Wedemayer, G. J., Patten, P. A., Wang, L. H., Schultz, P. G., and Stevens, R. C. (1997). Structural insights into the evolution of an antibody combining site. *Science* **276,** 1665–1669.

Whitlow, M., Howard, A. J., Wood, J. F., Voss, E. W., Jr., and Hardman, K. D. (1995). 1.85 Å structure of anti-fluorescein 4-4-20 Fab. *Prot. Eng.* **8,** 749–761.

Wiens, G. D., Roberts, V. A., Whitcomb, E. A., O'Hare, T., Stenzel-Poore, M. P., and Rittenberg, M. B. (1998). Harmful somatic mutations: Lessons from the dark side. *Immunol. Rev.* **162,** 197–209.

Woo, C. J., Martin, A., and Scharff, M. D. (2003). Induction of somatic hypermutation is associated with modifications in immunoglobulin variable region chromatin. *Immunity* **19,** 479–489.

Yin, J., Mundorff, E. C., Yang, P. L., Wendt, K. U., Hanway, D., Stevens, R. C., and Schultz, P. G. (2001). A comparative analysis of the immunological evolution of antibody 28B4. *Biochemistry* **40,** 10764–10773.

Yoshikawa, K., Okazaki, I. M., Eto, T., Kinoshita, K., Muramatsu, M., Nagaoka, H., and Honjo, T. (2002). AID enzyme-induced hypermutation in an actively transcribed gene in fibroblasts. *Science* **296,** 2033–2036.

Yu, Q., Konig, R., Pillai, S., Chiles, K., Kearney, M., Palmer, S., Richman, D., Coffin, J. M., and Landau, N. R. (2004). Single-strand specificity of APOBEC3G accounts for minus-strand deamination of the HIV genome. *Nat. Struct. Mol. Biol.* **11,** 435–442.

Zaccai, G. (2000). How soft is a protein a protein dynamic force constant measured by neutron scattering. *Science* **288,** 1604–1607.

Zimmermann, J., Oakman, E. L., Thorpe, I., Shi, X., Abbyad, P., Brooks, I. C., Boxer, S. A., and Romesberg, F. E. (2006). Antibody evolution constrains conformational heterogeneity by tailoring protein dynamics. *Proc. Natl. Acad. Sci. USA* **103,** 13722–13727.

Evolution of the Immunoglobulin Heavy Chain Class Switch Recombination Mechanism

Jayanta Chaudhuri,[¶,1] Uttiya Basu,[*,†,‡,1] Ali Zarrin,[*,†,‡] Catherine Yan,[*,†,‡] Sonia Franco,[*,†,‡] Thomas Perlot,[*,†,‡] Bao Vuong,[¶] Jing Wang,[*,†,‡] Ryan T. Phan,[*,†,‡] Abhishek Datta,[*,†,‡] John Manis,[§] and Frederick W. Alt[*,†,‡]

*The Howard Hughes Medical Institute, The Children's Hospital, Harvard Medical School, Boston, Massachusetts
†The CBR Institute for Biomedical Research, Harvard Medical School, Boston, Massachusetts
‡Department of Genetics, Harvard Medical School, Boston, Massachusetts
§Joint Program in Transfusin Medicine, Department of Pathology, Children's Hospital, Harvard Medical School, Boston, Massachusetts
¶Immunology Program, Memorial Sloan Kettering Cancer Center, New York, New York

Abstract 157
1. Overview of Genetic Alterations in B Lymphocytes 158
2. Activation-Induced Cytidine Deaminase 162
3. Role of Germ Line Transcription and Switch Regions in CSR 169
4. Posttranscriptional Regulation of AID 180
5. Mechanisms Involved in Synapsis of AID Initiated DSBs in Widely
   Separated S Regions 184
6. General DNA Repair Systems in the Joining Phase of CSR 189
7. Evolution of CSR 197
   References 198

Abstract

To mount an optimum immune response, mature B lymphocytes can change the class of expressed antibody from IgM to IgG, IgA, or IgE through a recombination/deletion process termed immunoglobulin heavy chain (IgH) class switch recombination (CSR). CSR requires the activation-induced cytidine deaminase (AID), which has been shown to employ single-stranded DNA as a substrate in vitro. IgH CSR occurs within and requires large, repetitive sequences, termed S regions, which are parts of germ line transcription units (termed "C_H genes") that are composed of promoters, S regions, and individual IgH constant region exons. CSR requires and is directed by germ line transcription of participating C_H genes prior to CSR. AID deamination of cytidines in S regions appears to lead to S region double-stranded breaks (DSBs) required to initiate CSR. Joining of two broken S regions to complete CSR exploits the activities of general DNA DSB repair mechanisms. In this chapter, we discuss our current knowledge of the function of S regions, germ line transcription,

[1]These authors contributed equally.

AID, and DNA repair in CSR. We present a model for CSR in which transcription through S regions provides DNA substrates on which AID can generate DSB-inducing lesions. We also discuss how phosphorylation of AID may mediate interactions with cofactors that facilitate access to transcribed S regions during CSR and transcribed variable regions during the related process of somatic hypermutation (SHM). Finally, in the context of this CSR model, we further discuss current findings that suggest synapsis and joining of S region DSBs during CSR have evolved to exploit general mechanisms that function to join widely separated chromosomal DSBs.

1. Overview of Genetic Alterations in B Lymphocytes

B lymphocytes are critical components of the mammalian immune system as they can generate antibodies against almost any foreign pathogen. This enormous diversity is achieved by the unique ability of a B cell (and a T cell) to somatically modify its genome. Somatic diversification of immunoglobulin genes in B cells occurs in several developmental stages and involves three distinct processes. First, developing B cells in fetal liver and adult bone marrow assemble the variable regions of the immunoglobulin heavy (IgH) and light (IgL) chain genes from component variable (V), diversity (D), and joining (J) gene segments by the process of V(D)J recombination. This site-directed recombination reaction is initiated by the lymphoid-specific RAG-1 and RAG-2 endonuclease and completed by components of the nonhomologous end-joining (NHEJ) machinery (Dudley *et al.*, 2005; Jung and Alt, 2004; Jung *et al.*, 2006; Schatz and Spanopoulou, 2005). Productive V(D)J recombination at the IgH locus leads to the generation of a transcription unit in which the complete variable region exon lies upstream of a series of Cμ heavy chain (HC) constant region exons. Processing of the resulting primary transcripts generates a mature mRNA that encodes the V(D)J-Cμ protein known as a μHC (Fig. 1). The μHC pairs with a κ or λ light chain (LC) synthesized from a productively recombined κ or λ locus to form an IgM molecule, which leads to the generation of a surface IgM$^+$ B cells. The mature IgM$^+$ B cell then migrates to the secondary lymphoid organs such as the spleen and lymph nodes, where it may encounter a cognate antigen and be activated to undergo two additional diversification reactions, namely IgH class switch recombination (CSR) (Chaudhuri and Alt, 2004; Dudley *et al.*, 2005; Honjo *et al.*, 2002; Kenter, 2005; Maizels, 2005; Manis *et al.*, 2002b; Min and Selsing, 2005; Stavnezer, 1996) and somatic hypermutation (SHM) (Goodman *et al.*, 2007; Li *et al.*, 2004; Martomo and Gearhart, 2006; Neuberger *et al.*, 2005; Papavasiliou and Schatz, 2002a).

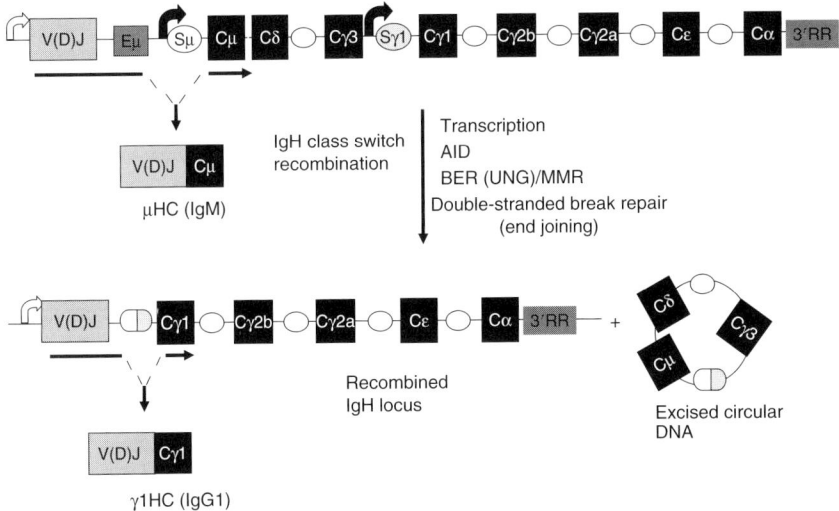

Figure 1 IgH CSR. The assembled V(D)J variable region segment together with Cμ (or Cδ) exons constitutes a transcription unit (arrows depict promoters) which synthesizes a μHC that pairs with a κ or λ LC to generate an IgM-expressing mature B cell. On encountering antigens in the peripheral lymphoid compartments, B cells undergo IgH class switching. CSR replaces Cμ with one of the downstream C_H genes so that a new antibody isotype (IgG1 is shown) can be expressed. CSR occurs between repetitive S region sequences (ovals) that precede each C_H gene and requires transcription, AID and components of several DNA repair pathways including BER, MMR, end-joining, and general DNA DSB response proteins. UNG, a component of BER plays an essential role in CSR downstream of AID activity. The IgH enhancers Eμ and 3′ regulatory region (3′RR) are shown. The 3′ regulatory region is represented as 3′RR. See text for more details.

CSR is a process that, within a clonal B-cell lineage, allows the assembled V(D)J exon to be expressed first with Cμ exons and then with one of several sets of downstream C_H exons (referred to as C_H genes) (Honjo and Kataoka, 1978). Thus, CSR allows production of different IgH isotypes or antibody classes (e.g., IgG, IgE, and IgA), which are determined by the different IgH constant region genes (e.g., Cγ, Cε, and Cα), with maintenance of the same variable region antigen-binding specificity. The C_H region of the HC molecule determines the effector function of the antibody molecule, for example where the antibody goes in the body or what types of downstream antigen elimination pathways are activated once cognate antigen is bound (Chaudhuri and Alt, 2004; Honjo et al., 2002). The mouse IgH locus consists of eight C_H genes (Chaudhuri and Alt, 2004; Honjo and Kataoka, 1978; Stavnezer, 1996), each of which is preceded by long switch (S) regions. Unrearranged C_H genes are also organized into germ line transcription units in which transcription is initiated from a promoter lying upstream of individual S regions (see below). CSR is a deletional recombination event that occurs via the introduction of DNA double-stranded breaks (DSBs) into two participating S regions followed by joining of the broken S regions to each other accompanied by deletion of all of the intervening sequences, including the various C_H genes (Cory and Adams, 1980; Iwasato et al., 1990; Matsuoka et al., 1990; von Schwedler et al., 1990). Thus, CSR juxtaposes the expressed V(D)J exon to a new, downstream C_H gene (Fig. 1).

We have learned that the initiation of the normal CSR process has several required components, including S regions, transcription through the participating S regions, and activation-induced cytidine deaminase (AID) (Chaudhuri and Alt, 2004; Honjo et al., 2002) (Fig. 2). The functions of each of these components will be discussed in detail below. In our current model for the initiation of CSR, germ line transcription is required to allow AID to access targeted S regions and, thereby, to generate lesions that are ultimately turned into DSBs. This model for CSR also suggests that once DSBs are generated in two S regions, that, at least in large part, they are synapsed (e.g., brought

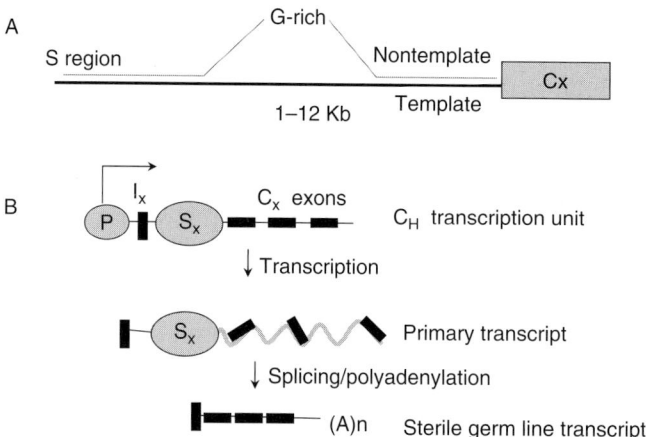

Figure 2 Basic requirements for the initiation of IgH CSR. (A) Switch regions are characterized by repetitive DNA sequences with a G-rich nontemplate strand. (B) C_H genes are transcription units with transcription initiating from a cytokine-inducible promoter (P) upstream of an I exon. The primary transcript undergoes splicing to remove the S region (S_x) and is polyadenylated, but the mature product, referred to as germ line transcript, does not encode a protein. (C) The activated B-cell-specific protein AID is essential for CSR and somatic hypermutation as outlined in the text.

together over large distances) and joined by general DNA repair processes with the actual joining employing forms of general cellular DNA end-joining and DNA repair pathways (Zarrin et al., 2007). We will also discuss briefly the synapsis and joining pathways employed for CSR.

The mechanism by which CSR is initiated is intimately related to that of SHM, and, as we discuss later, CSR well may have evolved from SHM. For comparison to CSR in this chapter, we provide here only a very brief introduction to SHM. More detailed discussions of SHM can be found elsewhere (Goodman et al., 2007; Li et al., 2004; Neuberger et al., 2005; Odegard and Schatz, 2006). SHM introduces point mutations, and sometimes, small insertions and deletions, at a very high rate ($\sim 10^{-3}$ to 10^{-4} per bp per generation) into the variable region exons of both IgH and IgL genes to allow selection of B cells that generate mutated variable regions that have increased affinity for antigen (Crews et al., 1981; Griffiths et al., 1984; McKean et al., 1984; Rajewsky, 1996; Sablitzky et al., 1985). SHM can occur throughout the assembled variable region exon; however, a majority of the mutations are focused to the so-called RGYW "hot spot" sequence (where R = purine, Y = pyrimidine, and W = A or T nucleotide) (Rogozin and Diaz, 2004; Rogozin and Kolchanov, 1992). While other nomenclature is used, for example the RGYW complementary sequence WRCY or the subset WRC (Goodman et al., 2007; Pham et al., 2003; Yu et al., 2004), we will use RGYW as a generic term to cover all SHM hot spot motifs.

RGYW motifs are particularly abundant in the complementarity determining regions of IgH and IgL variable region genes that encode the antigen-binding domains (Wagner et al., 1995). SHM requires AID and transcription through the assembled variable region exons, with mutations being observed from 100 to 200 bp from the promoter and extending 1.5- to 2-kb downstream of it, sparing the constant regions (Gearhart and Bogenhagen, 1983; Lebecque and Gearhart, 1990; Pech et al., 1981; Rada et al., 1994; Rothenfluh et al., 1995; Winter et al., 1997). In transgenic SHM substrate studies, variable region exons or their promoters could be replaced with various other sequences (Michael et al., 2002; Peters and Storb, 1996; Tumas-Brundage and Manser, 1997; Yelamos et al., 1995) and non-Ig promoters (Betz et al., 1994; Tumas-Brundage and Manser, 1997), respectively, without markedly affecting the mutability of the sequence, indicating that the primary sequence of the V genes are not unique in ability to target the SHM machinery. SHM can also function to varying degrees on certain non-Ig genes (Gordon et al., 2003; Muschen et al., 2000; Muto et al., 2006; Pasqualucci et al., 1998, 2001; Shen et al., 1998). At this time, the precise sequence requirements and *cis*-acting elements that target SHM *in vivo* have not been defined fully. Potential factors that influence targeting of SHM have been discussed elsewhere (Odegard and

Schatz, 2006; Yang, 2007) and will be covered only in part here, mainly in the context of the topic of factors that help target AID activity in CSR.

2. Activation-Induced Cytidine Deaminase

The discovery of AID represented a huge advance in our understanding of mechanisms of immunoglobulin gene diversification (Muramatsu et al., 1999, 2000). AID was discovered in a subtractive hybridization screen for genes that are upregulated in a B-cell line (CH12-F3) undergoing CSR (Muramatsu et al., 1999). AID is a 24-kDa protein expressed almost exclusively in activated B cells (Muramatsu et al., 1999). Targeted deletion of AID in mice or mutations of the gene in hyper IgM patients led to a complete block in both CSR and SHM (Muramatsu et al., 2000; Revy et al., 2000). While the function of AID in CSR and SHM is a subject of debate (see below), the most widely accepted view is that AID functions as a single-stranded (ss)-specific DNA deaminase that catalyzes the deamination of cytidine residues in transcribed S regions and V genes during CSR and SHM, respectively (see below; Goodman et al., 2007). In this regard, biochemical data indicates that efficient deamination of chromosomal DNA by AID may rely, at least in part, on structural features of transcribed double-stranded (ds) DNA substrates that allow them to form ssDNA structures or on additional factors that interact with AID to promote its access to transcribed dsDNA substrates (Chaudhuri et al., 2004; see below). The deaminated DNA then appears to be processed by components of several DNA repair pathways, that for CSR lead to the generation of DSBs required to initiate CSR. In chicken B cells, AID also is required to initiate the gene conversion process that is involved in diversifying assembled Ig variable region genes in this species (Arakawa et al., 2002; Harris et al., 2002b; Yang, 2007).

2.1. AID Is the Major Specific Factor for CSR and SHM

In addition to being absolutely required for initiation of CSR and SHM, ectopic AID expression in nonlymphoid cells promoted CSR and SHM of artificial substrates, indicating that AID is also sufficient to induce these processes in nonlymphoid cells (Martin et al., 2002; Okazaki et al., 2002, 2003; Wang et al., 2004; Yoshikawa et al., 2002). However, in these studies, the rate of CSR was low, the spectrum of SHM was limited (primarily transition mutations at G:C bases), and there was no target or region specificity, as several transcribed genes were found to be mutated independent of chromosomal location. Thus, while current studies clearly identify AID as the key factor for B-cell-specific initiation of CSR and SHM, reminiscent of the key role of the RAG endonuclease in initiating V(D)J recombination in developing lymphocytes (Jung et al., 2006), the possibility remains that other B-cell-specific factors, yet to be identified, may still function to mediate efficiency and specificity of CSR and SHM in vivo.

2.2. AID Is Required Upstream of DNA Lesions

Several studies suggested that AID is required for the generation of DNA lesions in S regions. First, foci of phosphorylated histone H2AX (γH2AX), which normally form around chromosomal DNA DSBs (Rogakou et al., 1998), were observed around S regions in an AID-dependent fashion (Petersen et al., 2001). Second, DSBs detected by ligation-mediated PCR (LM-PCR) in S regions of B cells undergoing CSR (Wuerffel et al., 1997) were found to be AID dependent (Catalan et al., 2003; Schrader et al., 2005). In addition, S region somatic mutations, which may be related to AID function in initiation of CSR, are abrogated in AID-deficient mice (Nagaoka et al., 2002; Petersen et al., 2001). Also internal deletions of S regions, that most likely reflect joining of DSBs on individual S regions during CSR (see below), are largely AID dependent (Dudley et al., 2002). We note, however, that LM-PCR assays were reported to detect AID-independent DNA breaks in V genes leading to the suggestion that AID may have functions downstream of DSBs (Bross and Jacobs, 2003; Papavasiliou and Schatz, 2002b; Zan et al., 2003); however, it is not clear that these DSBs actually represent lesions directly related to SHM (Faili et al., 2002). Thus, the generally accepted view is that AID is required upstream of the cleavage reaction in CSR.

2.3. DNA Deamination Versus Putative RNA Editing Activities of AID

The role of AID in generating DNA lesions in S regions has been a subject of intense debate and significant controversy. Early on, both DNA and RNA were proposed to be potential substrates of AID with respect to SHM and CSR (Martin et al., 2002; Muramatsu et al., 2000; Neuberger and Scott, 2000; Petersen-Mahrt et al., 2002; Tian and Alt, 2000a). Here, we will discuss current evidence in support of each model. Evidence argued to support an RNA editing model for AID activity will be presented first and is covered in more detail elsewhere (Muramatsu et al., 2007). Subsequently, evidence in support of the DNA deamination model will be presented along with a critical evaluation of data that has been proposed to argue against the DNA deamination model.

2.4. The RNA Editing Hypothesis

There are two major lines of evidence that have been used to argue for the hypothesis that AID effects CSR via RNA editing. The original line of evidence for RNA editing was based on the homology of AID to an RNA editing cytidine deaminase APOBEC1 (Muramatsu et al., 1999). In this regard, AID was proposed to edit a cellular mRNA to generate a new mRNA that encodes a novel endonuclease required to activate CSR and SHM (Muramatsu et al., 2000). This proposal was later extended to include the proposal that there are specific SHM and CSR mRNA targets of AID, based on observations that certain mutations in AID block CSR but not SHM and vice versa (Shinkura et al., 2004; Ta et al., 2003). Thus, it was argued that AID could associate with particular proteins so that the resulting complex edits one mRNA that encodes a factor required for SHM and another mRNA that encodes a factor required for CSR (Honjo et al., 2005). To date, however, no SHM or CSR-specific AID cofactor or mRNA substrates have been identified. Moreover, it is now clear that APOBEC1 is a fairly recent evolutionary arrival and is apparently derived from AID. The only other descendants of AID whose function is known are the APOBEC3 family, members of which deaminate the DNA of retroviral replication intermediates (Conticello et al., 2007; Gourzi et al., 2006; Petersen-Mahrt, 2005; Rosenberg and Papavasiliou, 2007).

A second line of evidence that has been argued to support the RNA editing hypothesis versus a DNA deamination model of AID activity was based on the observation that *de novo* protein synthesis is required for generation of AID-dependent binding of γH2AX to the IgH S regions in activated B cells (Begum et al., 2004b) and for CSR (Doi et al., 2003). However, an alternative explanation of these findings, that would not be inconsistent with the DNA deamination model, is that CSR requires highly labile proteins that function downstream of deamination to generate DSBs.

Thus, the RNA-editing model is still based largely on a presumed analogy with APOBEC1 function, without direct evidence in its support. In particular, no biochemical RNA editing activity has been described for AID. However, it is conceivable that if AID does indeed edit a particular RNA, the specific RNA sequence and/or specific cofactors would be required to demonstrate the editing activity. Finally, to date, no one has found any edited mRNA sequences that encode the putative SHM and CSR lesion-generating enzymes.

2.5. The DNA Deamination Model for AID Function

The DNA deamination model forms the basis for much of our current thinking and understanding of how AID initiates the CSR and SHM reactions. Thus, the basic tenets of this proposal, as put forward by Neuberger and colleagues for

SHM and CSR (Petersen-Mahrt et al., 2002), are outlined below. There is also a significant body of data that relates the AID deamination models to potential functions of AID in initiating gene conversion as a mechanism to diversify chicken variable region genes that is discussed in detail elsewhere (Arakawa et al., 2002; Harris et al., 2002b; Yamazoe et al., 2004; Yang, 2007).

It has been proposed that AID functions in SHM to convert dC to dU in variable region exons (Petersen-Mahrt et al., 2002). Subsequently, during DNA replication, dU is read as dT by DNA polymerase, resulting in transition mutations that change dC:dG base pairs to dA/dT base pairs. In addition, dU in DNA can be converted into an abasic site by removal of uracil base by uracil DNA glycosylase (UNG), an isoform of which, UNG2, is expressed highly in proliferating B cells (Kavli et al., 2005). This reaction is normally an early step in the repair of mismatches by the base excision repair (BER) pathway. However, if UNG activity, instead, is directly followed by replication across the abasic site, then any of the four nucleotides could be inserted, thereby leading to both transition (purine to purine, pyrimidine to pyrimidine) and transversion (purine to pyrimidine and vice versa) mutations at dC:dG bases. Finally, the mismatch repair (MMR) pathway also could process the dU:dG mismatch. The Msh2/Msh6 mismatch recognition complex, and its associated proteins such as Pms2/Mlh1 and exonuclease 1 (EXO1), can introduce nicks or single-stranded gaps distal to the initial site of deamination (Li et al., 2004). Subsequently, gap-filling by recruited error-prone polymerases, such as polymerase eta (Wilson et al., 2005), could lead to additional mutations. Thus, AID-mediated DNA deamination of dCs, followed by activities of UNG and MMR proteins, theoretically can explain the entire spectrum of mutations observed during SHM *in vivo* (Petersen-Mahrt et al., 2002).

For CSR, the DNA deamination model predicts that UNG activity followed by activity of the apurinic/apyrimidinic endonuclease (APE1), another normal BER component, will create a nick in S region DNA (Petersen-Mahrt et al., 2002). Two closely spaced nicks on opposite strands of S regions could then lead to a DNA DSB. In addition, gaps and nicks created by MMR proteins as described for SHM, if overlapping on opposite strands of S region DNA, could also lead to DSBs in S regions (Chaudhuri and Alt, 2004; Li et al., 2004; Min and Selsing, 2005). More details about the role of S regions as substrates for generating multiple AID-initiated DSBs required for CSR will be discussed below. However, we note that several key aspects of the DNA deamination model as applied to CSR remain to be elucidated, in particular, the mechanism by which AID-initiated lesions are turned into DSBs rather than just being repaired by the BER or MMR pathways (see below). A very intriguing question is why these lesions are turned into mutations in variable region exons during SHM and DSBs (as well as mutations) in S regions during CSR. One simple possibility may be just the increased density of AID target motifs in S regions versus variable regions (Chaudhuri and Alt, 2004); while another, not mutually exclusive, possibility could be the existence of specific cofactors that might direct one process versus the other (Barreto et al., 2003; Shinkura et al., 2004; Ta et al., 2003). Evidence relevant to consideration of the DNA deamination model of AID function is discussed in the next section.

2.6. Experimental Findings Relevant to Consideration of the DNA Deamination Model for AID Function

2.6.1. AID Mutates DNA in Bacteria

The first evidence in support of the DNA deamination model was based on the observation that enforced expression of AID in *Escherichia coli*, which is not expected to harbor an mRNA substrate for AID, led to mutations of several bacterial genes (Petersen-Mahrt et al., 2002; Ramiro et al., 2003). It is to be noted, however, that DNA deamination activity appears to be a function of all polynucleotide cytidine deaminases, as other members of this family, including APOBEC3 and even APOBEC1, had similar mutagenic activities in bacteria (Harris et al., 2002a). Still, the finding that AID can mutate DNA in bacteria (Petersen-Mahrt et al., 2002) provided the impetus to test and prove whether AID indeed functions by deaminating DNA during CSR and SHM. Below, we describe the various experimental approaches employed to test predictions of the DNA deamination model and also discuss results that have been presented in the context of challenging some of the interpretations of these findings.

2.6.2. AID Is an ssDNA-Specific Cytidine Deaminase In Vitro

Biochemical assays, using either recombinant or purified B-cell AID, showed that AID efficiently deaminates dC to dU on ssDNA but not ds DNA (Branstetter et al., 2003; Chaudhuri et al., 2003, 2004; Dickerson et al., 2003; Pham et al., 2003; Sohail et al., 2003; Yu et al., 2004). More details about biochemical analyses of AID activity in relationship to transcription of dsDNA substrates will be discussed below and elsewhere (Goodman et al., 2007). Notably, RGYW SHM hot spot motifs served as preferred sites for deamination *in vitro* (Chaudhuri et al., 2004; Pham et al., 2003; Yu et al., 2004). Therefore, the *in vitro* biochemical activity of AID provides a striking recapitulation of the *in vivo* targets for SHM and CSR. In this regard, in addition to variable region exons, mammalian S regions and *Xenopus* S regions, the latter of which unlike mammalian S regions cannot form R-loop structures that are AID targets (see below), are very rich in RGWY sequences (Zarrin et al., 2004). Thus, the matching pattern of biochemical activity of AID with its *in vivo* SHM and CSR target sequence preferences provides very strong support that AID directly works on DNA substrates *in vivo*. The alternative RNA editing view would need to make the cumbersome argument that AID edits two different transcripts to generate two different DNA-modifying enzymes with the same general DNA substrate specificity as found, by biochemical analyses, for AID itself.

2.6.3. Binding of AID to S Regions

When overexpressed as a tagged protein in B cells, AID was found to specifically localize to Sγ and Sε regions via chromatin immunoprecipitation (ChIP) assays performed with B cells activated for CSR (Nambu *et al.*, 2003). The association of AID with S regions strongly supported the notion that AID functions directly on DNA. However, this conclusion was questioned by another study that argued tagged AID did not go to the Sμ region based on ChIP analyses of activated B cells (Begum *et al.*, 2004a). However, subsequent studies, in which ChIP experiments were carried out on the authentic endogenous AID protein in primary B cells activated for CSR, revealed a clear and definitive correlation between activation-dependent transcriptional activation of specific C_H genes and AID binding to the appropriate downstream regions (Chaudhuri *et al.*, 2004), confirming the earlier findings with the tagged AID proteins (Nambu *et al.*, 2003). Thus, in splenic B cells activated with lipopolysaccarides (LPS) (that directs CSR to IgG2b, see below), AID associated primarily with Sγ2b as opposed to Sγ1, while in B cells activated with LPS + interleukin 4 (IL-4) (that promote CSR to IgG1, see below), AID was bound primarily to Sγ1 as opposed to Sγ2b. In studies of the normal cellular AID protein, binding of AID to Sμ was also clearly observed (Chaudhuri and Alt, unpublished observations). Thus, the association of AID with appropriate CSR target sequences in activated B cells strongly supports the notion that AID acts directly on DNA *in vivo*.

2.6.4. UNG/MMR Mutations Alter the Spectrum of SHM and Severely Impair CSR

Genetic studies have provided very strong support for the DNA deamination model. Inhibition or mutation of UNG in chickens, mice, and humans leads to a pronounced skewing of SHM to transitions at dC (Di Noia and Neuberger, 2002; Imai *et al.*, 2003; Rada *et al.*, 2002b; see also, Durandy *et al.*, 2007), as would be expected if most of the mutations incorporated are due to replication at dU. Furthermore, UNG deficiency led to a severe block in CSR in mice and humans (Imai *et al.*, 2003; Rada *et al.*, 2002b). Moreover, the majority of residual

CSR activity in UNG-deficient mice could be eliminated in UNG/Msh2-double-deficient B cells, indicating that both UNG-related and MMR pathways contribute to CSR (Rada et al., 2004). In addition, in the double mutant, SHM was primarily restricted to transition mutations at dG:dC base pairs as one would predict if all mutations are generated due to replication at dG:dU bases (Rada et al., 2004). It is very difficult to explain the skewing of the SHM pattern and the severe block in CSR without invoking the presence of dU in DNA. This evidence provided very strong support for the DNA deamination model. In this regard, the unrelated uracil-excision enzyme SMUG1 can restore CSR to UNG-deficient B cells (Di Noia et al., 2006) suggesting that the CSR defect caused by UNG deficiency somehow results from a failure to recognize/excise uracil rather than some speculative nonuracil-related function of UNG.

2.6.5. Studies That Have Challenged the Proposed Function of UNG in CSR

Several studies have challenged the proposed role of UNG in CSR. First, using accumulation of γH2AX as a marker for DSBs, it was shown that inhibition of UNG (using a specific inhibitor Ugi) did not impair DNA cleavage at the IgH locus in B cells undergoing CSR (Begum et al., 2004a). Second, UNG mutants that had apparently lost their U-removal activity rescued CSR in UNG-deficient B cells (Begum et al., 2004a). Finally, B-cell hybridomas derived from UNG-deficient or UNG/Msh2-double-deficient mice revealed similar levels of internal deletions in Sμ (a marker for AID-dependent DSBs in S regions, see below) as observed in wild-type B-cell hybridomas (Begum et al., 2006). These observations led to the proposal that the U-removal activity of UNG is dispensable for the generation of the DSBs in S regions. Instead, UNG was proposed to participate in an as yet undefined step in CSR downstream of DNA DSBs (Begum et al., 2004a). Since one of the basic tenets of DNA deamination model proposes UNG-mediated removal of AID-created dU residues prior to DSBs, the above results were interpreted as requiring a reevaluation of the DNA model (Honjo et al., 2005). However, even if this interesting hypothesis that UNG has a novel function downstream of DSBs was proven correct, it would not directly argue against the DNA deamination model for CSR. Moreover, there are several alternative interpretations of these findings outlined in this paragraph that do not invoke a completely novel role of UNG in CSR.

It is possible that UNG inhibition does lead to decreased DSBs in S regions; however, the decrease may not be readily apparent in an indirect DSB assay such as accumulation of γH2AX molecules. In this regard, a single DSB can cause the nucleation of γH2AX over megabases of DNA (Rogakou et al., 1999).

Indeed, a more direct LM-PCR assay revealed significantly reduced S region DSBs in UNG-deficient B cells from human patients and mice (Imai et al., 2003; Schrader et al., 2005). Another explanation offered for the finding of catalytically impaired UNG mutants that support CSR is that they still bind DNA dU-DNA and, in this way, may lead to a replication block severe enough to force resolution via MMR pathway (Lee et al., 2004a). It has also been argued that the UNG catalytic mutants analyzed may have low levels of residual U-removal activity (Stivers, 2004). Thus, overexpression of such hypomorphic mutants in the retroviral transduction experiments (Begum et al., 2004a) might result in sufficient UNG activity to restore CSR in UNG-deficient B cells. Another apparent set of contradictory findings involved a human UNG mutant that is severely defective in supporting CSR in a patient (Imai et al., 2003) but which was found to complement the CSR defect of UNG-deficient mouse B cells (Begum et al., 2004a). However, this difference appears to be explained by differential degradation of this mutant AID in human cells versus when overexpressed in UNG-deficient mouse cells (Durandy et al., 2007; Kavli et al., 2005). Also the observed internal deletions within Sµ in UNG or UNG/Msh2-deficient B cells might be explained by accumulation of AID-mediated deaminated residues in the mutant B cells that are channeled into DSBs and deletions on fusion via expression of UNG and/or Msh2 that is present in the hybridoma fusion partner.

2.7. AID Function: Conclusions

There is strong, direct genetic, and biochemical data to support the proposal that AID-mediated DNA deamination is an obligatory step in CSR and SHM. On the other hand, support for an RNA-based model essentially rests on drawing a parallel with apolipoprotein B RNA editing by APOBEC1. Thus, given the compelling body of evidence that supports AID function in CSR via DNA deamination, we will only focus on this working model of AID function in the remaining chapter.

3. Role of Germ Line Transcription and Switch Regions in CSR

3.1. Overview

Most current evidence supports the model that transcription through S regions provides DNA structures that allows AID to initiate CSR on genomic dsDNA. Here, we will review the current evidence that bears on the potential functions that S regions serve in the CSR along with a summary of findings that implicated a role for transcription in regulating and mechanistically targeting CSR.

Then, we will discuss our current understanding about how transcription of S regions makes them accessible to the CSR initiating activities of AID.

3.2. Organization of the IgH C_H Locus

The mouse IgH locus consists of eight sets of C_H exons that are arranged as 5'VDJ-Cµ-Cδ-Cγ3-Cγ1-Cγ2b-Cγ2a-Cε-Cα (Chaudhuri and Alt, 2004; Stavnezer, 1996) (Fig. 1). Each set of C_H exons (except Cδ) is preceded by a 1- to 10-kb long switch (S) regions that are composed of repetitive sequences. In mammals, S regions are unusually G-rich on the template strand and are primarily composed of tandem repetitive sequences within which certain motifs, such as TGGGG, GGGGT, GGGCT, GAGCT, and AGCT, predominate (Davis et al., 1980; Dunnick et al., 1980; Kataoka et al., 1981; Nikaido et al., 1982; Obata et al., 1981; Sakano et al., 1980; Takahashi et al., 1980) (Fig. 2A). The length and the distribution of the individual repetitive sequences vary among different S regions. Sµ is exceptionally high in the degree of repetitiveness and enriched in the GAGCT motifs, with the short AGCT palindrome representing the canonical form of the RGYW motif. Sγ1, at about 10 kb, is the largest S region. The Sγ1 sequence, like other Sγ sequences, carries multiple repeats of a characteristic 49-bp unit that among other features is also rich in RGYW (including AGCT) motifs (Obata et al., 1981). Notably, S regions precede all C_H genes that undergo CSR, although in some species the S region sequences can be quite divergent (see below). In addition, the vast majority of CSR junctions occur within (and occasionally just beyond) the S regions (Dunnick et al., 1993; Kinoshita et al., 1999). Thus, it has been reasonably assumed for decades that S regions are the main targets of CSR.

3.3. S Region Function in CSR

Formal proof for the role of S regions in CSR came from gene targeted mutation and replacement experiments. Thus, deletion of the majority of Sµ led to a severe block in CSR to all downstream C_H genes (Khamlichi et al., 2004; Luby et al., 2001). Likewise, deletion of Sγ1 led to a nearly complete block in CSR to IgG1 but left CSR to other downstream C_H genes intact (Shinkura et al., 2003). In addition, at least for the Sγ1, there is a direct correlation between length of the Sγ1 49-bp repeat sequence and its ability to promote CSR, as shown by replacing endogenous Sγ1 with varying lengths of the core Sγ1 49-bp repeat units (Zarrin et al., 2005). As CSR to IgG1 is the most frequent form of CSR in mice and Sγ1 is by far the longest S region, the observed correlation between repetitive S region length and CSR frequency may imply that S region length, at least in part, may have evolved to modulate CSR frequency (Zarrin et al., 2005). Finally, it must be noted that the decrease in CSR associated with S region deletions or truncations does not prove a specific role for S region sequences per se in CSR, as it remained possible that any sufficiently long spacer sequence would be sufficient. However, additional gene replacement studies showed that non-S region sequences that lacked unusual characteristics of S regions (e.g., repeat structure, G/C rich structure, and so on) did not support CSR, strongly supporting the notion that S region structure, and not just having a certain length of intronic sequence flanking C_H genes, is important for mediating CSR (Shinkura et al., 2003; Zarrin et al., 2005). Together, these experiments provide compelling evidence that S region sequences evolved to serve as specialized targets for the CSR.

3.4. The Role of Germ Line C_H Gene Transcription in Targeting CSR

The germ line C_H genes (except $C\delta$) are organized into characteristic transcription units (Fig. 2) whose induction directly correlates with CSR potential of the associated S region (Manis et al., 2002b). Germ line transcripts that were considered "sterile" because they did not encode any detectable protein were first noted to occur for Abelson murine leukemia virus (A-MuLV) transformed pre-B cells that had an inherent capacity to switch from μ to $\gamma 2b$ expression in culture; the transcripts also were considered to be germ line based on the fact that they lacked V_H sequences and "sterile" in that they did not encode proteins that cross-reacted with anti-$\gamma 2b$ antibodies (Alt et al., 1982a,b; Yancopoulos et al., 1986). Similarly, a B-cell lymphoma line (I.29) was found to transcribe several C_H genes, again in an apparently germ line fashion, prior to CSR (Stavnezer-Nordgren and Sirlin, 1986). The transcription of germ line C_H regions in cell lines that were predisposed to switch to those IgH isotypes led to the proposal that germ line transcription of particular C_H genes rendered them "accessible" for CSR (Stavnezer-Nordgren and Sirlin, 1986; Stavnezer et al., 1988; Yancopoulos et al., 1986). This suggested mechanism of control was analogous to that previously suggested for differential control of Ig and TCR gene V(D)J recombination via accessibility to a common V(D)J recombinase (Yancopoulos and Alt, 1985, 1986). As we will discuss, this accessibility mechanism for controlling CSR has been born out by studies of AID function and we now know far more about how transcription of germ line C_H genes renders them accessible for AID function and CSR than we do about how germ line V, D, and J segments become accessible to the RAG endonuclease and V(D)J recombination.

Cloning and sequencing of a "germ line" transcript of the $C\mu$ gene provided the first structure of a germ line C_H transcript (Lennon and Perry, 1985).

The Cμ transcript was found to be initiated from the intronic enhancer region between J_H and Cμ and the primary transcript was spliced to generate a "mature" transcript in which a novel noncoding exon was attached to the Cμ exons. This transcript did not have any open reading frames that could encode a Cμ-containing protein, agreeing with the notion that it was sterile (Lennon and Perry, 1985). Subsequently, cloning and sequencing of a germ line Cγ2b transcript derived from an A-MuLV transformant and comparing it to the structure of the genomic region encompassing the corresponding genomic sequences revealed a similar structure to that of the germ line Cμ transcript (Lutzker and Alt, 1988). Subsequent studies of other germ line C_H transcripts in mice and humans showed that all of the downstream C_H genes were organized into similar transcription units (Manis et al., 2002b; Stavnezer, 2000) (Fig. 2B). In particular, germ line C_H transcripts are initiated from a promoter that lies just upstream of a noncoding 5' exon referred to as an "intervening" or I exon (Lutzker and Alt, 1988), proceed through the S region sequence, and are terminated/polyadenylated downstream at normal positions downstream of the C_H exons. The primary C_H transcripts undergo splicing which fuses the I exon to the C_H exons and removes intronic sequences including S regions. However, the processed germ line transcripts are "sterile" because they lack an open reading frame and fail to encode any detectable protein (Manis et al., 2002b). The inability of the germ line C_H transcripts to encode proteins and the correlation of their expression with CSR potential provided the first support for the notion that they might function mechanistically to target CSR (discussed further below).

Treatment of B cells with various combinations of activators and cytokines induces them to switch to particular IgH isotypes (Snapper et al., 1988b). For example, treatment of splenic B cells with bacterial LPS induces switching to IgG2b (and IgG3) (Kearney and Lawton, 1975); while also treating LPS-stimulated splenic B cells with IL-4 inhibits switching to IgG2b and induces switching to IgG1 and IgE (Calvert et al., 1983; Kearney et al., 1976; Snapper et al., 1988a). In this regard, studies of normal LPS or LPS + IL-4 treated splenic B cells showed that germ line transcription through the Sγ2b and Cγ2b sequences was induced prior to actual CSR recombination to Sγ2b; while treatment of normal splenic B cells with LPS + IL-4 inhibited induction of γ2b germ line transcription and CSR to γ2b, while promoting germ line transcription of and CSR to Cγ1 and Cε (Lutzker and Alt, 1988; Rothman et al., 1988; Stavnezer et al., 1988). Similar findings were made for other C_H genes and/or cytokines (Esser and Radbruch, 1989; Jabara et al., 1993; Kepron et al., 1989; Mandler et al., 1993; Severinson et al., 1990; Stavnezer, 1995), and subsequent studies showed that downstream germ line I region promoters had elements that allowed them to be specifically activated by particular cytokines

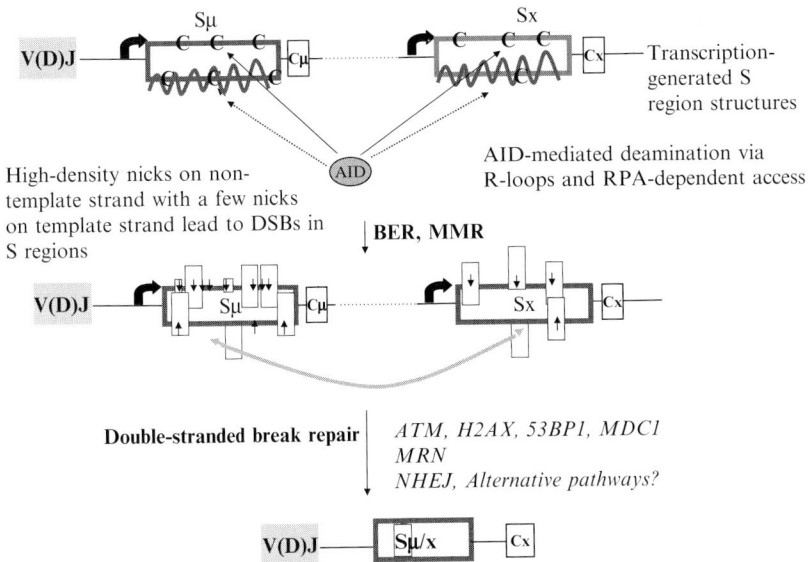

Figure 3 Overall model for CSR. Transcription through S regions generates higher-order RNA–DNA structures, including R-loops, that probably allow both RPA-dependent and -independent access to the nontemplate strand of S regions. The activities of BER and MMR proteins convert the deaminated residues into nicks, and closely spaced nicks on opposite strands of DNA are converted into DSBs. The mechanism that allows AID deamination on the template strand is not well understood, but it is possible that a high density of breaks on the nontemplate strand coupled with a few breaks on the bottom strand is sufficient to generate DSBs. The DSBs between Sμ and a downstream S region are synapsed, probably by components of the general DSB response pathway, including ATM, the Mre11/Nbs1/Rad50 (MRN) complex, 53BP1, and MDC1. Subsequently, the DNA breaks are ligated, by the NHEJ or other alternative pathways discussed in the text. See text for more details.

(Manis *et al.*, 2002b; Stavnezer, 2000). Of note, the germ line Cμ transcripts appear constitutive and not specifically responsive to any form of B-cell activation or cytokine, perhaps in accord with the fact that Sμ is the donor in all types of CSR to downstream C_H genes (Li *et al.*, 1994). Therefore, these studies provided strong support that induction of germ line transcription through particular C_H genes was somehow linked to determining accessibility for CSR in response to normal physiological stimuli (Figs. 1 and 3). Finally, while not discussed further here, the conserved structural organization and splicing patterns of all germ line C_H units also suggest the possibility that transcripts themselves or splicing *per se* may have some role in the CSR process, a possibility with some experimental support (Lorenz *et al.*, 1995) but which mechanistically has remained unclear.

Direct evidence for the mechanistic requirement for germ line transcription in CSR came from gene-targeting studies. Deletion of I exon promoters severely impaired CSR to the corresponding IgH isotypes (Jung et al., 1993; Lorenz et al., 1995; Zhang et al., 1993). Moreover, replacement of I exon promoters with heterologous constitutive promoters activated CSR to particular C_H genes under conditions where CSR to that C_H gene would not normally be induced (Bottaro et al., 1994; Jung et al., 1993; Kuzin et al., 2000; Lorenz et al., 1995; Qiu et al., 1999; Seidl et al., 1998; Zhang et al., 1993); these studies provided the most direct evidence that germ line transcription per se and not just elements deleted with the germ line promoters somehow targeted CSR. Finally, other studies showed that the integrity of elements at the 3′ end of the IgH locus, referred to as the 3′IγH regulatory region (Fig. 1; reviewed in Birshtein et al., 1997), were necessary for the induction of germ line transcription from the various downstream C_H genes (Cogne et al., 1994; Pinaud et al., 2001) and led to a "promoter" competition models to, in part, explain how different stimulatory treatments could turn off as well as turn on different germ line promoters and, as a result, CSR to particular C_H genes (Cogne et al., 1994; Manis et al., 2002b). Together, these studies also led to the notion that induction of germ line transcription through S regions might somehow be directly mechanistically involved in targeting the CSR process and not just a correlate of S region "accessibility." In contrast, it is commonly thought that germ line V segment transcription may not be required for V(D)J recombinational accessibility (Cobb et al., 2006; Jung et al., 2006; Sen and Oltz, 2006).

3.5. Mechanisms by Which Transcription Through S Regions Promotes CSR

The role of germ line transcription was a subject of intense speculation. Transcription was proposed to be required for several nonmutually exclusive steps in CSR, including modifying chromatin configuration (Stavnezer-Nordgren and Sirlin, 1986), providing accessibility to enzymes required for CSR (Stavnezer et al., 1988; Yancopoulos et al., 1986), or generating DNA structures that allow access to a CSR recombinase (Daniels and Lieber, 1995b; Lutzker et al., 1988; Reaban et al., 1994; Stavnezer et al., 1988; Tian and Alt, 2000b). While none of these proposed mechanisms are mutually exclusive, it now appears that transcription through S regions functions, at least in large part, to provide AID access chromosomal S regions during CSR.

3.5.1. R-Loops

As mentioned above, mammalian S regions consist of 1- to 12-kb-long DNA sequences that are characterized by a G-rich nontemplate strand and the presence of repeat sequences that, in the mouse, can vary in length between

5 bp (Sμ) and 80 bp (Sα). By virtue of the G-richness of the nontemplate strand, transcription through S regions leads to the generation of higher order DNA structures in which the transcribed RNA stably hybridizes to the template strand (Daniels and Lieber, 1995a, 1996; Mizuta et al., 2003; Reaban and Griffin, 1990; Reaban et al., 1994; Tian and Alt, 2000b). More detailed studies showed that the transcription of mammalian S regions *in vitro* leads to the generation of stable R-loops in which the nascent transcript hybridizes to the template strand and displaces the nontemplate strand as an ssDNA loop (Tian and Alt, 2000b; Yu et al., 2003) (Figs. 2 and 3). Moreover, stable R-loops have also been shown to form on transcription of S regions *in vivo* (Yu et al., 2003). The looped-out nontemplate strand can also assume additional structures such as stem-loops from the abundant palindromic repeats (Tashiro et al., 2001) or can form G4 DNA in which four DNA strands associate via Hoogsteen bonding between planar arrays of G-residues (Dempsey et al., 1999; Larson et al., 2005; Sen and Gilbert, 1988).

Genetic support that R-loops may influence CSR came from the observation that inversion of the endogenous 12-kb Sγ1 inhibited R-loop formation *in vitro* and was accompanied by a significant decrease (to 25% of WT levels) in CSR to IgG1 in activated mutant B cells *in vivo* (Shinkura et al., 2003). Furthermore, a 1-kb synthetic G-rich sequence that could form R-loops when transcribed *in vitro*, but which had no S region motifs, could replace Sγ1 to mediate CSR to IgG1, albeit at significantly lower levels than the 12-kb full length Sγ1 sequence (Shinkura et al., 2003). Strikingly, the ability of the synthetic sequence, like the endogenous Sγ1 sequence, to mediate CSR was orientation dependent, with CSR observed only in the orientation that favored R-loop formation (G-rich on the nontemplate strand) (Shinkura et al., 2003).

AID is an ssDNA deaminase with no activity on dsDNA (Bransteitter et al., 2003; Chaudhuri et al., 2003; Dickerson et al., 2003; Sohail et al., 2003). As most DNA in cells is in a duplex form, the mechanism by which AID can gain efficient access to dsDNA *in vivo* has also been a topic of considerable interest. The observation that transcribed S regions display ssDNA substrates in the context of R-loops, both *in vivo* and *in vitro* (Tian and Alt, 2000b; Yu et al., 2003), suggested that AID could potentially gain access to S region DNA via such structures. The finding that purified AID efficiently deaminates ssDNA, but not dsDNA, *in vitro* also supports the proposed function for R-loops in the context of CSR. Moreover, purified AID did not deaminate T7 *in vitro* transcribed dsDNA sequences (such as V_H genes) that do not form R-loops but did efficiently deaminate nontemplate strands of an *in vitro* transcribed dsDNA substrates, including S regions, that could form R-loops (Chaudhuri et al., 2003). In agreement with the proposed function of the R-loop, the *in vitro* studies showed that AID only efficiently deaminated the transcribed dsDNA when it was transcribed in the R-loop forming but not in the reverse, non-R-loop forming orientation (Chaudhuri et al., 2003). Thus, these findings suggested that mammalian S regions may have evolved the capability to generate R-loops on transcription as one means of optimizing AID access to double-stranded chromosomal S region DNA and provided the first clear mechanistic link between S regions, germ line transcription, and AID activity in the context of CSR (Chaudhuri et al., 2003, 2004). Yet, these findings did not explain how AID accesses variable region exons, during SHM, since transcribed variable region exons are not predicted to and were not found experimentally to form R-loops. Additional studies of this issue revealed that AID access to S regions also likely employs additional mechanisms beyond R-loop formation (Fig. 3) as outlined below.

3.5.2. RPA Functions as a Cofactor to Allow AID to Access Certain Transcribed dsDNA Sequences That Do Not Form R-Loops

The R-loop mechanism does not provide an explanation as to how AID gains access to transcribed variable regions during SHM, which are not G-rich on their nontranscribed strand and which do not have a clear-cut propensity to form R-loops. To determine if cofactors could allow AID deamination of substrates that do not form R-loops, an *in vitro* assay was established that measured AID-mediated deamination of transcribed synthetic dsDNA substrates that consisted of repeated RGYW motifs (Chaudhuri et al., 2004). Such substrates do not form R-loops when transcribed *in vitro*. These studies identified the trimeric, ssDNA-binding protein, RPA, as a potential cofactor that allowed AID to efficiently deaminate transcribed DNA, including the RGYW synthetic sequences and several tested variable region exons (Chaudhuri et al., 2004) (Fig. 4). In this context, RPA interacts with AID purified from B cells via its 32-kDa subunit (the trimeric RPA complex consists of 17-, 32-, and 70-kDa subunits) and the AID/RPA complex, but not the two proteins separately, binds well to transcribed RGYW containing DNA *in vitro*, and leads to deaminations that occur near the known SHM hot spot motifs (Chaudhuri et al., 2004). As AID preferentially deaminates RGYW sequences *in vitro* (Pham et al., 2003; Yu et al., 2004), and RPA can bind to ssDNA bubbles as small as four nucleotides (Matsunaga et al., 1996), the AID/RPA complex was proposed to bind to and stabilizes ssDNA in the context of transcription bubbles, thus providing ssDNA substrate for AID-mediated deamination (Chaudhuri et al., 2004) (Fig. 4).

While both AID and Ig gene SHM are found in bony fish, CSR is first observed evolutionarily in amphibians including *Xenopus*, suggesting that CSR evolved after SHM (Mussmann et al., 1997; Stavnezer and Amemiya, 2004). Notably, the S regions of *Xenopus* are long, repetitive sequences that are

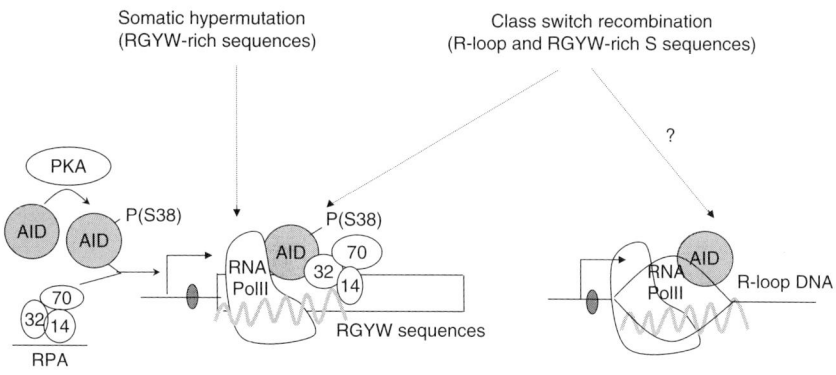

Figure 4 Model for access of AID to DNA during SHM and CSR. Phosphorylation of AID on Ser38 (P-Ser38) by PKA allows interaction with the 32-kDa subunit of the ssDNA-binding protein RPA. The AID/RPA complex can bind to and stabilize ssDNA in the context of small transcription bubbles of transcribed RGYW containing SHM substrates, allowing AID-mediated DNA deamination. Deamination of ssDNA in R-loops formed on transcription of S regions during CSR is probably RPA independent. However, S regions are also rich in RGYW sequences and RPA-dependent AID deamination could provide an additional mechanism to target S regions during CSR. See text for more details.

actually A/T rich and would not be predicted to form R-loops on transcription, a prediction that was confirmed by *in vitro* transcription studies (Zarrin *et al.*, 2004). The fact that *Xenopus* S regions are not R-loop forming structures raised the possibility that either amphibian AID gained access to transcribed dsDNA S region targets by a different mechanism than mammalian AID or that there were other mechanisms that can target AID, even to mammalian S regions. The latter possibility gained further support from the finding that the inverted Sγ1 sequences, that do not form readily detectable R-loops on transcription, possess residual CSR activity *in vivo*. Strikingly, the A/T rich *Xenopus* Sμ region was able to replace mouse Sγ1 to promote substantial CSR to IgG1 in mouse B cells *in vivo* (Zarrin *et al.*, 2004). Analysis of CSR junctions showed that *Xenopus* Sμ-mediated CSR in mice occurred primarily within AGCT sequences (a subset of the RGYW motif) that are present at a high density in the 3′ portion of the *Xenopus* Sμ employed and that when this sequence was inverted *in vivo*, CSR junctions tracked with the AGCT motifs (Zarrin *et al.*, 2004). Notably, the dense AGCT motifs within the *Xenopus* Sμ were also the preferred sites of deamination by the AID/RPA complex when this sequence was transcribed *in vitro*, regardless of orientation (Zarrin *et al.*, 2004).

These findings support the notion that CSR activities of AID may have evolved from SHM functions of AID (Barreto et al., 2005a; Wakae et al., 2006), the latter of which may rely in part on ability of AID to access sequences rich in transcribed SHM motifs in the context of a complex with RPA (Fig. 4; see below). In this regard, the RGYW SHM motifs may also serve as primordial motifs for the targeting of AID/RPA during CSR (Zarrin et al., 2004). Moreover, because mammalian S regions are particularly rich in RGYW sequences, these motifs are likely to have a role for AID targeting during CSR in mammals (see below; Fig. 3).

3.6. Open Questions Regarding AID Access to Transcribed dsDNA

3.6.1. Template Versus Nontemplate Strand Activities

The generation of DSBs in S regions calls for AID activity on both the nontemplate and the template strand of DNA, as has been observed (Xue et al., 2006). The issue of AID targeting both DNA strands is also pertinent for SHM where mutations occur on both DNA strands. Neither AID nor the AID/RPA complex (see below) deaminated the template strand of transcribed substrates *in vitro* (Chaudhuri et al., 2003, 2004; Pham et al., 2003; Ramiro et al., 2003), thereby raising the question as to how deamination of both strands is achieved *in vivo*. For CSR, if a high density of nicks were generated on the nontemplate strand, only a few nicks would need to be generated on the template strand to make DSBs (Chaudhuri and Alt, 2004). In the context of an R-loop mechanism, AID might act on the ssDNA exposed at the transition between duplex DNA and the R-loop structure or RNaseH-mediated collapse of R-loop structures could lead to missalignment of repeats on opposite strands, resulting in ssDNA loops on both DNA strands (Yu and Lieber, 2003). Another possibility, for both SHM and CSR, is that there are other, as yet undefined, factors that allow AID to target both strands of transcribed DNA. It is also possible that bidirectional transcription through V genes or S regions could serve to target both strands. In this context, antisense transcription through rearranged variable region exons and S regions has been observed in naive and activated B cells from wild-type mice and in B-cell lines (Perlot and Alt, unpublished observations; Ronai et al., 2007). Finally, it has been proposed that AID itself can target both DNA strands either in the context of supercoiled DNA (in the absence of transcription) (Shen and Storb, 2004) or in the context of transcription with *E. coli*. RNA polymerase (Besmer et al., 2006). In the latter context, it is conceivable that transcription by mammalian RNA polymerase may generate access to AID or the AID/RPA complex differently that what is found for the T7 RNA polymerase used in prior studies.

3.6.2. Targeting of AID Activity

A matter of continued debate is the mechanism that allows specific targeting of AID to the Ig locus during CSR and SHM (Barreto *et al.*, 2005b; Chaudhuri and Alt, 2004; Li *et al.*, 2004; Longerich *et al.*, 2006; Odegard and Schatz, 2006). The specificity of AID on S regions could potentially be explained by the uniqueness of S region sequence that predispose them to form higher order structures that could be targeted by AID (Chaudhuri *et al.*, 2003). The targeting of V genes during SHM, however, does not appear to rely on specialized structures, as the V genes could be replaced with non-Ig genes in the context of transgenic SHM passenger gene substrates without obvious effect on mutation rate (Betz *et al.*, 1994; Tumas-Brundage and Manser, 1997). Of all the transcribed genes analyzed in a B cell, the V genes and only a very small number of non-Ig genes (BCL6, CD95, mb1, B29) have been found to be mutated (Gordon *et al.*, 2003; Pasqualucci *et al.*, 1998; Peng *et al.*, 1999; Shen *et al.*, 1998, 2000; Yang, 2007). Other non-Ig genes that do undergo mutations, for example the proto-oncogenes cMYC, RHO/TTF, and PIM1 (Gaidano *et al.*, 2003; Montesinos-Rongen *et al.*, 2004; Pasqualucci *et al.*, 2001), probably represent misstargeted AID activity. Studies with ectopically expressed AID in transgenes have extended the range of genes and cell types in which AID was shown to function *in vivo* (Kotani *et al.*, 2005; Okazaki *et al.*, 2003).

What then allows AID to specifically target the Ig locus during SHM. It is possible that AID is recruited to the transcribing Ig locus via interaction with other protein(s) that interact specifically with *cis*-elements of the Ig locus. In this regard, transgenic studies on a rearranged Igκ locus suggested that two enhancers in the Igκ locus-iEκ (known as the intronic enhancer, located between Jκ5 and Cκ) and 3'Eκ (3' enhancers, located 9-kb 3' of Cκ) are required for SHM of a transgenic Igκ substrate (O'Brien *et al.*, 1987; Sharpe *et al.*, 1991). However, mutational studies of the enhancers in the endogenous locus gave somewhat different results as mice lacking 3'Ek (van der Stoep *et al.*, 1998) or iEk (Inlay *et al.*, 2006) individually did exhibit major alterations in the frequency of SHM, although more subtle differences were not ruled out. In addition, deletion of either the core Eμ enhancer or the 3'IgH enhancer does not appear to substantially impair SHM (Perlot *et al.*, 2005; Ronai *et al.*, 2005). In light of these findings, it will be necessary to further evaluate the putative roles of the enhancers in directing SHM and to assess whether there are additional endogenous elements that may have redundant activities (Odegard and Schatz, 2006). Overall, targeting of AID to the Ig locus could be due to a combination of several factors including transcription rate, presence of the *cis*-sequences in the DNA (such as transcription factor E2A-binding sites; Michael *et al.*, 2003), and the concentration of RGYW hot spot sequences. In the latter context, it has been shown that efficiency of deamination by the AID/RPA complex is proportional to the density of RGYW (or AGCT) sequences *in vitro* (Chaudhuri *et al.*, 2004) and possibly *in vivo* (Zarrin *et al.*, 2004).

Elucidating the mechanism of AID specificity is of utmost relevance to our understanding of the ontogeny of mature B-cell lymphomas. Overexpression of AID converts it into a general mutator (Martin *et al.*, 2002; Okazaki *et al.*, 2003; Yoshikawa *et al.*, 2002), and deregulated AID activity has been implicated in the ontogeny of mature B-cell lymphomas that form the most common lymphoid malignancies in humans. A large number of diffuse large B-cell lymphomas (DLBCLs) as well as AIDS-related non-Hodgkins lymphoma harbor multiple mutations in several proto-oncogenes including *BCL-6* and *cMYC*, with a mutation pattern reminiscent of that observed during SHM of V genes (Pasqualucci *et al.*, 2001). Such aberrant SHM possibly results from a loss of AID target specificity and could thus be a major contributing factor toward DLBCL pathogenesis. Furthermore, a direct role for AID in the generation of MYC-IgH translocations has been shown in murine models B-cell malignancies (Ramiro *et al.*, 2004, 2006; Unniraman *et al.*, 2004).

It is clear that AID activity has to be stringently harnessed to prevent its loss of specificity and it is, thus, not surprising that AID expression and activity is regulated at multiple levels. These include transcription (Muramatsu *et al.*, 1999) (i.e., AID is expressed only in activated B cells), intracellular localization (Rada *et al.*, 2002a) (i.e., AID is primarily found in the cytoplasm, although it acts on DNA in the nucleus), and now, as described in detail below, AID phosphorylation has emerged as a major mode of regulating AID activity (Basu *et al.*, 2005; Chaudhuri *et al.*, 2004; McBride *et al.*, 2006; Pasqualucci *et al.*, 2006). Finally, it must be remembered that a further level in which AID activity could be controlled is via repair of deaminated cytidines via normal BER or MMR activities, as opposed to further, apparently, aberrant processing of these residues to initiate SHM or CSR. Thus, a further form of control might involve channeling AID-induced lesions into a normal repair pathway versus a pathway that leads to mutations and DSBs (Di Noia *et al.*, 2006). In this regard, the potentially high level of the latter pathway in B cells might also reflect specific factors.

4. Posttranscriptional Regulation of AID

4.1. Nuclear Versus Cytoplasmic Localization

Multiple reports indicate that the majority of AID present in B cells is sequestered in the cytoplasm of B cells (Basu *et al.*, 2005; Pasqualucci *et al.*, 2004; Rada *et al.*, 2002a; Schrader *et al.*, 2005). Considering that AID directly deaminates DNA at the Ig locus, the cytoplasmic sequestration of AID may be a mechanism to harness its activity. In this regard, AID shuttling between the nucleus and the cytoplasm may be required for optimal regulation of CSR and SHM. AID possesses a defined nuclear localization signal (NLS) at its N-terminus, in addition to a nuclear export signal (NES) at its C-terminus (McBride et al., 2004). Mutation of either of these motifs leads to the abrogation of nucleocytoplasmic shuttling of AID (Barreto et al., 2003; McBride et al., 2004; Shinkura et al., 2004). Recent work also indicated that increased cellular AID levels in mouse B cells led to decreased CSR (Muto et al., 2006). How the cellular level of the AID protein would alter AID activity in CSR is unclear. Perhaps, higher cytoplasmic AID levels may inhibit AID nuclear entry. Notably, phosphorylated AID also appears to be preferentially present in the nucleus of B cells as opposed to the cytoplasm (Basu et al., 2005; McBride et al., 2006). Moreover, studies that employed an antibody that recognizes a major form of phosphorylated AID (see below) have shown that phosphorylated AID is enriched in the chromatin-bound AID fraction (McBride et al., 2006). Thus, phosphorylation-dependent interaction of AID with RPA may promote chromatin association of AID in B cells and, thereby, also contribute to its activity and nuclear localization.

4.2. AID Phosphorylation

Initial clues that AID may be phosphorylated were derived from *in vitro* deamination assays on transcribed SHM substrates (Chaudhuri et al., 2004). It was observed that while AID purified from B cells could efficiently deaminate transcribed dsDNA SHM substrates in an RPA-dependent fashion, AID isolated from ectopically expressing 293 cells could neither interact with RPA nor efficiently promote deamination of transcribed dsDNA *in vitro* (Chaudhuri et al., 2004). Metabolic labeling of activated splenic B cells with ^{32}P-orthophosphate revealed that AID is much more highly phosphorylated in activated B cells than in the line of 293 cells employed for these studies. Significantly, phosphatase treatment of B-cell AID led to a concomitant decrease in the ability of AID to mediate RPA-dependent deamination of transcribed SHM substrates, associated with a failure of dephosphorylated AID to interact with RPA (Chaudhuri et al., 2004).

Mass spectrometric studies revealed that a portion of AID purified from B cells is phosphorylated at two sites, Ser38 and Tyr184 (Basu et al., 2005; McBride et al., 2006). Notably, Ser38 in AID exists in the context of a cAMP-dependent protein kinase A (PKA) consensus motif. In this regard, AID can be phosphorylated *in vitro* by PKA at Ser38 and coexpression of PKA with AID in fibroblast cells led to phosphorylation of AID at Ser38 (Basu et al., 2005;

Pasqualucci et al., 2006). Nonphosphorylated AID that has been phosphorylated by PKA in vitro gains ability to bind RPA and mediate dsDNA deamination of transcribed SHM substrates (Basu et al., 2005). Notably, through use of an antibody that detects AID phosphorylated at Ser38, AID ectopically expressed in certain nonlymphoid cell lines was found to be phosphorylated to the same level as AID in activated B cells (McBride et al., 2006). The difference between this result and the lack of phosphorylation observed in 293 cells observed in an earlier study (Chaudhuri et al., 2004) most likely reflects cell type differences. As PKA is a ubiquitous kinase, it would not be surprising that there are cell type and growth condition variations that can alter its activity.

Mutation of AID(Ser38) to alanine AID(Ser38A) markedly decreased ability to phosphorylate AID in vitro by PKA and, correspondingly, impaired ability of AID to interact with RPA and mediate deamination of a transcribed SHM substrate in vitro (Basu et al., 2005). However, the Ser38A mutation had no observed effect on the ssDNA deamination activity of AID(Ser38A) in vitro, indicating that this mutation did not affect the basic catalytic activity of the AID protein. Significantly, AID(Ser38A), expressed from retroviral vectors, was markedly reduced (10–20% of wild-type levels) in ability to restore CSR activity to AID-deficient B cells stimulated to undergo CSR in culture (Basu et al., 2005; McBride et al., 2006; Pasqualucci et al., 2006), consistent with proposal that phosphorylation of AID at Ser38 plays an important role in allowing AID to function at optimal efficiency to effect CSR in vivo (Basu et al., 2005). Pharmacological inhibition of PKA in B cells also decreased CSR, whereas conditional deletion of the regulatory subunit of PKA, so as to constitutively activate PKA, led to increased CSR (Pasqualucci et al., 2006), providing additional in vivo evidence for the relevance of AID phosphorylation by PKA. Thus, work from multiple laboratories has strongly supported the model that AID phosphorylation is important for augmenting ability of AID to function in CSR, likely through an RPA-mediated mechanism for accessing transcribed S regions (Fig. 4).

In the types of retroviral transduction assays used to measure CSR activity of AID(Ser38A) mutants, expression of the transduced protein can significantly exceed wild-type levels in B cells (Ramiro et al., 2006). Thus, for hypomorphic mutants, such as AID(Ser38A) which retain baseline catalytic activity in CSR, sufficient overexpression could potentially mask the effect of mutations that just decrease the overall activity of the protein in the CSR process. For example, given that the Ser38A mutant AID retained full catalytic activity on ssDNA, residual CSR activity observed for the mutant protein within the retroviral transduction studies might reflect CSR occurring via a non-RPA-dependent (e.g., R-loop) mechanism (Basu et al., 2005; Longerich et al., 2006).

In this regard, one study, in contrast to the findings of others outlined above, reported that the AID(Ser38A) mutation had little effect on CSR in a similar retroviral overexpression assay (Wang et al., 2006). A potential explanation for this apparent discrepancy, supported by preliminary data (Basu et al., 2007), is that retroviral expression vectors employed for the latter study may have led to even higher levels of AID expression than those obtained in the other studies and generated "saturating" expression levels of this hypomorphic mutant. Finally, because AID may be expressed at levels greater than those of the endogenous AID protein in all of the reported retroviral overexpression type assays used to measure ability of the mutant proteins to affect CSR, it remains possible that integrity of the Ser38A residue may prove even more important than estimated. In this regard, the relative contribution of phosphorylation-independent versus phosphorylation-dependent mechanisms to CSR likely will be most accurately evaluated via knock-in approaches that would allow mutant protein expression to occur at normal physiological levels.

It is notable that AID of bony fish, which undergo SHM but not CSR, lacks a Ser38-equivalent PKA-phosphorylation site. Yet, expression of zebra fish AID (zAID) could substantially restore CSR to AID-deficient mouse B cells (Barreto et al., 2005a; Wakae et al., 2006). This intriguing observation opened up several possibilities, including (1) zAID does not require RPA interaction or phosphorylation at a Ser38-equivalent site to efficiently catalyze CSR; (2) zAID acts via RPA, but through phosphorylation at a different amino acid; and (3) zAID acts via RPA, but through a phosphorylation-independent pathway. In the latter context, it was speculated that a D44 residue in zAID might act as constitutive mimic of a phosphorylation site that allows constitutive RPA interaction (Basu et al., 2005). Indeed, preliminary studies suggest that zAID interacts constitutively with RPA and constitutively catalyzes transcription-dependent dsDNA deamination *in vitro*, with both activities being dependent on integrity of the D44 site (Basu and Alt, unpublished). In this regard, it will be of interest to determine whether mutation of D44 to an alanine impairs ability of zAID to mediate IgH CSR in B cells. If so, phosphorylation may have evolved in higher vertebrates as a means to regulate AID activity.

The potential role of AID phosphorylation in SHM also was assessed by a similar retroviral transduction approach (McBride et al., 2006). In these studies, AID(Ser38A) had significantly reduced capacity to mediate SHM on both physiological (Sμ in B cells) and artificial substrates (in fibroblasts) as compared to wild-type AID. On the basis of the biochemical studies, it seems quite possible that the strong effect of the Ser38A mutation on SHM may also be due to an inability of AID to access its targets, possibility due to a failure to bind RPA. Indeed, AID phosphorylated on Ser38 was highly enriched in the chromatin fraction (McBride et al., 2006). As for CSR, a more complete assessment of the potential influence of AID(Ser38A) mutation on SHM of endogenous V genes awaits the generation of B cells with a knock-in mutation.

5. Mechanisms Involved in Synapsis of AID Initiated DSBs in Widely Separated S Regions

5.1. Overview

The completion phase of CSR requires the close juxtaposition of DSBs in two S regions, referred to as synapsis, followed by their ligation. The mechanism that synapses DSBs in S regions, that exists as far as 200 kb apart, is only beginning to be understood. Germ line V, D, and J segments are flanked by short conserved recombination signal sequences (RSs) that are targets for the RAG endonuclease (Jung *et al.*, 2006). During V(D)J recombination in progenitor lymphocytes, an RAG complex binds RS sequences of two participating V, D, or J segments and introduces DSBs between the RSs and the flanking coding sequences. Such RAG cleavage occurs only in the context of a preformed synaptic complex (Jung *et al.*, 2006). Thus, it is thought that RAG itself may be involved in synapsis of V, D, and J segments for V(D)J recombination (Jung *et al.*, 2006). Subsequent to cleavage, V, D, and J DSBs are joined by the NHEJ pathway of DNA DSB repair (Bassing *et al.*, 2002b; Rooney *et al.*, 2004), and RAG appears to be involved in shepherding broken V, D, and J segments specifically into the NHEJ pathway (Lee *et al.*, 2004b). By analogy, it seemed possible that AID and/or S regions may play specific roles in the synapsis and joining processes of CSR. However, as we discuss below, recent work suggests that mechanisms of S region synapsis and joining may predominantly exploit general cellular mechanisms and, at least in part, not rely on AID or S regions *per se*.

5.2. CSR Versus Internal S Region Deletions as Mechanisms to Resolve S Region DSBs

In contrast to RAG activity on V, D, and J segments, AID activity on S regions does not require coordinate interaction between two S regions, as AID can deaminate single S regions *in vitro* (Chaudhuri *et al.*, 2004). Moreover, constitutively transcribed S regions randomly integrated into the genome of a pro-B-cell line undergo high rate of AID-dependent internal deletions (Dudley *et al.*, 2002). In this regard, internal deletions in S regions have been extensively used in the interpretation of data related to synapsis. Internal deletions are readily observed in the endogenous Sμ region in splenic B cells or B-cell lines activated in culture to undergo CSR (Alt *et al.*, 1982a; Dudley *et al.*, 2002; Gu *et al.*, 1993; Yancopoulos *et al.*, 1986). Such internal deletions are thought to reflect joining of two DSBs within Sμ regions, perhaps in the absence of, or synapsis with, a DSB in a downstream S region (Dudley et al., 2002) (Fig. 5). In addition, Sμ also undergoes mutations at a high rate, again possibly reflecting AID activity on S regions independent of CSR (Nagaoka et al., 2002; Petersen et al., 2001). Given that S region mutations and internal deletions are AID dependent (Dudley et al., 2002; Nagaoka et al., 2002; Petersen et al., 2001; Schrader et al., 2005), they probably represent the same general process as CSR, although this has never been formally proven.

While internal deletions in Sμ can be readily detected, those in the downstream S regions are observed less frequently (Dudley et al., 2002; Reina-San-Martin et al., 2003, 2004, 2007; Schrader et al., 2003). One possible explanation for this observation is that Sμ may be a preferred AID substrate due to its sequence and/or proximity to the strong IgH intronic enhancer Eμ, with targeting of AID to downstream S regions constituting the rate-limiting step of CSR. In this scenario, Sμ would be the target of a higher level of DSBs, with some occurring simultaneously, than occurs in downstream S regions. Thus, a significant proportion of simultaneous Sμ breaks may be resolved via short-range intra-S recombinations leading to internal deletions (Fig. 5). This possibility

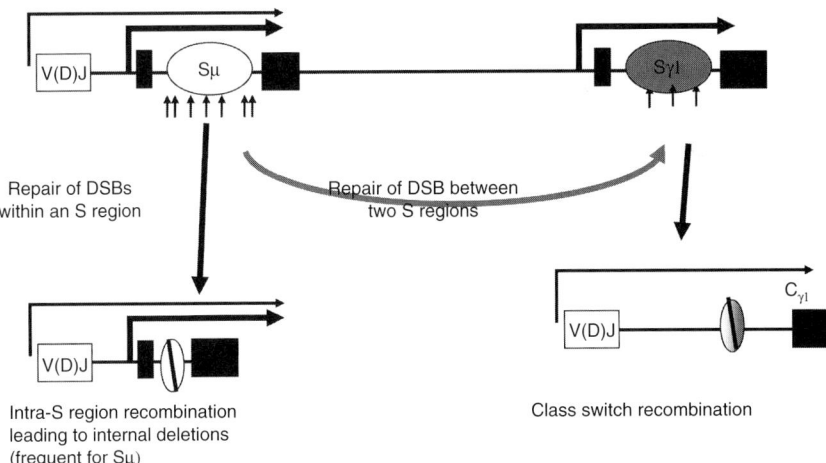

Figure 5 Internal Sμ deletions versus long-range CSR. In addition to productive CSR by long-range DSB repair between two distal S regions, B cells stimulated to undergo CSR also undergo a high rate of internal deletions in Sμ. Such intra-S recombination probably represents resolution of two DSBs (arrows) within Sμ. CSR represents resolution of two DSBs in different S regions. While internal deletions are readily observed in Sμ, those in the downstream S regions are less frequent, possible reasons for which are discussed in the text. See text for more details.

is consistent with the observation that when Sµ was inhibited from being a donor, internal deletions in Sγ1 could be readily detected (Gu et al., 1993). However, it must be acknowledged that there are other possible explanations for the appearance of increased internal Sµ deletions versus downstream S region deletions, including different efficiencies or mechanisms (e.g., internal deletion versus simple rejoining) of repair of one versus the other. In the latter context, only deletions visible via Southern blotting have generally been assayed in prior studies for internal deletions. It is conceivable that DSBs in downstream S regions may occur more frequently but be repaired via smaller internal deletions/rearrangements, as have been observed in the sequence of an Sγ2b region downstream of an Sµ junction (Yancopoulos et al., 1986). In this regard, it was shown that both the acceptor and donor S regions in B cells undergoing CSR accumulate mutations with comparable frequency in B cells undergoing CSR (Xue et al., 2006).

5.3. CSR Has Adopted a General Repair Mechanism to Join/Synapse Distant DSBs

At least three different, not necessarily mutually exclusive, models have been put forward to explain how distal DNA DSBs are synapsed during CSR. First, by analogy to RAG proteins, AID itself may have a direct role in synapsis by binding to two participating S regions and bringing them together by its ability to dimerize (Prochnow et al., 2006; Wang et al., 2006). Certain C-terminal mutations in AID impair CSR without affecting SHM or Sµ mutations, suggesting that AID activity and targeting to Sµ is intact (Barreto et al., 2003) and that the C-terminal portion of AID, itself or by recruiting other proteins, could contribute to such a synaptic role. Second, S regions themselves have been proposed to be involved in synapsis. For example, colocalization of transcribed S regions to transcription complexes assembled at the IgH locus may aid in the juxtaposition of S regions (Manis et al., 2002b). In addition, an S region function in synapsis might also involve the binding of MMR complex Msh2/Msh6 to transcribed S regions and to itself (Larson et al., 2005). Formation of S region higher order structures has been implicated in synapsis (Dempsey et al., 1999; Larson et al., 2005). Finally, DNA damage response proteins, such as ATM, 53BP1, and H2AX, have been proposed to facilitate synapsis and joining of distal DSBs by mediating changes in chromatin structure and potentially by physically anchoring distal DSBs (see below) (Bassing and Alt, 2004a; Reina-San-Martin et al., 2003). The first evidence in support of the latter hypothesis came from observations that mutations in these proteins lead to CSR defects, without obviously affecting the rate of large internal Sµ deletions that were visible via Southern blotting of IgM$^+$ hybridomas made from activated B cells (Reina-San-Martin et al., 2003, 2004, 2007).

To elucidate potential mechanisms of synapsis during CSR, a novel system was established to test whether "recombinational IgH switching" could be established without S regions or AID when DSBs are artificially generated in place of S regions (Fig. 6) (Zarrin et al., 2007). To accomplish this, S regions were replaced with cassettes containing an 18-bp target to generate for the rare-cutting yeast homing endonuclease I-SceI that recognizes its targets and introduces staggered DSBs (Colleaux et al., 1988; Rouet et al., 1994). B cells were generated via gene targeted mutation in ES cells in which the entire endogenous mouse Sγ1 sequence was replaced by two I-SceI sites separated by a 500-bp fragment of DNA that is inert with respect to ability to catalyze CSR in vivo. Replacement of Sγ1 with this cassette led to an essential inhibition of CSR to IgG1 on the mutant allele. However, on expression of I-SceI endonuclease from a retrovirus in activated mutant B cells, switching to IgG1 was stimulated to levels that in some experiments approached the lower range of wild-type levels (Zarrin et al., 2007). Characterization of recombination junctions revealed that Sμ was fused to one or the other I-SceI sites, consistent with the direct dependence of IgH class switching to IgG1 on I-SceI expression

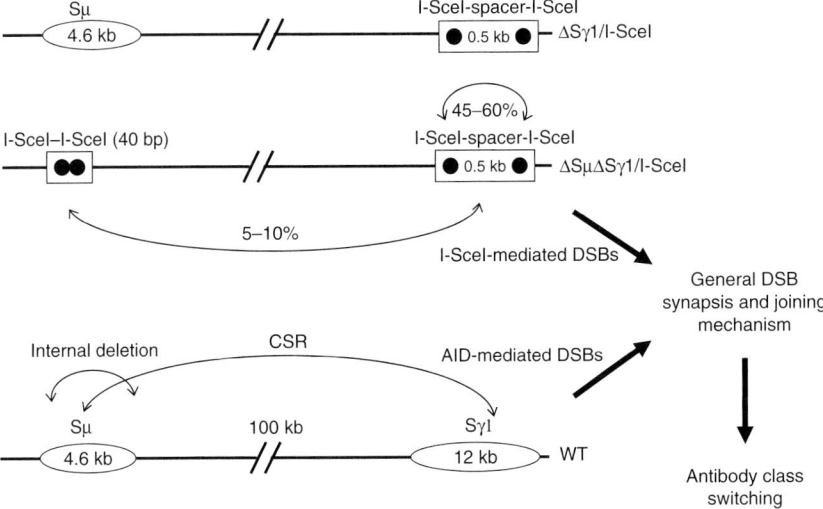

Figure 6 I-SceI-dependent class switching and a model for the role of general DNA repair during IgH CSR. In the absence of S regions and AID, the frequency of I-SceI-mediated DSBs can promote class switching. Short-range recombinations (0.5 kb apart) are joined more frequently (45–60%) than DSBs that are 100 kb away (5–10%). These results (discussed in details in the text) suggest that CSR utilizes the general DNA DSB repair pathway to synapse and join distal S region breaks during CSR. See text for more details. This figure is adapted from Zarrin et al. (2007).

in this system. These findings provided strong evidence that a DSB in an S region could bypass some of the requirements for an S region, at least for switching to Sγ1. Moreover, the findings showed that AID-initiated DSBs in the Sμ region, apparently unlike RAG generated DSBs during V(D)J recombination, can be joined efficiently to DSBs generated by an entirely different mechanism. This finding may also be relevant for mechanisms that lead to chromosomal translocations involving AID-initiated DSBs in S regions (Zarrin et al., 2007).

In the experiments described above, only the downstream acceptor Sγ1 region was replaced with an I-SceI site and AID was still present. To formally test potential roles of S regions, B cells were generated in which I-SceI replaced both the Sγ1 and Sμ sequences. The two I-SceI sites that replaced Sμ were only 40 bp apart, compared to the 500 bp that separated the I-SceI sites in Sγ1; however, these two pairs of I-SceI sites in the place of Sμ and Sγ1 were about 100 kb apart within the IgH locus (Fig. 6). The double mutant B cells showed essentially complete loss of ability to switch to IgG1 on the mutant allele that, again, was rescued to substantial levels via retroviral introduction of I-SceI endonuclease expression, showing that S region sequences were not necessary. In fact, I-SceI-dependent switching to IgG1 in B cells in which both Sμ and Sγ1 had been replaced with I-SceI sites occurred at levels as high or higher than in B cells with a full-length endogenous Sμ and a 1-kb Sγ1 (Zarrin et al., 2005, 2007). To address the requirement for AID, IgM$^+$ hybridomas were generated from B cells harboring Sμ and Sγ1 replacements. As expected from earlier studies, these hybridomas did not express detectable AID or germ line transcripts of the Cγ1 locus; nevertheless, infection with I-SceI retrovirus led to a substantial level of class switching to IgG1 (Zarrin et al., 2007). Thus, it would appear that neither S regions nor germ line transcription (within the level detectable by this assay) are required for a relatively high level of recombinational IgH class switching mediated by two I-SceI generated DSBs in the IgH locus. These studies do not rule out roles for either AID or S regions in the joining phase of CSR, for example to promote the most efficient degree of synapsis and joining. However, the surprisingly high rate of recombinational IgH switching mediated via I-SceI DSBs in absence of these factors reveals an unanticipated general repair process that promotes the joining of widely separated IgH locus DSBs. Therefore, S regions and germ line S region transcription may have evolved, at least in large part, to provide structures for AID recognition and deamination en route to generation of DSBs with more general mechanisms leading to synapsis and joining (Fig. 6).

The I-SceI model system also allowed a comparative assessment of efficiency of joining between short-range (500-bp internal deletions) and long-range

(100-kb IgH class switching events) I-SceI-generated DSBs. Surprisingly, long-range DSBs were joined at a rate that was as much as 10–20% of the frequency of short-range joins between the two I-SceI sites in the downstream cassette. This pattern is somewhat reminiscent of internal deletions versus long-range CSR events observed in normal activated B cells (Figs. 5 and 6). These results led to the proposal that S regions may have evolved as structures to allow generation of a sufficiently high level of AID-initiated DSBs that CSR would be ensured by a general mechanism that promotes a relatively high frequency of long-range joins between DSBs within a chromosome with respect to the frequency of short-range joins or simple rejoining of a single DSB (Zarrin et al., 2007). However, the question remains as to what mechanisms lead to the frequent synapsis and joining of chromosomal DSBs that are 100 kb or more apart. It is possible that there are features of the IgH locus structure in activated B cells that put S regions in proximity to promote such joining (Chaudhuri and Jasin, 2007; Zarrin et al., 2007). On the other hand, it is also possible that aspects of the normal DSB response, including the generation of repair foci over large (greater than 100 kb) distances may function to join widely separated general DSBs (Zarrin et al., 2007).

6. General DNA Repair Systems in the Joining Phase of CSR

6.1. DNA Damage Response

In mammalian cells, DSBs can be introduced into a cell due to external insults such as exposure to ionizing radiation (IR), metabolic processes such as oxidative stress, as well as via developmentally regulated processes which include V(D)J recombination and CSR in lymphocytes (Bassing and Alt, 2004b). If left unrepaired, DSBs can cause cell death or can give rise to potentially oncogenic translocations (Bassing and Alt, 2004b; Franco et al., 2006a; Xu, 2006). Mammalian cells have therefore evolved a complex network to sense, signal, and repair DSBs. There are two major characterized pathways of DSB repair in mammalian cells. Homologous recombination is a postreplicative repair process that requires large regions of homology and provides accurate repair. The other major known mammalian repair pathway is NHEJ which joins ends that lack homologies or have only short homologies (Bogue et al., 1997, 1998; Li et al., 1995; Roth et al., 1985) and appears to be most important in prereplicative phases of the cell cycle when HR is not operative (Mills et al., 2004). Joining of DSBs via either of these pathways first involves the activation of a DNA damage response, which involves a large number of different proteins. There have been several comprehensive reviews of the DNA damage response (Bassing and Alt, 2004b; Burma et al., 2006; Franco et al., 2006a;

Povirk, 2006; Stucki and Jackson, 2006; Xu, 2006) and it is also covered more extensively by another chapter in this volume (Ramiro et al., 2007). Here, we will introduce the DNA damage response as it pertains to the mechanism of CSR.

The exact sequence of events that lead to the recognition of a DSB and the assembly of proteins that effect cell cycle arrest and mediate repair is still emerging. One of the earliest responders to DSBs is the MRN complex (Lee and Paull, 2005) that consists of the proteins Mre11, RAD50, and Nbs1 (Carney et al., 1998). The MRN complex associates with DSBs immediately following DNA damage (Lee and Paull, 2005) and recruits ATM, which is a serine/threonine kinase. ATM is considered to be one of the master regulators of the DSB response, via direct interaction between the C-terminal domain of Nbs1 and ATM (Falck et al., 2005). ATM is a member of a large family of PI3-related kinases that include ATR (ATM and RAD3-related) and DNA-PKcs (DNA-dependent catalytic subunit catalytic subunit) (Shiloh, 2003). ATM and the related kinases can phosphorylate a large number of DNA repair and cell cycle checkpoint proteins, including the G1 checkpoint protein p53, as wells as Nbs1 (Falck et al., 2005), H2AX (Burma et al., 2001; Paull et al., 2000), 53BP1 (Anderson et al., 2001; Rappold et al., 2001), and MDC1 (Lou et al., 2006). Activation of these downstream molecules leads to ATM-dependent cell cycle arrest in response to DSBs and the subsequent repair of the damage (Fig. 7).

An early and critical event in the ATM-dependent response to DSBs is the phosphorylation of DSB-proximal H2AX molecules on Ser139 to form γH2AX (Rogakou et al., 1998). H2AX phosphorylation leads to the rapid, hierarchical assembly of several repair factors, including MDC1, 53BP1, and NBS1, which via their ability to bind to γH2AX form multiprotein complexes or foci at sites of DNA damage (Kobayashi et al., 2002; Stewart et al., 2003; Stucki et al., 2005; Ward et al., 2003a). Although H2AX phosphorylation is not required for the initial recruitment of these factors to the DSB (Celeste et al., 2003b), it is necessary for the formation of normal, extended repair foci (Bassing et al., 2002a; Celeste et al., 2003a). Recent studies have highlighted a complex interplay between DSB repair factors and chromatin conformation around DNA breaks. For example, 53BP1 can be recruited to DSBs via its interaction with methylated lysine 79 of histone H3, a chromatin mark that may be exposed during chromatin remodeling following DNA damage (Huyen et al., 2004). Likewise, chromatin-bound MDC1 facilitates the recruitment of additional molecules of ATM to the DSB. Such recruitment then leads to phosphorylation of H2AX molecules that are distal to the initial site of lesion, and generates a positive feedback loop that promotes the stable association of DNA damage response factors in large domains or foci that can spread up to a megabase on either side of the DSB (Lou et al., 2006; Stucki and Jackson, 2006).

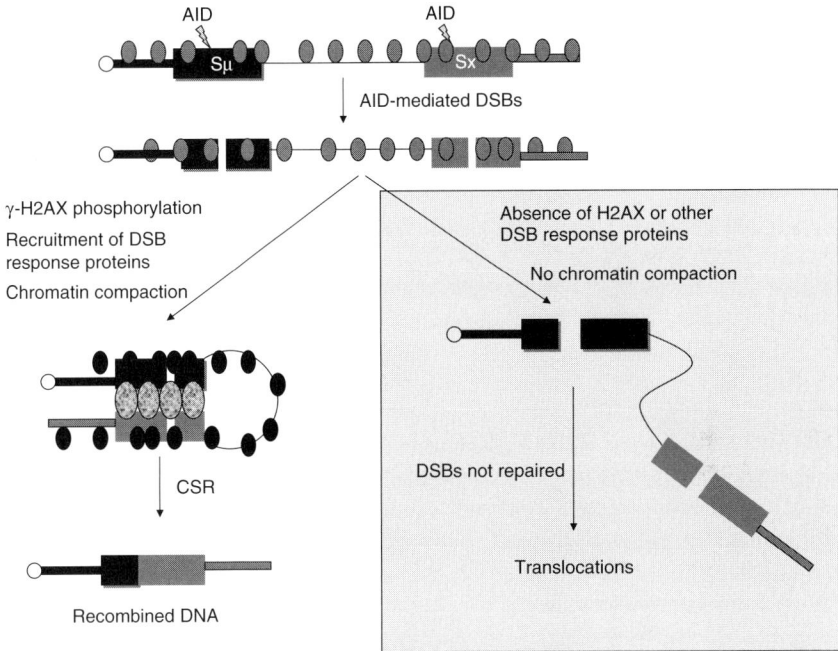

Figure 7 S region synapsis and roles of DSB response proteins during CSR. AID-dependent generation of DSBs induces modifications and mobilization of the DSB response pathway including the phosphorylation of the histone H2AX (gray ovals) to generate γH2AX (black ovals). Recruitment of several DSB response proteins (ATM, MRN complex, MDC1, 53BP1) (speckled ovals) to the break alters chromatin structure which may facilitate synapsis between two distal DSBs, and hold broken S regions together for repair. In the absence of the DNA damage response proteins such as H2AX (as shown), the breaks are not held together and thus not repaired. Such broken S regions frequently participate in translocations. See text for details.

The formation of repair foci with the accumulated DSB response proteins may allow enforcement of cell cycle checkpoints while, potentially, simultaneously providing a molecular bridge between DNA ends, preventing their dissociation until repair ensues (Bassing and Alt, 2004a; Franco et al., 2006a; Stucki and Jackson, 2006; Xu, 2006). In keeping with this notion, mice and cells deficient for ATM, 53BP1, Nbs1, Mdc1, and H2AX share a number of phenotypes potentially related to DSB repair deficiency, including IR sensitivity, DNA repair defects, and genomic instability (Bassing et al., 2002a, 2003; Kracker et al., 2005; Morales et al., 2003; Reina-San-Martin et al., 2005; Ward et al., 2003b). Moreover, studies of CSR and V(D)J recombination have suggested that these proteins may have a direct influence on DNA DSB repair via end joining (Bredemeyer et al., 2006; Franco et al., 2006b).

6.2. DSB Response Proteins in CSR

Cumulative evidence suggests that the general response to deleterious DSBs also is operative at AID-initiated DSBs during CSR (Fig. 7). The first evidence to support a role for the DSB response in CSR came from the finding that AID-dependent foci of γH2AX and NBS1 accumulate at the IgH locus of B cells activated *in vitro* (Petersen *et al.*, 2001). In addition, mice deficient for ATM, H2AX, MDC1, NBS1, or 53BP1 are impaired, to variable extents, for CSR (Franco *et al.*, 2006b; Kracker *et al.*, 2005; Lahdesmaki *et al.*, 2004; Manis *et al.*, 2004; Petersen *et al.*, 2001; Reina-San-Martin *et al.*, 2003, 2004, 2005; Ward *et al.*, 2004). In contrast, these DSB response factors are not required for SHM, a process that can occur without DSB intermediates (Manis *et al.*, 2004; Reina-San-Martin *et al.*, 2003). Moreover, mice that are doubly deficient for H2AX and p53 routinely develop B-cell lymphomas, a subset of which has S region translocations (Bassing *et al.*, 2003). How DSB response factors function in general chromosomal DSB repair and more specifically during CSR is not fully understood, but it could be by simply altering chromatin structure around DSBs to allow repair factor access. Alternatively, but not mutually exclusively, it could function by forming large complexes that would hold broken ends together or even help bring more widely separated ends together. In this context, it was proposed that the formation of H2AX-dependent foci of DSB response proteins, most of which also bind each other and/or DNA, might represent an "anchoring" activity that holds DSBs together in a synaptic complex to facilitate their ligation by end joining (Bassing and Alt, 2004a) (Fig. 7). Similar arguments have been made with respect to HR where phosphorylated histone H2A in yeast binds cohesin (Shroff *et al.*, 2004; Unal *et al.*, 2004).

Quantification of the frequency of AID-dependent chromosomal breaks within the IgH locus in single B cells activated for CSR has provided direct support of role of DSB response proteins in the end-joining phase of IgH CSR (Franco *et al.*, 2006b; Ramiro *et al.*, 2006). Specifically, analyses of H2AX-, MDC1-, ATM-, 53BP1-, or NBS1-deficient B cells activated for CSR via two color fluorescence *in situ* hybridization (FISH) with probes from upstream and downstream regions of the IgH locus revealed large numbers of metaphases containing chromosomal breaks within one and sometimes both IgH loci (Franco *et al.*, 2006b; Ramiro *et al.*, 2006) (Fig. 8). Such IgH locus chromosomal breaks were *bona fide* AID-dependent breaks, as they were fully rescued by AID-deficiency *in vivo* (Franco *et al.*, 2006b). Moreover, a substantial percentage of IgH locus breaks observed in these backgrounds participated in chromosomal translocations (Franco *et al.*, 2006b; Ramiro *et al.*, 2006). Therefore, the DSB response plays a major role in preventing DSBs introduced during IgH CSR, as well as general DSBs, from separating and

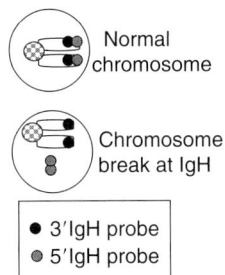

Figure 8 FISH assay commonly used to detect chromosome aberrations in the absence of DSB response proteins. FISH probes that detect the 5' or 3' regions of the IgH locus (gray or black ovals, respectively) can detect unrepaired DSBs in the IgH locus. The striped oval represents the centromere.

progressing into chromosomal breaks and translocations (Franco et al., 2006b). These findings provided strong support for the notion that the DSB response is required to support normal end joining (Bassing and Alt, 2004a; Franco et al., 2006a). Similar conclusions were subsequently made for the role of ATM in V(D)J recombination (Bredemeyer et al., 2006), although the DSB response may not turn out to be as important overall in V(D)J recombination due to the role of RAG proteins in synapsis and/or channeling DSBs into NHEJ (Bassing and Alt, 2004b).

Notably, while ATM-, H2AX-, and 53BP1-deficient B cells had a relatively major impairment in CSR, they still appeared to accumulate internal Sμ deletions at normal or (for 53BP1, see below) increased frequency subsequent to activation, leading to the suggestion that such factors also may somehow be involved in long-range S region synapsis but are not necessary for shorter range deletions (Reina-San-Martin et al., 2003, 2004, 2007). In contrast to H2AX-, MDC1-, or ATM-deficient B cells which have only a partial impairment of CSR, 53BP1-deficient B cells are severely impaired for CSR (Franco et al., 2006b; Kracker et al., 2005; Lahdesmaki et al., 2004; Manis et al., 2004; Petersen et al., 2001; Reina-San-Martin et al., 2003, 2004, 2005; Ward et al., 2004). Yet, IgH FISH analyses demonstrated that the frequency of chromosomal breaks within the IgH locus does not differ significantly from those observed in H2AX- or ATM-deficient B cells (Franco et al., 2006b). Moreover, activated 53BP1-deficient B cells proliferate and activate efficiently (Manis et al., 2004; Ward et al., 2004), and 53BP1-deficient cells and mice show only modest growth retardation and moderate cellular genomic instability (Manis et al., 2004; Ward et al., 2004). This group of findings led to the proposal that 53BP1 may have novel functions in CSR (Franco et al., 2006a). In this context,

53BP1-deficient B cells exhibit markedly increased levels of internal deletions versus normal long-range CSR events, raising the intriguing possibility that 53BP1 might have a particularly important function in long-range synapsis (Reina-San-Martin et al., 2007), although it will be important, as discussed for UNG experiments above, to ensure that such deletions happened in normal B cells as opposed to in hybridomas postfusion.

The requirement for DSB response factors to mediate normal levels of CSR, to suppress AID-dependent IgH locus translocations, and to promote long-range CSR reactions versus internal deletions has led to the suggestion that the DSB response may be a key factor involved in promoting the higher than expected joining frequency of widely separated chromosomal IgH locus DSBS (Bassing and Alt, 2004a; Zarrin et al., 2007). To address this model, there are many questions that need to be answered. One would be whether the joining of widely separated versus proximal I-SceI-generated DSBs within the IgH locus would be altered in DSB response factor-deficient cells in a manner observed for internal S region deletions versus CSR events. Another would be whether joining of DSBs separated by 100 kb or more occurred at loci other than the IgH locus and in cells other than activated B cells. Yet another question would be the distance at which DSBs could be separated and still show increased frequency of joining. Moreover, one must ask why mammalian cells would have evolved mechanisms to mediate these long-range interactions in the first place, as opposed to resolving DSBs exclusively through religation of the broken DNA ends. In this context, the frequency of joining I-SceI-generated DSBs separated by 100 kb in the IgH locus is orders of magnitude greater than that observed for translocations between I-SceI-generated DSBs on separate chromosomes (Weinstock et al., 2006). Given the greatly increased frequency of IgH locus translocations in DSB response-deficient B cells (Franco et al., 2006b; Ramiro et al., 2006), one notion would be that the long-range joining mechanisms might be a by-product of a mechanism that evolved to ensure DSB repair within a chromosome and suppress translocations (Bassing and Alt, 2004a; Zarrin et al., 2007).

6.3. End Joining

CSR joins lack major regions of homology and, therefore, are catalyzed by some form of DNA end-joining pathway. The NHEJ pathway has been the prime candidate. In this context, NHEJ joins ends that lack homology or ends that have very short homologies to form junctions reminiscent of those observed for CSR (Lieber et al., 2003; Rooney et al., 2004). NHEJ has seven known components (Fig. 9). Ku70 and Ku80 bind DSBs as a complex (Ku). Ku bound to DNA ends binds DNA-PKcs and activates it to form the DNA-PK holoenzyme (Lieber *et al.*, 2003; Rooney *et al.*, 2004). DNA-PK can phosphorylate Artemis to activate its endonuclease activity. XRCC4 and DNA Ligase 4 work together as a ligation complex which functions specifically in NHEJ (Lieber *et al.*, 2003; Rooney *et al.*, 2004). Cernunnos/XLF is a more recently identified NHEJ factor that appears to have some relationship to XRCC4 (Burma *et al.*, 2006; Sekiguchi and Ferguson, 2006). Ku70, Ku80, XRCC4, Ligase 4, and likely Cernunnos/XLF are conserved in evolution and are considered "core" NHEJ factors (Fig. 9). The activity of the NHEJ pathway has been characterized primarily in the context of V(D)J recombination. The RAG endonuclease generates V, D, and J coding ends as covalently sealed hairpins and RS ends a blunt 5′phosphorylated DSBs (Fig. 9). The "core" NHEJ factors are required for both coding and RS joins where they have functions ranging

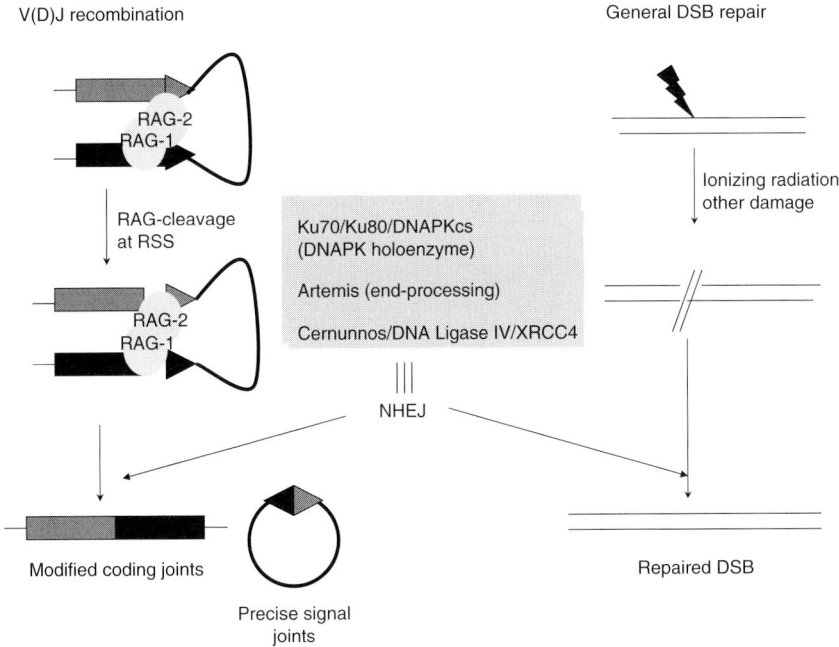

Figure 9 NHEJ is required for V(D)J recombination and for general DSB repair. The major components of the NHEJ pathway are shown. During V(D)J recombination, the RAG-1 and RAG2 proteins bind to and introduce DSBs at specific signal sequences (triangles) that flank the coding segments (rectangles). The RAG proteins cleave DNA mostly in the context of a preformed synaptic complex, and following cleavage, remain bound to the ends to shepherd in DNA repair proteins to ligate the DSBs. The NHEJ pathway also functions to join general DSBs. See text for more details.

from recognition of DSBs and recruitment of other factors to end ligation (Fig. 9) (Dudley *et al.*, 2005; Lieber *et al.*, 2003; Rooney *et al.*, 2004). In contrast, DNA-PKcs and Artemis are required for coding joins but are relatively dispensable for RS joins (Bogue *et al.*, 1998; Gao *et al.*, 1998a; Kurimasa *et al.*, 1999; Nicolas *et al.*, 1998; Rooney *et al.*, 2002; Taccioli *et al.*, 1998). In this context, the DNA-PKcs activated endonuclease activity of Artemis is necessary to open and process coding end hairpins (Ma *et al.*, 2002; Rooney *et al.*, 2002). It is thought that the various NHEJ factors play similar roles in the repair of general DSBs (Lieber *et al.*, 2003; Rooney *et al.*, 2004) (Fig. 9).

Evidence for a role for NHEJ components in CSR came from studies in which Ku 70 or Ku 80-deficient B cells were generated by rescuing B cell development with "knocked-in" productive V(D)J rearrangements at the IgH and Igκ loci (Casellas *et al.*, 1998; Manis *et al.*, 1998; Reina-San-Martin *et al.*, 2003). Notably, both Ku70 and Ku80 deficient B cells were completely deficient for ability to undergo CSR. However, interpretation of these results was complicated by the fact that Ku-deficient cells have proliferation defects (Manis *et al.*, 1998; Reina-San-Martin *et al.*, 2003) and that proliferation is also required for CSR (Hodgkin *et al.*, 1996). Therefore, cause and effect were not unequivocal. Notably, DNA-PKcs deficient B cells or B cells homozygous for the *scid* mutation (a point mutation in the DNA-PKcs catalytic domain) were severely impaired for CSR but did show residual CSR (Cook *et al.*, 2003; Manis *et al.*, 2002; Rolink *et al.*, 1996). In the case of DNA-PKcs deficient B cells, CSR to IgG1 occurred relatively normally (Manis *et al.*, 2002). On the other hand, Artemis deficient B cells show relatively normal CSR to all IgH isotypes (Rooney *et al.*, 2005). Preliminary analyses of DNA-PKcs-deficient and Artemis-deficient B cells for chromosome breaks by the IgH locus FISH method suggest that both might have some IgH breaks and translocations (Franco and Alt, unpublished data). Thus, while more detailed characterization of the nature of the Igh locus breaks in the Artemis and DNA-PKcs mutant cells will be required for unequivocal interpretations, it is possible that both components may be necessary for joining a fraction of IgH locus breaks that occur in B cells activated for CSR, consistent with the role of these factors in joining a subset of normal DSBs. Overall, it appears that NHEJ joins, at least, a subset of CSR DSBs. However, given that Ku70 and Ku80 and DNA-PKcs have functions outside of NHEJ (Chu *et al.*, 2000; Cohen *et al.*, 2004; Sekiguchi *et al.*, 2001), some of the CSR defects observed, in particular the complete defect in Ku-deficient B cells, might be due to effects on other processes.

XRCC4 and DNA Ligase 4 are absolutely required for coding and RS joining during V(D)J recombination (Frank *et al.*, 1998; Gao *et al.*, 1998b; Li and Alt, 1996; Taccioli *et al.*, 1993) and have no known functions outside of NHEJ.

A role for Ligase 4 in CSR was suggested by the finding that hypomorphic human Ligase 4 mutations affected CSR, in particular by leading to alterations of certain S region junctions such as increased use of microhomologies by some (Sμ to Sα) but not others (Sμ to Sγ) (Pan-Hammarstrom et al., 2005). However, it is not clear whether such alterations resulted from decreased or altered activity of Ligase 4 or increased contribution by some alternative pathway (Pan-Hammarstrom et al., 2005). To definitively assess the role of NHEJ in IgH CSR, it will be necessary to generate B cells completely deficient in XRCC4 or Ligase 4 by either IgH/Igκ V(D)J knock-in approach or by a conditional gene inactivation approach. Preliminary analyses of XRCC4 deficient B cells generated by such approaches suggested that they proliferated relatively normally and show signficant levels of CSR (C. Yan and F. Alt, unpublished data). It will now be of significant interest to employ IgH locus FISH assays to determine whether chromosomal breaks and translocations occur in such XRCC4-deficient B cells stimulated for CSR. In addition, it will be of substaintial interest to determine the nucleodide sequence of the junctions of CSR events that occur in XRCC4-deficient B cells. In mice, normal CSR junctions are roughly equally divided between blunt joins (no homologies at the ends) and joins with short micro-homologies. While an alternative end-joining pathway that appears to prefer micro-homologies is known to exist, the pathway does not function in V(D)J recombination in the absence of NHEJ and there has been little evidence that it can function to join chromosomal sequences other than translocations (Lee et al., 2004b; Zhu et al., 2002). In this context, it will be of great interest to determine whether this pathway can catalze chromosomal CSR in the absence of XRCC4 and, thereby, the classical NHEJ pathway.

7. Evolution of CSR

The process of SHM is an ancient reaction that exists in cartilaginous and bony fish (Cannon et al., 2004). Fish AID has been identified and the fish mutational hot spot (AGC/T triplet) is similar to that in mammals, suggesting that SHM in fish is most likely AID dependent. Fish, however, do not have S regions and do not undergo CSR; yet fish AID can mediate CSR in mammalian cells, indicating that the molecule has already acquired most of the activities required for CSR (Barreto et al., 2005a; Wakae et al., 2006). CSR first appeared in amphibians, with *Xenopus* B cells being able to switch from IgM to IgX (Stavnezer and Amemiya, 2004). Unlike mammals, *Xenopus* S regions are AT rich (Mussmann et al., 1997) and do not form R-loops (Zarrin et al., 2004). Therefore, CSR is probably mediated via the ability of AID, perhaps in conjunction with an RPA or a similar molecule, to target the AGCT sequence within *Xenopus* S regions in an SHM-like fashion (Zarrin et al., 2004). As completion of CSR employs general DSB repair mechanisms, including a mechanism to synapse widespread chromosomal DSBs, it appears that what may have been needed for the evolution of CSR was the appearance target sequences that could allow AID activities to generate DSBs. In this regard, primitive S regions, such as those in amphibians, may be composed of a high density of RGYW motifs, allowing an SHM form of AID access, with the density of AID deaminations predisposing to DSBs. Evolution of R-loop forming ability may have evolved later to maximize AID-initiated DSB activity. Thus, one might imagine that the evolution of CSR beyond fish may have simply required the evolution of primitive S regions from SHM motifs along with their continued evolutionary refinement over time into specialized structures that allow generation of sufficient AID DSBs to allow physiological CSR levels by general joining and synapsis mechanisms (Zarrin et al., 2007). While it is also possible that AID-specific cofactors evolved along the way to play a role in the diverse activities required for CSR, for example to direct the AID-induced lesions in to DSBs, the model outlined above is economical in that it would not require simultaneous evolution of S regions plus coevolution of AID-specific cofactors and/or potential AID structural modifications.

Acknowledgments

We thank Michael Neuberger for critically reviewing sections of this chapter. J.C. is a Damon Runyon Scholar, U.B. is a fellow of the Irvington Institute, A.D. is a Leukemia Research Foundation Fellow, R.T.P. is a fellow of the Cancer Research Institute, B.V. is supported by a training grant from the NIH. F.W.A is an investigator of the Howard Hughes Medical Institute. This work is supported by NIH grants CA92625, CA109901, and AI31541 to F.W.A.

References

Alt, F. W., Rosenberg, N., Casanova, R. J., Thomas, E., and Baltimore, D. (1982a). Immunoglobulin heavy-chain expression and class switching in a murine leukaemia cell line. *Nature* **296**, 325–331.
Alt, F. W., Rosenberg, N., Enea, V., Siden, E., and Baltimore, D. (1982b). Multiple immunoglobulin heavy-chain gene transcripts in Abelson murine leukemia virus-transformed lymphoid cell lines. *Mol. Cell. Biol.* **2**, 386–400.
Anderson, L., Henderson, C., and Adachi, Y. (2001). Phosphorylation and rapid relocalization of 53BP1 to nuclear foci upon DNA damage. *Mol. Cell Biol.* **21**, 1719–1729.
Arakawa, H., Hauschild, J., and Buerstedde, J. M. (2002). Requirement of the activation-induced deaminase (AID) gene for immunoglobulin gene conversion. *Science* **295**, 1301–1306.
Barreto, V., Reina-San-Martin, B., Ramiro, A. R., McBride, K. M., and Nussenzweig, M. C. (2003). C-terminal deletion of AID uncouples class switch recombination from somatic hypermutation and gene conversion. *Mol. Cell* **12**, 501–508.

Barreto, V. M., Pan-Hammarstrom, Q., Zhao, Y., Hammarstrom, L., Misulovin, Z., and Nussenzweig, M. C. (2005a). AID from bony fish catalyzes class switch recombination. *J. Exp. Med.* **202,** 733–738.

Barreto, V. M., Ramiro, A. R., and Nussenzweig, M. C. (2005b). Activation-induced deaminase: Controversies and open questions. *Trends Immunol.* **26,** 90–96.

Bassing, C. H., and Alt, F. W. (2004a). H2AX may function as an anchor to hold broken chromosomal DNA ends in close proximity. *Cell Cycle* **3,** e119–e123.

Bassing, C. H., and Alt, F. W. (2004b). The cellular response to general and programmed DNA double strand breaks. *DNA Repair (Amst.)* **3,** 781–796.

Bassing, C. H., Chua, K. F., Sekiguchi, J., Suh, H., Whitlow, S. R., Fleming, J. C., Monroe, B. C., Ciccone, D. N., Yan, C., Vlasakova, K., Livingston, D. M., Fergusson, D. O., *et al.* (2002a). Increased ionizing radiation sensitivity and genomic instability in the absence of histone H2AX. *Proc. Natl. Acad. Sci. USA* **99,** 8173–8178.

Bassing, C. H., Swat, W., and Alt, F. W. (2002b). The mechanism and regulation of chromosomal V(D)J recombination. *Cell* **109,** S45–S55.

Bassing, C. H., Suh, H., Ferguson, D. O., Chua, K. F., Manis, J., Eckersdorff, M., Gleason, M., Bronson, R., Lee, C., and Alt, F. W. (2003). Histone H2AX: A dosage-dependent suppressor of oncogenic translocations and tumors. *Cell* **114,** 359–370.

Basu, U., Chaudhuri, J., Alpert, C., Dutt, S., Ranganath, S., Li, G., Schrum, J. P., Manis, J. P., and Alt, F. W. (2005). The AID antibody diversification enzyme is regulated by protein kinase A phosphorylation. *Nature* **438,** 508–511.

Basu, U., Chaudhuri, J., Phan, R. T., Datta, A., and Alt, F. W. (2007). Regulation of activation induced deaminase via phosphorylation. *Adv. Exp. Med. Biol.* **596,** 129–137.

Begum, N. A., Kinoshita, K., Kakazu, N., Muramatsu, M., Nagaoka, H., Shinkura, R., Biniszkiewicz, D., Boyer, L. A., Jaenisch, R., and Honjo, T. (2004a). Uracil DNA glycosylase activity is dispensable for immunoglobulin class switch. *Science* **305,** 1160–1163.

Begum, N. A., Kinoshita, K., Muramatsu, M., Nagaoka, H., Shinkura, R., and Honjo, T. (2004b). *De novo* protein synthesis is required for activation-induced cytidine deaminase-dependent DNA cleavage in immunoglobulin class switch recombination. *Proc. Natl. Acad. Sci. USA* **101,** 13003–13007.

Begum, N. A., Izumi, N., Nishikori, M., Nagaoka, H., Shinkura, R., and Honjo, T. (2007). Requirement of non-canonical activity of uracil DNA glycosylase for class switch recombination. *J. Biol. Chem.* **282,** 731–742.

Besmer, E., Market, E., and Papavasiliou, F. N. (2006). The transcription elongation complex directs activation-induced cytidine deaminase-mediated DNA deamination. *Mol. Cell. Biol.* **26,** 4378–4385.

Betz, A. G., Milstein, C., Gonzalez-Fernandez, A., Pannell, R., Larson, T., and Neuberger, M. S. (1994). Elements regulating somatic hypermutation of an immunoglobulin kappa gene: Critical role for the intron enhancer/matrix attachment region. *Cell* **77,** 239–248.

Birshtein, B. K., Chen, C., Saleque, S., Michaelson, J. S., Singh, M., and Little, R. D. (1997). Murine and human 3′IγH regulatory sequences. *Curr. Top. Microbiol. Immunol.* **224,** 73–80.

Bogue, M. A., Wang, C., Zhu, C., and Roth, D. B. (1997). V(D)J recombination in Ku86-deficient mice: Distinct effects on coding, signal, and hybrid joint formation. *Immunity* **7,** 37–47.

Bogue, M. A., Jhappan, C., and Roth, D. B. (1998). Analysis of variable (diversity) joining recombination in DNA dependent protein kinase (DNA-PK)-deficient mice reveals DNA-PK-independent pathways for both signal and coding joint formation. *Proc. Natl. Acad. Sci. USA* **95,** 15559–15564.

Bottaro, A., Lansford, R., Xu, L., Zhang, J., Rothman, P., and Alt, F. W. (1994). S region transcription per se promotes basal IgE class switch recombination but additional factors regulate the efficiency of the process. *EMBO J.* **13**, 665–674.

Bransteitter, R., Pham, P., Scharff, M. D., and Goodman, M. F. (2003). Activation-induced cytidine deaminase deaminates deoxycytidine on single-stranded DNA but requires the action of RNase. *Proc. Natl. Acad. Sci. USA* **100**, 4102–4107.

Bredemeyer, A. L., Sharma, G. G., Huang, C. Y., Helmink, B. A., Walker, L. M., Khor, K. C., Nuskey, B., Sullivan, K. E., Pandita, T. K., Bassing, C. H., and Sleckman, B. P. (2006). ATM stabilizes DNA double-strand-break complexes during V(D)J recombination. *Nature* **442**, 466–470.

Bross, L., and Jacobs, H. (2003). DNA double strand breaks occur independent of AID in hypermutating Ig genes. *Clin. Dev. Immunol.* **10**, 83–89.

Burma, S., Chen, B. P., Murphy, M., Kurimasa, A., and Chen, D. J. (2001). ATM phosphorylates histone H2AX in response to DNA double-strand breaks. *J. Biol. Chem.* **276**, 42462–42467.

Burma, S., Chen, B. P., and Chen, D. J. (2006). Role of non-homologous end joining (NHEJ) in maintaining genomic integrity. *DNA Repair (Amst.)* **5**, 1042–1048.

Calvert, J. E., Kim, M. F., Gathings, W. E., and Cooper, M. D. (1983). Differentiation of B lineage cells from liver of neonatal mice: Generation of immunoglobulin isotype diversity in vitro. *J. Immunol.* **131**, 1693–1697.

Cannon, J. P., Haire, R. N., Rast, J. P., and Litman, G. W. (2004). The phylogenetic origins of the antigen-binding receptors and somatic diversification mechanisms. *Immunol. Rev.* **200**, 12–22.

Carney, J. P., Maser, R. S., Olivares, H., Davis, E. M., Le Beau, M., Yates, J. R., III, Hays, L., Morgan, W. F., and Petrini, J. H. (1998). The hMre11/hRad50 protein complex and Nijmegen breakage syndrome: Linkage of double-strand break repair to the cellular DNA damage response. *Cell* **93**, 477–486.

Casellas, R., Nussenzweig, A., Wuerffel, R., Pelanda, R., Reichlin, A., Suh, H., Qin, X. F., Besmer, E., Kenter, A., Rajewsky, K., et al. (1998). Ku80 is required for immunoglobulin isotype switching. *EMBO J.* **17**, 2404–2411.

Catalan, N., Selz, F., Imai, K., Revy, P., Fischer, A., and Durandy, A. (2003). The block in immunoglobulin class switch recombination caused by activation-induced cytidine deaminase deficiency occurs prior to the generation of DNA double strand breaks in switch mu region. *J. Immunol.* **171**, 2504–2509.

Celeste, A., Difilippantonio, S., Difilippantonio, M. J., Fernandez-Capetillo, O., Pilch, D. R., Sedelnikova, O. A., Eckhaus, M., Ried, T., Bonner, W. M., and Nussenzweig, A. (2003a). H2AX haploinsufficiency modifies genomic stability and tumor susceptibility. *Cell* **114**, 371–383.

Celeste, A., Fernandez-Capetillo, O., Kruhlak, M. J., Pilch, D. R., Staudt, D. W., Lee, A., Bonner, R. F., Bonner, W. M., and Nussenzweig, A. (2003b). Histone H2AX phosphorylation is dispensable for the initial recognition of DNA breaks. *Nat. Cell Biol.* **5**, 675–679.

Chaudhuri, J., and Alt, F. W. (2004). Class-switch recombination: Interplay of transcription, DNA deamination and DNA repair. *Nat. Rev. Immunol.* **4**, 541–552.

Chaudhuri, J., and Jasin, M. (2007). Antibodies get a break. *Science* **315**, 335–336.

Chaudhuri, J., Tian, M., Khuong, C., Chua, K., Pinaud, E., and Alt, F. W. (2003). Transcription-targeted DNA deamination by the AID antibody diversification enzyme. *Nature* **422**, 726–730.

Chaudhuri, J., Khuong, C., and Alt, F. W. (2004). Replication protein A interacts with AID to promote deamination of somatic hypermutation targets. *Nature* **430**, 992–998.

Chu, W., Gong, X., Li, Z., Takabayashi, K., Ouyang, H., Chen, Y., Lois, A., Chen, D. J., Li, G. C., Karin, M., and Raz, E. (2000). DNA-PKcs is required for activation of innate immunity by immunostimulatory DNA. *Cell* **103**, 909–918.

Cobb, R. M., Oestreich, K. J., Osipovich, O. A., and Oltz, E. M. (2006). Accessibility control of V(D)J recombination. *Adv. Immunol.* **91,** 45–109.

Cogne, M., Lansford, R., Bottaro, A., Zhang, J., Gorman, J., Young, F., Cheng, H. L., and Alt, F. W. (1994). A class switch control region at the 3' end of the immunoglobulin heavy chain locus. *Cell* **77,** 737–747.

Cohen, H. Y., Lavu, S., Bitterman, K. J., Hekking, B., Imahiyerobo, T. A., Miller, C., Frye, R., Ploegh, H., Kessler, B. M., and Sinclair, D. A. (2004). Acetylation of the C terminus of Ku70 by CBP and PCAF controls Bax-mediated apoptosis. *Mol. Cell* **13,** 627–638.

Colleaux, L., D'Auriol, L., Galibert, F., and Dujon, B. (1988). Recognition and cleavage site of the intron-encoded omega transposase. *Proc. Natl. Acad. Sci. USA* **85,** 6022–6026.

Conticello, S. G., Langlois, M., Yang, Z., and Neuberger, M. S. (2007). DNA deamination in immunity: AID in the context of its APOBEC relatives. *Adv. Immunol.* **94,** 37–73.

Cook, A. J., Oganesian, L., Harumal, P., Basten, A., Brink, R., and Jolly, C. J. (2003). Reduced switching in SCID B cells is associated with altered somatic mutation of recombined S regions. *J. Immunol.* **171,** 6556–6564.

Cory, S., and Adams, J. M. (1980). Deletions are associated with somatic rearrangement of immunoglobulin heavy chain genes. *Cell* **19,** 37–51.

Crews, S., Griffin, J., Huang, H., Calame, K., and Hood, L. (1981). A single VH gene segment encodes the immune response to phosphorylcholine: Somatic mutation is correlated with the class of the antibody. *Cell* **25,** 59–66.

Daniels, G. A., and Lieber, M. R. (1995a). RNA:DNA complex formation upon transcription of immunoglobulin switch regions: Implications for the mechanism and regulation of class switch recombination. *Nucleic Acids Res.* **23,** 5006–5011.

Daniels, G. A., and Lieber, M. R. (1995b). Strand specificity in the transcriptional targeting of recombination at immunoglobulin switch sequences. *Proc. Natl. Acad. Sci. USA* **92,** 5625–5629.

Daniels, G. A., and Lieber, M. R. (1996). Transcription targets recombination at immunoglobulin switch sequences in a strand-specific manner. *Curr. Top. Microbiol. Immunol.* **217,** 171–189.

Davis, M. M., Kim, S. K., and Hood, L. E. (1980). DNA sequences mediating class switching in alpha-immunoglobulins. *Science* **209,** 1360–1365.

Dempsey, L. A., Sun, H., Hanakahi, L. A., and Maizels, N. (1999). G4 DNA binding by LR1 and its subunits, nucleolin and hnRNP D, A role for G-G pairing in immunoglobulin switch recombination. *J. Biol. Chem.* **274,** 1066–1071.

Di Noia, J., and Neuberger, M. S. (2002). Altering the pathway of immunoglobulin hypermutation by inhibiting uracil-DNA glycosylase. *Nature* **419,** 43–48.

Di Noia, J. M., Rada, C., and Neuberger, M. S. (2006). SMUG1 is able to excise uracil from immunoglobulin genes: Insight into mutation versus repair. *EMBO J.* **25,** 585–595.

Dickerson, S. K., Market, E., Besmer, E., and Papavasiliou, F. N. (2003). AID mediates hypermutation by deaminating single stranded DNA. *J. Exp. Med.* **197,** 1291–1296.

Doi, T., Kinoshita, K., Ikegawa, M., Muramatsu, M., and Honjo, T. (2003). Inaugural article: De novo protein synthesis is required for the activation-induced cytidine deaminase function in class-switch recombination. *Proc. Natl. Acad. Sci. USA* **100,** 2634–2638.

Dudley, D. D., Manis, J. P., Zarrin, A. A., Kaylor, L., Tian, M., and Alt, F. W. (2002). Internal IgH class switch region deletions are position-independent and enhanced by AID expression. *Proc. Natl. Acad. Sci. USA* **99,** 9984–9989.

Dudley, D. D., Chaudhuri, J., Bassing, C. H., and Alt, F. W. (2005). Mechanism and control of V(D)J recombination versus class switch recombination: Similarities and differences. *Adv. Immunol.* **86,** 43–112.

Dunnick, W., Rabbitts, T. H., and Milstein, C. (1980). An immunoglobulin deletion mutant with implications for the heavy-chain switch and RNA splicing. *Nature* **286,** 669–675.

Dunnick, W., Hertz, G. Z., Scappino, L., and Gritzmacher, C. (1993). DNA sequences at immunoglobulin switch region recombination sites [published erratum appears in Nucleic Acids Res 1993 May 11;21(9):2285]. *Nucleic Acids Res.* **21,** 365–372.

Durandy, A., Taubenheim, N., Peron, S., and Fischer, A. (2007). Pathophysiology of B cell intrinsic immunoglobulin class switch recombination deficiencies. *Adv. Immunol.* **94,** 275–306.

Esser, C., and Radbruch, A. (1989). Rapid induction of transcription of unrearranged S gamma 1 switch regions in activated murine B cells by interleukin 4. *EMBO J.* **8,** 483–488.

Faili, A., Aoufouchi, S., Flatter, E., Gueranger, Q., Reynaud, C. A., and Weill, J. C. (2002). Induction of somatic hypermutation in immunoglobulin genes is dependent on DNA polymerase iota. *Nature* **419,** 944–947.

Falck, J., Coates, J., and Jackson, S. P. (2005). Conserved modes of recruitment of ATM, ATR and DNA-PKcs to sites of DNA damage. *Nature* **434,** 605–611.

Franco, S., Alt, F. W., and Manis, J. P. (2006a). Pathways that suppress programmed DNA breaks from progressing to chromosomal breaks and translocations. *DNA Repair (Amst.)* **5,** 1030–1041.

Franco, S., Gostissa, M., Zha, S., Lombard, D. B., Murphy, M. M., Zarrin, A. A., Yan, C., Tepsuporn, S., Morales, J. C., Adams, M. M., Lou, Z., Bassing, C. H., *et al.* (2006b). H2AX prevents DNA breaks from progressing to chromosome breaks and translocations. *Mol. Cell* **21,** 201–214.

Frank, K. M., Sekiguchi, J. M., Seidl, K. J., Swat, W., Rathbun, G. A., Cheng, H. L., Davidson, L., Kangaloo, L., and Alt, F. W. (1998). Late embryonic lethality and impaired V(D)J recombination in mice lacking DNA ligase IV. *Nature* **396,** 173–177.

Gaidano, G., Pasqualucci, L., Capello, D., Berra, E., Deambrogi, C., Rossi, D., Maria Larocca, L., Gloghini, A., Carbone, A., and Dalla-Favera, R. (2003). Aberrant somatic hypermutation in multiple subtypes of AIDS-associated non-Hodgkin lymphoma. *Blood* **102,** 1833–1841.

Gao, Y., Chaudhuri, J., Zhu, C., Davidson, L., Weaver, D. T., and Alt, F. W. (1998a). A targeted DNA-PKcs-null mutation reveals DNA-PK-independent functions for KU in V(D)J recombination. *Immunity* **9,** 367–376.

Gao, Y., Sun, Y., Frank, K. M., Dikkes, P., Fujiwara, Y., Seidl, K. J., Sekiguchi, J. M., Rathbun, G. A., Swat, W., Wang, J., Bronson, R. T., Malynn, B. A., *et al.* (1998b). A critical role for DNA end-joining proteins in both lymphogenesis and neurogenesis. *Cell* **95,** 891–902.

Gearhart, P. J., and Bogenhagen, D. F. (1983). Clusters of point mutations are found exclusively around rearranged antibody variable genes. *Proc. Natl. Acad. Sci. USA* **80,** 3439–3443.

Griffiths, G. M., Berek, C., Kaartinen, M., and Milstein, C. (1984). Somatic mutation and the maturation of immune response to 2-phenyl oxazolone. *Nature* **312,** 271–275.

Goodman, M. F., Scharff, M. D., and Romesberg, F. E. (2007). AID-initiated purposeful mutations in immunoglobulin genes. *Adv. Immunol.* **94,** 127–155.

Gordon, M. S., Kanegai, C. M., Doerr, J. R., and Wall, R. (2003). Somatic hypermutation of the B cell receptor genes B29 (Igbeta, CD79b) and mb1 (Igalpha, CD79a). *Proc. Natl. Acad. Sci. USA* **100,** 4126–4131.

Gourzi, P., Leonova, T., and Papavasiliou, F. N. (2006). A role for activation-induced cytidine deaminase in the host response against a transforming retrovirus. *Immunity* **24,** 779–786.

Gu, H., Zou, Y. R., and Rajewsky, K. (1993). Independent control of immunoglobulin switch recombination at individual switch regions evidenced through Cre-loxP-mediated gene targeting. *Cell* **73,** 1155–1164.

Harris, R. S., Petersen-Mahrt, S. K., and Neuberger, M. S. (2002a). RNA editing enzyme APOBEC1 and some of its homologs can act as DNA mutators. *Mol. Cell* **10,** 1247–1253.
Harris, R. S., Sale, J. E., Petersen-Mahrt, S. K., and Neuberger, M. S. (2002b). AID is essential for immunoglobulin V gene conversion in a cultured B cell line. *Curr. Biol.* **12,** 435–438.
Hodgkin, P. D., Lee, J. H., and Lyons, A. B. (1996). B cell differentiation and isotype switching is related to division cycle number. *J. Exp. Med.* **184,** 277–281.
Honjo, T., and Kataoka, T. (1978). Organization of immunoglobulin heavy chain genes and allelic deletion model. *Proc. Natl. Acad. Sci. USA* **75,** 2140–2144.
Honjo, T., Kinoshita, K., and Muramatsu, M. (2002). Molecular mechanism of class switch recombination: Linkage with somatic hypermutation. *Annu. Rev. Immunol.* **20,** 165–196.
Honjo, T., Nagaoka, H., Shinkura, R., and Muramatsu, M. (2005). AID to overcome the limitations of genomic information. *Nat. Immunol.* **6,** 655–661.
Huyen, Y., Zgheib, O., Ditullio, R. A., Jr., Gorgoulis, V. G., Zacharatos, P., Petty, T. J., Sheston, E. A., Mellert, H. S., Stavridi, E. S., and Halazonetis, T. D. (2004). Methylated lysine 79 of histone H3 targets 53BP1 to DNA double-strand breaks. *Nature* **432,** 406–411.
Imai, K., Slupphaug, G., Lee, W. I., Revy, P., Nonoyama, S., Catalan, N., Yel, L., Forveille, M., Kavli, B., Krokan, H. E., Ochs, H. D., Fischer, A., *et al.* (2003). Human uracil-DNA glycosylase deficiency associated with profoundly impaired immunoglobulin class-switch recombination. *Nat. Immunol.* **4,** 1023–1028.
Inlay, M. A., Gao, H. H., Odegard, V. H., Lin, T., Schatz, D. G., and Xu, Y. (2006). Roles of the Ig kappa light chain intronic and 3′ enhancers in Igk somatic hypermutation. *J. Immunol.* **177,** 1146–1151.
Iwasato, T., Shimizu, A., Honjo, T., and Yamagishi, H. (1990). Circular DNA is excised by immunoglobulin class switch recombination. *Cell* **62,** 143–149.
Jabara, H. H., Loh, R., Ramesh, N., Vercelli, D., and Geha, R. S. (1993). Sequential switching from mu to epsilon via gamma 4 in human B cells stimulated with IL-4 and hydrocortisone. *J. Immunol.* **151,** 4528–4533.
Jung, D., and Alt, F. W. (2004). Unraveling V(D)J recombination: Insights into gene regulation. *Cell* **116,** 299–311.
Jung, D., Giallourakis, C., Mostoslavsky, R., and Alt, F. W. (2006). Mechanism and control of V(D)J recombination at the immunoglobulin heavy chain locus. *Annu. Rev. Immunol.* **24,** 541–570.
Jung, S., Rajewsky, K., and Radbruch, A. (1993). Shutdown of class switch recombination by deletion of a switch region control element. *Science* **259,** 984–987.
Kataoka, T., Miyata, T., and Honjo, T. (1981). Repetitive sequences in class-switch recombination regions of immunoglobulin heavy chain genes. *Cell* **23,** 357–368.
Kavli, B., Andersen, S., Otterlei, M., Liabakk, N. B., Imai, K., Fischer, A., Durandy, A., Krokan, H. E., and Slupphaug, G. (2005). B cells from hyper-IgM patients carrying UNG mutations lack ability to remove uracil from ssDNA and have elevated genomic uracil. *J. Exp. Med.* **201,** 2011–2021.
Kearney, J. F., and Lawton, A. R. (1975). B lymphocyte differentiation induced by lipopolysaccharide. I. Generation of cells synthesizing four major immunoglobulin classes. *J. Immunol.* **115,** 671–676.
Kearney, J. F., Cooper, M. D., and Lawton, A. R. (1976). B cell differentiation induced by lipopolysaccharide. IV. Development of immunoglobulin class restriction in precursors of IgG-synthesizing cells. *J. Immunol.* **117,** 1567–1572.
Kenter, A. L. (2005). Class switch recombination: An emerging mechanism. *Curr. Top. Microbiol. Immunol.* **290,** 171–199.

Kepron, M. R., Chen, Y. W., Uhr, J. W., and Vitetta, E. S. (1989). IL-4 induces the specific rearrangement of gamma 1 genes on the expressed and unexpressed chromosomes of lipopolysaccharide-activated normal murine B cells. *J. Immunol.* **143,** 334–339.

Khamlichi, A. A., Glaudet, F., Oruc, Z., Denis, V., Le Bert, M., and Cogne, M. (2004). Immunoglobulin class-switch recombination in mice devoid of any S mu tandem repeat. *Blood* **103,** 3828–3836.

Kinoshita, K., Lee, C. G., Tashiro, J., Muramatsu, M., Chen, X. C., Yoshikawa, K., and Honjo, T. (1999). Molecular mechanism of immunoglobulin class switch recombination. *Cold Spring Harb. Symp. Quant. Biol.* **64,** 217–226.

Kobayashi, J., Tauchi, H., Sakamoto, S., Nakamura, A., Morishima, K., Matsuura, S., Kobayashi, T., Tamai, K., Tanimoto, K., and Komatsu, K. (2002). NBS1 localizes to gamma-H2AX foci through interaction with the FHA/BRCT domain. *Curr. Biol.* **12,** 1846–1851.

Kotani, A., Okazaki, I. M., Muramatsu, M., Kinoshita, K., Begum, N. A., Nakajima, T., Saito, H., and Honjo, T. (2005). A target selection of somatic hypermutations is regulated similarly between T and B cells upon activation-induced cytidine deaminase expression. *Proc. Natl. Acad. Sci. USA* **102,** 4506–4511.

Kracker, S., Bergmann, Y., Demuth, I., Frappart, P. O., Hildebrand, G., Christine, R., Wang, Z. Q., Sperling, K., Digweed, M., and Radbruch, A. (2005). Nibrin functions in Ig class-switch recombination. *Proc. Natl. Acad. Sci. USA* **102,** 1584–1589.

Kurimasa, A., Ouyang, H., Dong, L. J., Wang, S., Li, X., Cordon-Cardo, C., Chen, D. J., and Li, G. C. (1999). Catalytic subunit of DNA-dependent protein kinase: Impact on lymphocyte development and tumorigenesis. *Proc. Natl. Acad. Sci. USA* **96,** 1403–1408.

Kuzin, I. I., Ugine, G. D., Wu, D., Young, F., Chen, J., and Bottaro, A. (2000). Normal isotype switching in B cells lacking the I mu exon splice donor site: Evidence for multiple I mu-like germline transcripts. *J. Immunol.* **164,** 1451–1457.

Lahdesmaki, A., Taylor, A. M., Chrzanowska, K. H., and Pan-Hammarstrom, Q. (2004). Delineation of the role of the Mre11 complex in class switch recombination. *J. Biol. Chem.* **279,** 16479–16487.

Larson, E. D., Duquette, M. L., Cummings, W. J., Streiff, R. J., and Maizels, N. (2005). MutSalpha binds to and promotes synapsis of transcriptionally activated immunoglobulin switch regions. *Curr. Biol.* **15,** 470–474.

Lebecque, S. G., and Gearhart, P. J. (1990). Boundaries of somatic mutation in rearranged immunoglobulin genes: 5' boundary is near the promoter, and 3' boundary is approximately 1 kb from V(D)J gene. *J. Exp. Med.* **172,** 1717–1727.

Lee, G. S., Brandt, V. L., and Roth, D. B. (2004a). B cell development leads off with a base hit: dU:dG mismatches in class switching and hypermutation. *Mol. Cell* **16,** 505–508.

Lee, G. S., Neiditch, M. B., Salus, S. S., and Roth, D. B. (2004b). RAG proteins shepherd double-strand breaks to a specific pathway, suppressing error-prone repair, but RAG nicking initiates homologous recombination. *Cell* **117,** 171–184.

Lee, J. H., and Paull, T. T. (2005). ATM activation by DNA double-strand breaks through the Mre11-Rad50-Nbs1 complex. *Science* **308,** 551–554.

Lennon, G. G., and Perry, R. P. (1985). C mu-containing transcripts initiate heterogeneously within the IgH enhancer region and contain a novel 5'-nontranslatable exon. *Nature* **318,** 475–478.

Li, S. C., Rothman, P. B., Zhang, J., Chan, C., Hirsh, D., and Alt, F. W. (1994). Expression of I mu-C gamma hybrid germline transcripts subsequent to immunoglobulin heavy chain class switching. *Int. Immunol.* **6,** 491–497.

Li, Z., and Alt, F. W. (1996). Identification of the XRCC4 gene: Complementation of the DSBR and V(D)J recombination defects of XR-1 cells. *Curr. Top. Microbiol. Immunol.* **217**, 143–150.

Li, Z., Otevrel, T., Gao, Y., Cheng, H. L., Seed, B., Stamato, T. D., Taccioli, G. E., and Alt, F. W. (1995). The XRCC4 gene encodes a novel protein involved in DNA double-strand break repair and V(D)J recombination. *Cell* **83**, 1079–1089.

Li, Z., Woo, C. J., Iglesias-Ussel, M. D., Ronai, D., and Scharff, M. D. (2004). The generation of antibody diversity through somatic hypermutation and class switch recombination. *Genes Dev.* **18**, 1–11.

Lieber, M. R., Ma, Y., Pannicke, U., and Schwarz, K. (2003). Mechanism and regulation of human non-homologous DNA end-joining. *Nat. Rev. Mol. Cell Biol.* **4**, 712–720.

Longerich, S., Basu, U., Alt, F., and Storb, U. (2006). AID in somatic hypermutation and class switch recombination. *Curr. Opin. Immunol.* **18**, 164–174.

Lorenz, M., Jung, S., and Radbruch, A. (1995). Switch transcripts in immunoglobulin class switching. *Science* **267**, 1825–1828.

Lou, Z., Minter-Dykhouse, K., Franco, S., Gostissa, M., Rivera, M. A., Celeste, A., Manis, J. P., van Deursen, J., Nussenzweig, A., Paull, T. T., et al. (2006). MDC1 maintains genomic stability by participating in the amplification of ATM-dependent DNA damage signals. *Mol. Cell* **21**, 187–200.

Luby, T. M., Schrader, C. E., Stavnezer, J., and Selsing, E. (2001). The μ switch region tandem repeats are important, but not required, for antibody class switch recombination. *J. Exp. Med.* **193**, 159–168.

Lutzker, S., and Alt, F. W. (1988). Structure and expression of germ line immunoglobulin gamma 2b transcripts. *Mol. Cell. Biol.* **8**, 1849–1852.

Lutzker, S., Rothman, P., Pollock, R., Coffman, R., and Alt, F. W. (1988). Mitogen- and IL-4-regulated expression of germ-line Ig gamma 2b transcripts: Evidence for directed heavy chain class switching. *Cell* **53**, 177–184.

Ma, Y., Pannicke, U., Schwarz, K., and Lieber, M. R. (2002). Hairpin opening and overhang processing by an Artemis/DNA-dependent protein kinase complex in nonhomologous end joining and V(D)J recombination. *Cell* **108**, 781–794.

Maizels, N. (2005). Immunoglobulin gene diversification. *Annu. Rev. Genet.* **39**, 23–46.

Mandler, R., Chu, C. C., Paul, W. E., Max, E. E., and Snapper, C. M. (1993). Interleukin 5 induces S mu-S gamma 1 DNA rearrangement in B cells activated with dextran-anti-IgD antibodies and interleukin 4: A three component model for Ig class switching. *J. Exp. Med.* **178**, 1577–1586.

Manis, J. P., Gu, Y., Lansford, R., Sonoda, E., Ferrini, R., Davidson, L., Rajewsky, K., and Alt, F. W. (1998). Ku70 is required for late B cell development and immunoglobulin heavy chain class switching. *J. Exp. Med.* **187**, 2081–2089.

Manis, J. P., Dudley, D., Kaylor, L., and Alt, F. W. (2002a). IgH class switch recombination to IgG1 in DNA-PKcs-deficient B cells. *Immunity* **16**, 607–617.

Manis, J. P., Tian, M., and Alt, F. W. (2002b). Mechanism and control of class-switch recombination. *Trends Immunol.* **23**, 31–39.

Manis, J. P., Morales, J. C., Xia, Z., Kutok, J. L., Alt, F. W., and Carpenter, P. B. (2004). 53BP1 links DNA damage-response pathways to immunoglobulin heavy chain class-switch recombination. *Nat. Immunol.* **5**, 481–487.

Martin, A., Bardwell, P. D., Woo, C. J., Fan, M., Shulman, M. J., and Scharff, M. D. (2002). Activation-induced cytidine deaminase turns on somatic hypermutation in hybridomas. *Nature* **415**, 802–806.

Martomo, S. A., and Gearhart, P. J. (2006). Somatic hypermutation: Subverted DNA repair. *Curr. Opin. Immunol.* **18**, 243–248.

Matsunaga, T., Park, C. H., Bessho, T., Mu, D., and Sancar, A. (1996). Replication protein A confers structure-specific endonuclease activities to the XPF-ERCC1 and XPG subunits of human DNA repair excision nuclease. *J. Biol. Chem.* **271**, 11047–11050.

Matsuoka, M., Yoshida, K., Maeda, T., Usuda, S., and Sakano, H. (1990). Switch circular DNA formed in cytokine-treated mouse splenocytes: Evidence for intramolecular DNA deletion in immunoglobulin class switching. *Cell* **62**, 135–142.

McBride, K. M., Barreto, V., Ramiro, A. R., Stavropoulos, P., and Nussenzweig, M. C. (2004). Somatic hypermutation is limited by CRM1-dependent nuclear export of activation-induced deaminase. *J. Exp. Med.* **199**, 1235–1244.

McBride, K. M., Gazumyan, A., Woo, E. M., Barreto, V. M., Robbiani, D. F., Chait, B. T., and Nussenzweig, M. C. (2006). Regulation of hypermutation by activation-induced cytidine deaminase phosphorylation. *Proc. Natl. Acad. Sci. USA* **103**, 8798–8803.

McKean, D., Huppi, K., Bell, M., Staudt, L., Gerhard, W., and Weigert, M. (1984). Generation of antibody diversity in the immune response of BALB/c mice to influenza virus hemagglutinin. *Proc. Natl. Acad. Sci. USA* **81**, 3180–3184.

Michael, N., Martin, T. E., Nicolae, D., Kim, N., Padjen, K., Zhan, P., Nguyen, H., Pinkert, C., and Storb, U. (2002). Effects of sequence and structure on the hypermutability of immunoglobulin genes. *Immunity* **16**, 123–134.

Michael, N., Shen, H. M., Longerich, S., Kim, N., Longacre, A., and Storb, U. (2003). The E box motif CAGGTG enhances somatic hypermutation without enhancing transcription. *Immunity* **19**, 235–242.

Mills, K. D., Ferguson, D. O., Essers, J., Eckersdorff, M., Kanaar, R., and Alt, F. W. (2004). Rad54 and DNA Ligase IV cooperate to maintain mammalian chromatid stability. *Genes Dev.* **18**, 1283–1292.

Min, I. M., and Selsing, E. (2005). Antibody class switch recombination: Roles for switch sequences and mismatch repair proteins. *Adv. Immunol.* **87**, 297–328.

Mizuta, R., Iwai, K., Shigeno, M., Mizuta, M., Uemura, T., Ushiki, T., and Kitamura, D. (2003). Molecular visualization of immunoglobulin switch region RNA/DNA complex by atomic force microscope. *J. Biol. Chem.* **278**, 4431–4434.

Montesinos-Rongen, M., Van Roost, D., Schaller, C., Wiestler, O. D., and Deckert, M. (2004). Primary diffuse large B-cell lymphomas of the central nervous system are targeted by aberrant somatic hypermutation. *Blood* **103**, 1869–1875.

Morales, J. C., Xia, Z., Lu, T., Aldrich, M. B., Wang, B., Rosales, C., Kellems, R. E., Hittelman, W. N., Elledge, S. J., and Carpenter, P. B. (2003). Role for the BRCA1 C-terminal repeats (BRCT) protein 53BP1 in maintaining genomic stability. *J. Biol. Chem.* **278**, 14971–14977.

Muramatsu, M., Sankaranand, V. S., Anant, S., Sugai, M., Kinoshita, K., Davidson, N. O., and Honjo, T. (1999). Specific expression of activation-induced cytidine deaminase (AID), a novel member of the RNA-editing deaminase family in germinal center B cells. *J. Biol. Chem.* **274**, 18470–18476.

Muramatsu, M., Kinoshita, K., Fagarasan, S., Yamada, S., Shinkai, Y., and Honjo, T. (2000). Class switch recombination and hypermutation require activation-induced cytidine deaminase (AID), a potential RNA editing enzyme. *Cell* **102**, 553–563.

Muramatsu, M., Nagaoka, H., Shinkura, R., Begum, N. A., and Honjo, T. (2007). Discovery of activation-induced cytidine deaminase, the engraver of antibody memory. *Adv. Immunol.* **94**, 1–36.

Muschen, M., Re, D., Jungnickel, B., Diehl, V., Rajewsky, K., and Kuppers, R. (2000). Somatic mutation of the CD95 gene in human B cells as a side-effect of the germinal center reaction. *J. Exp. Med.* **192**, 1833–1840.

Mussmann, R., Courtet, M., Schwager, J., and Du Pasquier, L. (1997). Microsites for immunoglobulin switch recombination breakpoints from *Xenopus* to mammals. *Eur. J. Immunol.* **27**, 2610–2619.

Muto, T., Okazaki, I. M., Yamada, S., Tanaka, Y., Kinoshita, K., Muramatsu, M., Nagaoka, H., and Honjo, T. (2006). Negative regulation of activation-induced cytidine deaminase in B cells. *Proc. Natl. Acad. Sci. USA* **103**, 2752–2757.

Nagaoka, H., Muramatsu, M., Yamamura, N., Kinoshita, K., and Honjo, T. (2002). Activation-induced deaminase (AID)-directed hypermutation in the immunoglobulin smicro region: Implication of AID involvement in a common step of class switch recombination and somatic hypermutation. *J. Exp. Med.* **195**, 529–534.

Nambu, Y., Sugai, M., Gonda, H., Lee, C. G., Katakai, T., Agata, Y., Yokota, Y., and Shimizu, A. (2003). Transcription-coupled events associating with immunoglobulin switch region chromatin. *Science* **302**, 2137–2140.

Neuberger, M. S., and Scott, J. (2000). Immunology. RNA editing AIDs antibody diversification? *Science* **289**, 1705–1706.

Neuberger, M. S., Di Noia, J. M., Beale, R. C., Williams, G. T., Yang, Z., and Rada, C. (2005). Somatic hypermutation at A.T pairs: Polymerase error versus dUTP incorporation. *Nat. Rev. Immunol.* **5**, 171–178.

Nicolas, N., Moshous, D., Cavazzana-Calvo, M., Papadopoulo, D., de Chasseval, R., Le Deist, F., Fischer, A., and de Villartay, J. P. (1998). A human severe combined immunodeficiency (SCID) condition with increased sensitivity to ionizing radiations and impaired V(D)J rearrangements defines a new DNA recombination/repair deficiency. *J. Exp. Med.* **188**, 627–634.

Nikaido, T., Yamawaki-Kataoka, Y., and Honjo, T. (1982). Nucleotide sequences of switch regions of immunoglobulin C epsilon and C gamma genes and their comparison. *J. Biol. Chem.* **257**, 7322–7329.

O'Brien, R. L., Brinster, R. L., and Storb, U. (1987). Somatic hypermutation of an immunoglobulin transgene in kappa transgenic mice. *Nature* **326**, 405–409.

Obata, M., Kataoka, T., Nakai, S., Yamagishi, H., Takahashi, N., Yamawaki-Kataoka, Y., Nikaido, T., Shimizu, A., and Honjo, T. (1981). Structure of a rearranged gamma 1 chain gene and its implication to immunoglobulin class-switch mechanism. *Proc. Natl. Acad. Sci. USA* **78**, 2437–2441.

Odegard, V. H., and Schatz, D. G. (2006). Targeting of somatic hypermutation. *Nat. Rev. Immunol.* **6**, 573–583.

Okazaki, I. M., Kinoshita, K., Muramatsu, M., Yoshikawa, K., and Honjo, T. (2002). The AID enzyme induces class switch recombination in fibroblasts. *Nature* **416**, 340–345.

Okazaki, I. M., Hiai, H., Kakazu, N., Yamada, S., Muramatsu, M., Kinoshita, K., and Honjo, T. (2003). Constitutive expression of AID leads to tumorigenesis. *J. Exp. Med.* **197**, 1173–1181.

Pan-Hammarstrom, Q., Jones, A. M., Lahdesmaki, A., Zhou, W., Gatti, R. A., Hammarstrom, L., Gennery, A. R., and Ehrenstein, M. R. (2005). Impact of DNA ligase IV on nonhomologous end joining pathways during class switch recombination in human cells. *J. Exp. Med.* **201**, 189–194.

Papavasiliou, F. N., and Schatz, D. G. (2002a). Somatic hypermutation of immunoglobulin genes: Merging mechanisms for genetic diversity. *Cell* **109**, S35–S44.

Papavasiliou, F. N., and Schatz, D. G. (2002b). The activation-induced deaminase functions in a postcleavage step of the somatic hypermutation process. *J. Exp. Med.* **195**, 1193–1198.

Pasqualucci, L., Migliazza, A., Fracchiolla, N., William, C., Neri, A., Baldini, L., Chaganti, R. S., Klein, U., Kuppers, R., Rajewsky, K., et al. (1998). BCL-6 mutations in normal germinal center B cells: Evidence of somatic hypermutation acting outside Ig loci. Proc. Natl. Acad. Sci. USA **95**, 11816–11821.

Pasqualucci, L., Neumeister, P., Goossens, T., Nanjangud, G., Chaganti, R. S., Kuppers, R., and Dalla-Favera, R. (2001). Hypermutation of multiple proto-oncogenes in B-cell diffuse large-cell lymphomas. Nature **412**, 341–346.

Pasqualucci, L., Guglielmino, R., Houldsworth, J., Mohr, J., Aoufouchi, S., Polakiewicz, R., Chaganti, R. S., and Dalla-Favera, R. (2004). Expression of the AID protein in normal and neoplastic B cells. Blood **104**, 3318–3325.

Pasqualucci, L., Kitaura, Y., Gu, H., and Dalla-Favera, R. (2006). From the cover: PKA-mediated phosphorylation regulates the function of activation-induced deaminase (AID) in B cells. Proc. Natl. Acad. Sci. USA **103**, 395–400.

Paull, T. T., Rogakou, E. P., Yamazaki, V., Kirchgessner, C. U., Gellert, M., and Bonner, W. M. (2000). A critical role for histone H2AX in recruitment of repair factors to nuclear foci after DNA damage. Curr. Biol. **10**, 886–895.

Pech, M., Hochtl, J., Schnell, H., and Zachau, H. G. (1981). Differences between germ-line and rearranged immunoglobulin V kappa coding sequences suggest a localized mutation mechanism. Nature **291**, 668–670.

Peng, H. Z., Du, M. Q., Koulis, A., Aiello, A., Dogan, A., Pan, L. X., and Isaacson, P. G. (1999). Nonimmunoglobulin gene hypermutation in germinal center B cells. Blood **93**, 2167–2172.

Perlot, T., Alt, F. W., Bassing, C. H., Suh, H., and Pinaud, E. (2005). Elucidation of IgH intronic enhancer functions via germ-line deletion. Proc. Natl. Acad. Sci. USA **102**, 14362–14367.

Peters, A., and Storb, U. (1996). Somatic hypermutation of immunoglobulin genes is linked to transcription initiation. Immunity **4**, 57–65.

Petersen, S., Casellas, R., Reina-San-Martin, B., Chen, H. T., Difilippantonio, M. J., Wilson, P. C., Hanitsch, L., Celeste, A., Muramatsu, M., Pilch, D. R., Redon, C., Ried, T., et al. (2001). AID is required to initiate Nbs1/gamma-H2AX focus formation and mutations at sites of class switching. Nature **414**, 660–665.

Petersen-Mahrt, S. (2005). DNA deamination in immunity. Immunol. Rev. **203**, 80–97.

Petersen-Mahrt, S. K., Harris, R. S., and Neuberger, M. S. (2002). AID mutates E. coli suggesting a DNA deamination mechanism for antibody diversification. Nature **418**, 99–103.

Pham, P., Bransteitter, R., Petruska, J., and Goodman, M. F. (2003). Processive AID-catalysed cytosine deamination on single-stranded DNA simulates somatic hypermutation. Nature **424**, 103–107.

Pinaud, E., Khamlichi, A. A., Le Morvan, C., Drouet, M., Nalesso, V., Le Bert, M., and Cogne, M. (2001). Localization of the 3′ IgH locus elements that effect long-distance regulation of class switch recombination. Immunity **15**, 187–199.

Povirk, L. F. (2006). Biochemical mechanisms of chromosomal translocations resulting from DNA double-strand breaks. DNA Repair (Amst) **5**, 1199–1212.

Prochnow, C., Bransteitter, R., Klein, M. G., Goodman, M. F., and Chen, X. S. (2007). The APOBEC-2 crystal structure and functional implications for the deaminase AID. Nature **445**, 447–451.

Qiu, G., Harriman, G. R., and Stavnezer, J. (1999). Ialpha exon-replacement mice synthesize a spliced HPRT-C(alpha) transcript which may explain their ability to switch to IgA. Inhibition of switching to IgG in these mice. Int. Immunol. **11**, 37–46.

Rada, C., Gonzalez-Fernandez, A., Jarvis, J. M., and Milstein, C. (1994). The 5′ boundary of somatic hypermutation in a V kappa gene is in the leader intron. Eur. J. Immunol. **24**, 1453–1457.

Rada, C., Jarvis, J. M., and Milstein, C. (2002a). AID-GFP chimeric protein increases hypermutation of Ig genes with no evidence of nuclear localization. *Proc. Natl. Acad. Sci. USA* **99**, 7003–7008.
Rada, C., Williams, G. T., Nilsen, H., Barnes, D. E., Lindahl, T., and Neuberger, M. S. (2002b). Immunoglobulin isotype switching is inhibited and somatic hypermutation perturbed in UNG-deficient mice. *Curr. Biol.* **12**, 1748–1755.
Rada, C., Di Noia, J. M., and Neuberger, M. S. (2004). Mismatch recognition and uracil excision provide complementary paths to both Ig switching and the A/T-focused phase of somatic mutation. *Mol. Cell* **16**, 163–171.
Rajewsky, K. (1996). Clonal selection and learning in the antibody system. *Nature* **381**, 751–758.
Ramiro, A. R., Stavropoulos, P., Jankovic, M., and Nussenzweig, M. C. (2003). Transcription enhances AID-mediated cytidine deamination by exposing single-stranded DNA on the nontemplate strand. *Nat. Immunol.* **4**, 452–456.
Ramiro, A. R., Jankovic, M., Eisenreich, T., Difilippantonio, S., Chen-Kiang, S., Muramatsu, M., Honjo, T., Nussenzweig, A., and Nussenzweig, M. C. (2004). AID is required for c-myc/IgH chromosome translocations *in vivo*. *Cell* **118**, 431–438.
Ramiro, A. R., Jankovic, M., Callen, E., Difilippantonio, S., Chen, H. T., McBride, K. M., Eisenreich, T. R., Chen, J., Dickins, R. A., Lowe, S. W., *et al.* (2006). Role of genomic instability and p53 in AID-induced c-myc-Igh translocations. *Nature* **440**(7080), 105–109.
Ramiro, A. R., San-Martin, B. R., McBride, K., Jankovic, M., Barreto, V., Nussenzweig, A., and Nussenzweig, M. C. (2007). The role of activation induced deaminase in antibody diversification and chromosome translocations. *Adv. Immunol.* **94**, 75–107.
Rappold, I., Iwabuchi, K., Date, T., and Chen, J. (2001). Tumor suppressor p53 binding protein 1 (53BP1) is involved in DNA damage-signaling pathways. *J. Cell Biol.* **153**, 613–620.
Reaban, M. E., and Griffin, J. A. (1990). Induction of RNA-stabilized DNA conformers by transcription of an immunoglobulin switch region. *Nature* **348**, 342–344.
Reaban, M. E., Lebowitz, J., and Griffin, J. A. (1994). Transcription induces the formation of a stable RNA.DNA hybrid in the immunoglobulin alpha switch region. *J. Biol. Chem.* **269**, 21850–21857.
Reina-San-Martin, B., Difilippantonio, S., Hanitsch, L., Masilamani, R. F., Nussenzweig, A., and Nussenzweig, M. C. (2003). H2AX is required for recombination between immunoglobulin switch regions but not for intra-switch region recombination or somatic hypermutation. *J. Exp. Med.* **197**, 1767–1778.
Reina-San-Martin, B., Chen, H. T., Nussenzweig, A., and Nussenzweig, M. C. (2004). ATM is required for efficient recombination between immunoglobulin switch regions. *J. Exp. Med.* **200**, 1103–1110.
Reina-San-Martin, B., Nussenzweig, M. C., Nussenzweig, A., and Difilippantonio, S. (2005). Genomic instability, endoreduplication, and diminished Ig class-switch recombination in B cells lacking Nbs1. *Proc. Natl. Acad. Sci. USA* **102**, 1590–1595.
Reina-San-Martin, B., Chen, J., Nussenzweig, A., and Nussenzweig, M. C. (2007). Enhanced intra-switch region recombination during immunoglobulin class switch recombination in 53BP1(−/−) B cells. *Eur. J. Immunol.* **37**, 235–239.
Revy, P., Muto, T., Levy, Y., Geissmann, F., Plebani, A., Sanal, O., Catalan, N., Forveille, M., Dufourcq-Labelouse, R., Gennery, A., Tezcan, I., Ersoy, F., *et al.* (2000). Activation-induced cytidine deaminase (AID) deficiency causes the autosomal recessive form of the Hyper-IgM syndrome (HIGM2). *Cell* **102**, 565–575.
Rogakou, E. P., Pilch, D. R., Orr, A. H., Ivanova, V. S., and Bonner, W. M. (1998). DNA double-stranded breaks induce histone H2AX phosphorylation on serine 139. *J. Biol. Chem.* **273**, 5858–5868.

Rogakou, E. P., Boon, C., Redon, C., and Bonner, W. M. (1999). Megabase chromatin domains involved in DNA double-strand breaks *in vivo*. *J. Cell Biol.* **146**, 905–916.

Rogozin, I. B., and Diaz, M. (2004). Cutting edge: DGYW/WRCH is a better predictor of mutability at G:C bases in Ig hypermutation than the widely accepted RGYW/WRCY motif and probably reflects a two-step activation-induced cytidine deaminase-triggered process. *J. Immunol.* **172**, 3382–3384.

Rogozin, I. B., and Kolchanov, N. A. (1992). Somatic hypermutagenesis in immunoglobulin genes. II. Influence of neighbouring base sequences on mutagenesis. *Biochim. Biophys. Acta* **1171**, 11–18.

Rolink, A., Melchers, F., and Andersson, J. (1996). The SCID but not the RAG-2 gene product is required for S mu-S epsilon heavy chain class switching. *Immunity* **5**, 319–330.

Ronai, D., Iglesias-Ussel, M. D., Fan, M., Shulman, M. J., and Scharff, M. D. (2005). Complex regulation of somatic hypermutation by cis-acting sequences in the endogenous IgH gene in hybridoma cells. *Proc. Natl. Acad. Sci. USA* **102**, 11829–11834.

Ronai, D., Iglesias-Ussel, M. D., Fan, M., Li, Z., Martin, A., and Scharff, M. D. (2007). Detection of chromatin-associated single-stranded DNA in regions targeted for somatic hypermutation. *J. Exp. Med.* **204**, 181–190.

Rooney, S., Sekiguchi, J., Zhu, C., Chen, H. L., Manis, J. P., Whitlow, S., Devido, J., Foy, D., Lombard, D., and Alt, F. W. (2002). "Leaky" Scid phenotype associated with defective V(D)J coding end processing in Artemis-deficient mice. *Mol. Cell* **10**, 1379–1390.

Rooney, S., Chaudhuri, J., and Alt, F. W. (2004). The role of the non-homologous end-joining pathway in lymphocyte development. *Immunol. Rev.* **200**, 115–131.

Rooney, S., Alt, F. W., Sekiguchi, J., and Manis, J. P. (2005). Artemis-independent functions of DNA-dependent protein kinase in Ig heavy chain class switch recombination and development. *Proc. Natl. Acad. Sci. USA* **102**, 2471–2475.

Rosenberg, B. R., and Papavasiliou, F. N. (2007). Beyond SHM and CSR: AID and related cytidine deaminases in the host response to viral infection. *Adv. Immunol.* **94**, 215–244.

Roth, D. B., Porter, T. N., and Wilson, J. H. (1985). Mechanisms of nonhomologous recombination in mammalian cells. *Mol. Cell. Biol.* **5**, 2599–2607.

Rothenfluh, H. S., Blanden, R. V., and Steele, E. J. (1995). Evolution of V genes: DNA sequence structure of functional germline genes and pseudogenes. *Immunogenetics* **42**, 159–171.

Rothman, P., Lutzker, S., Cook, W., Coffman, R., and Alt, F. W. (1988). Mitogen plus interleukin 4 induction of C epsilon transcripts in B lymphoid cells. *J. Exp. Med.* **168**, 2385–2389.

Rouet, P., Smih, F., and Jasin, M. (1994). Introduction of double-strand breaks into the genome of mouse cells by expression of a rare-cutting endonuclease. *Mol. Cell. Biol.* **14**, 8096–8106.

Sablitzky, F., Weisbaum, D., and Rajewsky, K. (1985). Sequence analysis of non-expressed immunoglobulin heavy chain loci in clonally related, somatically mutated hybridoma cells. *EMBO J.* **4**, 3435–3437.

Sakano, H., Maki, R., Kurosawa, Y., Roeder, W., and Tonegawa, S. (1980). Two types of somatic recombination are necessary for the generation of complete immunoglobulin heavy-chain genes. *Nature* **286**, 676–683.

Schatz, D. G., and Spanopoulou, E. (2005). Biochemistry of V(D)J recombination. *Curr. Top. Microbiol. Immunol.* **290**, 49–85.

Schrader, C. E., Bradley, S. P., Vardo, J., Mochegova, S. N., Flanagan, E., and Stavnezer, J. (2003). Mutations occur in the Ig Smu region but rarely in Sgamma regions prior to class switch recombination. *EMBO J.* **22**, 5893–5903.

Schrader, C. E., Linehan, E. K., Mochegova, S. N., Woodland, R. T., and Stavnezer, J. (2005). Inducible DNA breaks in Ig S regions are dependent on AID and UNG. *J. Exp. Med.* **202**, 561–568.

Seidl, K. J., Bottaro, A., Vo, A., Zhang, J., Davidson, L., and Alt, F. W. (1998). An expressed neo(r) cassette provides required functions of the 1gamma2b exon for class switching. *Int. Immunol.* **10**, 1683–1692.

Sekiguchi, J. M., and Ferguson, D. O. (2006). DNA double-strand break repair: A relentless hunt uncovers new prey. *Cell* **124**, 260–262.

Sekiguchi, J., Ferguson, D. O., Chen, H. T., Yang, E. M., Earle, J., Frank, K., Whitlow, S., Gu, Y., Xu, Y., Nussenzweig, A., and Alt, F. W. (2001). Genetic interactions between ATM and the nonhomologous end-joining factors in genomic stability and development. *Proc. Natl. Acad. Sci. USA* **98**, 3243–3248.

Sen, D., and Gilbert, W. (1988). Formation of parallel four-stranded complexes by guanine-rich motifs in DNA and its implications for meiosis. *Nature* **334**, 364–366.

Sen, R., and Oltz, E. (2006). Genetic and epigenetic regulation of IgH gene assembly. *Curr. Opin. Immunol.* **18**, 237–242.

Severinson, E., Fernandez, C., and Stavnezer, J. (1990). Induction of germ-line immunoglobulin heavy chain transcripts by mitogens and interleukins prior to switch recombination. *Eur. J. Immunol.* **20**, 1079–1084.

Sharpe, M. J., Milstein, C., Jarvis, J. M., and Neuberger, M. S. (1991). Somatic hypermutation of immunoglobulin kappa may depend on sequences $3'$ of C kappa and occurs on passenger transgenes. *EMBO J.* **10**, 2139–2145.

Shen, H. M., and Storb, U. (2004). Activation-induced cytidine deaminase (AID) can target both DNA strands when the DNA is supercoiled. *Proc. Natl. Acad. Sci. USA* **101**, 12997–13002.

Shen, H. M., Peters, A., Baron, B., Zhu, X., and Storb, U. (1998). Mutation of BCL-6 gene in normal B cells by the process of somatic hypermutation of Ig genes. *Science* **280**, 1750–1752.

Shen, H. M., Michael, N., Kim, N., and Storb, U. (2000). The TATA binding protein, c-Myc and survivin genes are not somatically hypermutated, while Ig and BCL6 genes are hypermutated in human memory B cells. *Int. Immunol.* **12**, 1085–1093.

Shiloh, Y. (2003). ATM and related protein kinases: Safeguarding genome integrity. *Nat. Rev. Cancer* **3**, 155–168.

Shinkura, R., Tian, M., Smith, M., Chua, K., Fujiwara, Y., and Alt, F. W. (2003). The influence of transcriptional orientation on endogenous switch region function. *Nat. Immunol.* **4**, 435–441.

Shinkura, R., Ito, S., Begum, N. A., Nagaoka, H., Muramatsu, M., Kinoshita, K., Sakakibara, Y., Hijikata, H., and Honjo, T. (2004). Separate domains of AID are required for somatic hypermutation and class-switch recombination. *Nat. Immunol.* **5**, 707–712.

Shroff, R., Arbel-Eden, A., Pilch, D., Ira, G., Bonner, W. M., Petrini, J. H., Haber, J. E., and Lichten, M. (2004). Distribution and dynamics of chromatin modification induced by a defined DNA double-strand break. *Curr. Biol.* **14**, 1703–1711.

Snapper, C. M., Finkelman, F. D., and Paul, W. E. (1988a). Differential regulation of IgG1 and IgE synthesis by interleukin 4. *J. Exp. Med.* **167**, 183–196.

Snapper, C. M., Finkelman, F. D., and Paul, W. E. (1988b). Regulation of IgG1 and IgE production by interleukin 4. *Immunol. Rev.* **102**, 51–75.

Sohail, A., Klapacz, J., Samaranayake, M., Ullah, A., and Bhagwat, A. S. (2003). Human activation-induced cytidine deaminase causes transcription-dependent, strand-biased C to U deaminations. *Nucleic Acids Res.* **31**, 2990–2994.

Stavnezer, J. (1995). Regulation of antibody production and class switching by TGF-beta. *J. Immunol.* **155**, 1647–1651.

Stavnezer, J. (1996). Immunoglobulin class switching. *Curr. Opin. Immunol.* **8**, 199–205.

Stavnezer, J. (2000). Molecular processes that regulate class switching. *Curr. Top. Microbiol. Immunol.* **245**, 127–168.

Stavnezer, J., and Amemiya, C. T. (2004). Evolution of isotype switching. *Semin. Immunol.* **16**, 257–275.

Stavnezer, J., Radcliffe, G., Lin, Y. C., Nietupski, J., Berggren, L., Sitia, R., and Severinson, E. (1988). Immunoglobulin heavy-chain switching may be directed by prior induction of transcripts from constant-region genes. *Proc. Natl. Acad. Sci. USA* **85**, 7704–7708.

Stavnezer-Nordgren, J., and Sirlin, S. (1986). Specificity of immunoglobulin heavy chain switch correlates with activity of germline heavy chain genes prior to switching. *EMBO J.* **5**, 95–102.

Stewart, G. S., Wang, B., Bignell, C. R., Taylor, A. M., and Elledge, S. J. (2003). MDC1 is a mediator of the mammalian DNA damage checkpoint. *Nature* **421**, 961–966.

Stivers, J. T. (2004). Comment on "Uracil DNA glycosylase activity is dispensable for immunoglobulin class switch." *Science* **306**, 2042.

Stucki, M., and Jackson, S. P. (2006). GammaH2AX and MDC1: Anchoring the DNA-damage-response machinery to broken chromosomes. *DNA Repair (Amst.)* **5**, 534–543.

Stucki, M., Clapperton, J. A., Mohammad, D., Yaffe, M. B., Smerdon, S. J., and Jackson, S. P. (2005). MDC1 directly binds phosphorylated histone H2AX to regulate cellular responses to DNA double-strand breaks. *Cell* **123**, 1213–1226.

Ta, V. T., Nagaoka, H., Catalan, N., Durandy, A., Fischer, A., Imai, K., Nonoyama, S., Tashiro, J., Ikegawa, M., Ito, S., Kinoshita, K., Muramatsu, M., *et al.* (2003). AID mutant analyses indicate requirement for class-switch-specific cofactors. *Nat. Immunol.* **4**, 843–848.

Taccioli, G. E., Rathbun, G., Oltz, E., Stamato, T., Jeggo, P. A., and Alt, F. W. (1993). Impairment of V(D)J recombination in double-strand break repair mutants. *Science* **260**, 207–210.

Taccioli, G. E., Amatucci, A. G., Beamish, H. J., Gell, D., Xiang, X. H., Torres Arzayus, M. I., Priestley, A., Jackson, S. P., Marshak Rothstein, S. P., Jeggo, P. A., and Herrera, V. L. (1998). Targeted disruption of the catalytic subunit of the DNA-PK gene in mice confers severe combined immunodeficiency and radiosensitivity. *Immunity* **9**, 355–366.

Takahashi, N., Kataoka, T., and Honjo, T. (1980). Nucleotide sequences of class-switch recombination region of the mouse immunoglobulin gamma 2b-chain gene. *Gene* **11**, 117–127.

Tashiro, J., Kinoshita, K., and Honjo, T. (2001). Palindromic but not G-rich sequences are targets of class switch recombination. *Int. Immunol.* **13**, 495–505.

Tian, M., and Alt, F. W. (2000a). RNA editing meets DNA shuffling. *Nature* **407**, 31–33.

Tian, M., and Alt, F. W. (2000b). Transcription-induced cleavage of immunoglobulin switch regions by nucleotide excision repair nucleases *in vitro*. *J. Biol. Chem.* **275**, 24163–24172.

Tumas-Brundage, K., and Manser, T. (1997). The transcriptional promoter regulates hypermutation of the antibody heavy chain locus. *J. Exp. Med.* **185**, 239–250.

Unal, E., Arbel-Eden, A., Sattler, U., Shroff, R., Lichten, M., Haber, J. E., and Koshland, D. (2004). DNA damage response pathway uses histone modification to assemble a double-strand break-specific cohesin domain. *Mol. Cell* **16**, 991–1002.

Unniraman, S., Fugmann, S. D., and Schatz, D. G. (2004). Immunology. UNGstoppable switching. *Science* **305**, 1113–1114.

van der Stoep, N., Gorman, J. R., and Alt, F. W. (1998). Reevaluation of 3′εκαππα function in stage- and lineage-specific rearrangement and somatic hypermutation. *Immunity* **8**, 743–750.

von Schwedler, U., Jack, H. M., and Wabl, M. (1990). Circular DNA is a product of the immunoglobulin class switch rearrangement. *Nature* **345**, 452–456.

Wagner, S. D., Milstein, C., and Neuberger, M. S. (1995). Codon bias targets mutation. *Nature* **376**, 732.

Wakae, K., Magor, B. G., Saunders, H., Nagaoka, H., Kawamura, A., Kinoshita, K., Honjo, T., and Muramatsu, M. (2006). Evolution of class switch recombination function in fish activation-induced cytidine deaminase, AID. *Int. Immunol.* **18**, 41–47.

Wang, C. L., Harper, R. A., and Wabl, M. (2004). Genome-wide somatic hypermutation. *Proc. Natl. Acad. Sci. USA* **101**, 7352–7356. Epub 2004 Apr 7329.

Wang, J., Shinkura, R., Muramatsu, M., Nagaoka, H., Kinoshita, K., and Honjo, T. (2006). Identification of a specific domain required for dimerization of activation-induced cytidine deaminase. *J. Biol. Chem.* **281**, 19115–19123.

Ward, I. M., Minn, K., Jorda, K. G., and Chen, J. (2003a). Accumulation of checkpoint protein 53BP1 at DNA breaks involves its binding to phosphorylated histone H2AX. *J. Biol. Chem.* **278**, 19579–19582.

Ward, I. M., Minn, K., van Deursen, J., and Chen, J. (2003b). p53 Binding protein 53BP1 is required for DNA damage responses and tumor suppression in mice. *Mol. Cell. Biol.* **23**, 2556–2563.

Ward, I. M., Reina-San-Martin, B., Olaru, A., Minn, K., Tamada, K., Lau, J. S., Cascalho, M., Chen, L., Nussenzweig, A., Livak, F., Nussenzweig, M. C., and Chen, J. (2004). 53BP1 is required for class switch recombination. *J. Cell Biol.* **165**, 459–464.

Weinstock, D. M., Elliott, B., and Jasin, M. (2006). A model of oncogenic rearrangements: Differences between chromosomal translocation mechanisms and simple double-strand break repair. *Blood* **107**, 777–780.

Wilson, T. M., Vaisman, A., Martomo, S. A., Sullivan, P., Lan, L., Hanaoka, F., Yasui, A., Woodgate, R., and Gearhart, P. J. (2005). MSH2-MSH6 stimulates DNA polymerase eta, suggesting a role for A:T mutations in antibody genes. *J. Exp. Med.* **201**, 637–645.

Winter, D. B., Sattar, N., Mai, J. J., and Gearhart, P. J. (1997). Insertion of 2 kb of bacteriophage DNA between an immunoglobulin promoter and leader exon stops somatic hypermutation in a kappa transgene. *Mol. Immunol.* **34**, 359–366.

Wuerffel, R. A., Du, J., Thompson, R. J., and Kenter, A. L. (1997). Ig Sgamma3 DNA-specifc double strand breaks are induced in mitogen-activated B cells and are implicated in switch recombination. *J. Immunol.* **159**, 4139–4144.

Xu, Y. (2006). DNA damage: A trigger of innate immunity but a requirement for adaptive immune homeostasis. *Nat. Rev. Immunol.* **6**, 261–270.

Xue, K., Rada, C., and Neuberger, M. S. (2006). The *in vivo* pattern of AID targeting to immunoglobulin switch regions deduced from mutation spectra in msh2−/− ung−/− mice. *J. Exp. Med.* **203**, 2085–2094.

Yamazoe, M., Sonoda, E., Hochegger, H., and Takeda, S. (2004). Reverse genetic studies of the DNA damage response in the chicken B lymphocyte line DT40. *DNA Repair (Amst.)* **3**, 1175–1185.

Yancopoulos, G. D., and Alt, F. W. (1985). Developmentally controlled and tissue-specific expression of unrearranged VH gene segments. *Cell* **40**, 271–281.

Yancopoulos, G. D., and Alt, F. W. (1986). Regulation of the assembly and expression of variable-region genes. *Annu. Rev. Immunol.* **4**, 339–368.

Yancopoulos, G. D., DePinho, R. A., Zimmerman, K. A., Lutzker, S. G., Rosenberg, N., and Alt, F. W. (1986). Secondary genomic rearrangement events in pre-B cells: VHDJH replacement by a LINE-1 sequence and directed class switching. *EMBO J.* **5**, 3259–3266.

Yang, S. Y. (2007). Targeting of AID-mediated sequence diversification by cis-acting determinants. *Adv. Immunol.* **94**, 109–125.

Yelamos, J., Klix, N., Goyenechea, B., Lozano, F., Chui, Y. L., Gonzalez-Fernandez, A., Pannell, R., Neuberger, M. S., and Milstein, C. (1995). Targeting of non-Ig sequences in place of the V segment by somatic hypermutation. *Nature* **376**, 225–229.

Yoshikawa, K., Okazaki, I. M., Eto, T., Kinoshita, K., Muramatsu, M., Nagaoka, H., and Honjo, T. (2002). AID enzyme-induced hypermutation in an actively transcribed gene in fibroblasts. *Science* **296**, 2033–2036.

Yu, K., and Lieber, M. R. (2003). Nucleic acid structures and enzymes in the immunoglobulin class switch recombination mechanism. *DNA Repair (Amst.)* **2**, 1163–1174.

Yu, K., Chedin, F., Hsieh, C. L., Wilson, T. E., and Lieber, M. R. (2003). R-loops at immunoglobulin class switch regions in the chromosomes of stimulated B cells. *Nat. Immunol.* **4**, 442–451.

Yu, K., Huang, F. T., and Lieber, M. R. (2004). DNA substrate length and surrounding sequence affect the activation-induced deaminase activity at cytidine. *J. Biol. Chem.* **279**, 6496–6500. Epub 2003 Nov 6425.

Zan, H., Wu, X., Komori, A., Holloman, W. K., and Casali, P. (2003). AID-dependent generation of resected double-strand DNA breaks and recruitment of Rad52/Rad51 in somatic hypermutation. *Immunity* **18**, 727–738.

Zarrin, A. A., Alt, F. W., Chaudhuri, J., Stokes, N., Kaushal, D., Du Pasquier, L., and Tian, M. (2004). An evolutionarily conserved target motif for immunoglobulin class-switch recombination. *Nat. Immunol.* **5**, 1275–1281.

Zarrin, A. A., Tian, M., Wang, J., Borjeson, T., and Alt, F. W. (2005). Influence of switch region length on immunoglobulin class switch recombination. *Proc. Natl. Acad. Sci. USA* **102**, 2466–2470.

Zarrin, A. A., Vecchio, C. D., Tseng, E., Gleason, M., Zarrin, P., Tian, M., and Alt, F. W. (2007). Antibody class switching mediated by yeast endonuclease generated DNA breaks. *Science* **315**, 377–381.

Zhang, J., Bottaro, A., Li, S., Stewart, V., and Alt, F. W. (1993). A selective defect in IgG2b switching as a result of targeted mutation of the I gamma 2b promoter and exon. *EMBO J.* **12**, 3529–3537.

Zhu, C., Mills, K. D., Ferguson, D. O., Lee, C., Manis, J., Fleming, J., Gao, Y., Morton, C. C., and Alt, F. W. (2002). Unrepaired DNA breaks in p53-deficient cells lead to oncogenic gene amplification subsequent to translocations. *Cell* **109**, 811–821.

Beyond SHM and CSR: AID and Related Cytidine Deaminases in the Host Response to Viral Infection

Brad R. Rosenberg and F. Nina Papavasiliou

Laboratory of Lymphocyte Biology, The Rockefeller University, New York, New York

Abstract	215
1. Introduction	215
2. Evolution of the AID/APOBEC Cytidine Deaminase Family	216
3. APOBEC3: A Subfamily of Antiviral Cytidine Deaminases	217
4. AID in the Host Response to Viral Infection	229
5. Concluding Remarks	235
References	237

Abstract

As the primary effector of immunoglobulin somatic hypermutation (SHM) and class switch recombination (CSR), activation-induced cytidine deaminase (AID) serves an important function in the adaptive immune response. Recent advances have demonstrated that AID and a group of closely related cytidine deaminases, the APOBEC3 proteins, also act in the innate host response to viral infection. Antiviral activity was first attributed to APOBEC3G as a potent inhibitor of HIV. It is now apparent that the targets of the APOBEC3 proteins extend beyond HIV, with family members acting against a wide variety of viruses as well as host-encoded retrotransposable genetic elements. Although it appears to function through a different mechanism, AID also possesses antiviral properties. Independent of its antibody diversification functions, AID protects against transformation by Abelson murine leukemia virus (Ab-MLV), an oncogenic retrovirus. Additionally, AID has been implicated in the host response to other pathogenic viruses. These emerging roles for the AID/APOBEC cytidine deaminases in viral infection suggest an intriguing evolutionary connection of innate and adaptive immune mechanisms.

1. Introduction

The immune system of mammals relies on a combination of innate and adaptive mechanisms to defend the host against a wide range of pathogens. In traditional classifications, innate immunity utilizes germ line-encoded pathogen recognition receptors to identify and respond to general nonself threats, while adaptive immunity employs combinatorial and mutational strategies to generate an exceedingly diverse set of antigen receptor specificities. With the identification and characterization of V(D)J recombination, it became apparent that the receptor diversity evident in lymphocytes is brought about by regulated alterations in somatic DNA. This strategy of modifying DNA to develop adaptive host defense was again observed with the elucidation of somatic hypermutation (SHM) and class switch recombination (CSR). Both of these processes are mediated by the cytidine deaminase *activation-induced cytidine deaminase* (AID). Recent work has shown that DNA editing for host defense is not an exclusive tool of the adaptive immune system, but plays important roles in the innate system as well. AID and its related family members, the *apolipoprotein B RNA-editing catalytic component* (APOBEC) proteins, have been implicated in protecting the host from a variety of exogenous and endogenous genetic hazards, most notably viral infection, genomic retrotransposition, and viral oncogenesis. This chapter examines recent work investigating the roles of AID and APOBEC cytidine deaminases in innate host defense.

2. Evolution of the AID/APOBEC Cytidine Deaminase Family

The members of the AID/APOBEC family of cytidine deaminases all share the capacity to deaminate cytidine to uracil in single-stranded polynucleotides. They also possess significant sequence homology. In mammals, this gene family includes AID, APOBEC1, APOBEC2, and APOBEC3. Additionally, in primates, the APOBEC3 gene has undergone considerable expansion; genes in this subfamily are designated alphabetically APOBEC3A–3H.

The first family member identified was APOBEC1. This enzyme was shown to possess cytidine deaminase activity with which it specifically edits apolipoprotein B mRNA transcripts (Navaratnam *et al.*, 1993; Teng *et al.*, 1993). Several years later, AID was discovered and recognized to share significant sequence homology with APOBEC1 (Muramatsu *et al.*, 1999). As the family's "founding member," APOBEC1 was viewed as the prototypical polynucleotide cytidine deaminase. However, it was speculated that AID (or another yet to be identified gene) evolutionarily predated APOBEC1 (Neuberger and Scott, 2000) and other potential family members. As new biological roles for the AID/APOBEC family have emerged, recent work has employed rigorous phylogenetic analysis to shed new light on the evolution and adaptation of these enzymes.

Despite the ubiquity of deaminases throughout biology, the AID/APOBEC family is present only in vertebrates (Conticello *et al.*, 2005). AID and APOBEC2 are the oldest members of the gene family, with the appearance of APOBEC1 and APOBEC3 occurring significantly later in mammalian evolution. In primates, members of the AID/APOBEC gene family have undergone rapid evolution and notably strong positive selection. Across primate species, the genomic sequences of APOBEC1, -3B, -3C, -3D, -3E, and -3G show a rapid accumulation of mutations that alter protein sequence relative to synonymous substitutions, indicating a strong positive selection for adaptive mutations (Sawyer et al., 2004). Evidence of strong positive selection is often observed in genes involved in host–pathogen interactions. One can easily envision an evolutionary scenario in which a particular gene evolves to restrict an endemic pathogen. The pathogen, subjected to selective pressure, evolves a countermeasure to overcome the host defense gene. With sufficiently dire consequences for both species, beneficial mutations are rapidly selected and the genetic conflict continues. Similar evolutionary struggles are likely responsible for the high rate of positive selection observed in AID/APOBEC family members. APOBEC3G exhibits the highest rate of positive selection among observably expressed AID/APOBEC genes (and one of the highest rates throughout the human genome), implying rapid evolution in response to strong selective pressure (Sawyer et al., 2004; Zhang and Webb, 2004). As discussed below, APOBEC3G does play an important role in defense against retroviruses. Similar innate immune functions and corresponding host–pathogen conflicts may be responsible for the adaptive positive selection apparent in other family members as well.

3. APOBEC3: A Subfamily of Antiviral Cytidine Deaminases

3.1. APOBEC3G Restricts HIV Infection

A function for APOBEC3G was first recognized in the study of a complex host–pathogen interaction: HIV infection of human cells. It was known for some time that the HIV gene product virion infectivity factor (Vif) is an important determinant of successful viral replication in certain cell types. Vif-deficient viruses are unable to propagate in "nonpermissive" cells (including T cells and macrophages) in which Vif-competent viruses can establish productive infections. Despite this extreme phenotype, the function of Vif remained elusive. Several heterokaryon cell fusion studies indicated that Vif probably acts by inhibiting a host antiviral mechanism present in nonpermissive cells (Madani and Kabat, 1998; Simon et al., 1998). This endogenous antiretroviral activity was pinpointed by Sheehy et al. (2002), who utilized subtractive cDNA cloning to identify a host defense gene absent from permissive cells: the cytidine deaminase APOBEC3G (originally named CEM15).

The proposed mechanism for APOBEC3G-mediated restriction of HIV is based on the protein's ability to package with newly formed viral particles and subsequently exert its cytidine deaminase activity (Harris et al., 2003; Lecossier et al., 2003; Mangeat et al., 2003; Mariani et al., 2003; Zhang et al., 2003). Early in infection, HIV reverse transcribes its RNA and integrates the resulting cDNA into the host genome. During the assembly of new HIV particles,

APOBEC3G associates with viral components and is incorporated into the virions. When released, these virions carry their APOBEC3G payload to naive cells. On infection, as the HIV RNA is reverse transcribed, APOBEC3G binds and deaminates cytidine residues throughout the newly synthesized first (−)-strand viral cDNA. This targeted hypermutation leads to two possible outcomes for the viral cDNA. The high dU content may recruit the uracil base-excision repair machinery or inherently destabilize viral cDNA, thereby leading to its degradation (Cullen, 2003; Gu and Sundquist, 2003). Alternatively (or additionally), second-strand synthesis and integration may proceed despite the mutations, resulting in a vastly crippled provirus unable to produce infectious virions. A schematic representation of this process appears in Fig. 1.

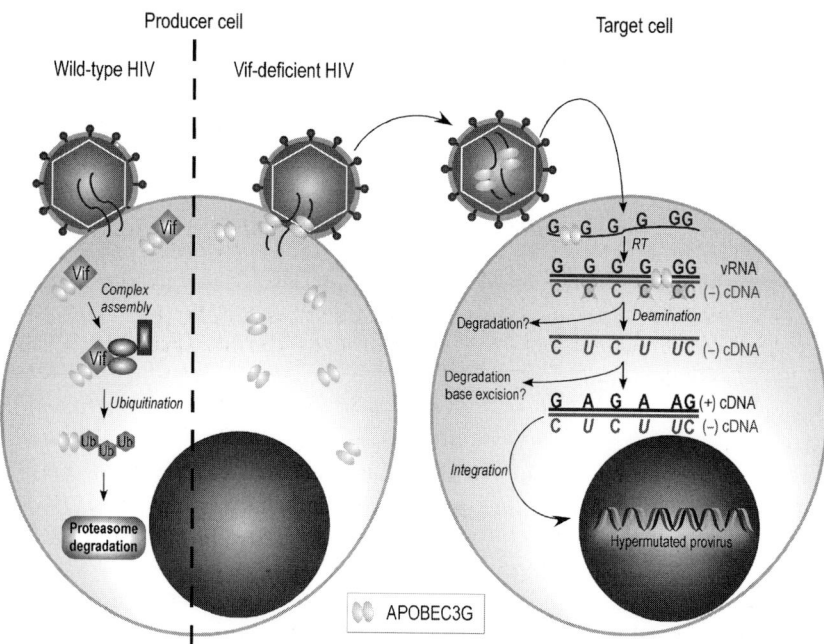

Figure 1 APOBEC3G in HIV infection. In the setting of wild-type HIV infection, HIV Vif associates with cellular APOBEC3G and targets it for ubiquitination and subsequent proteasomal degradation. However, infection with Vif-deficient HIV allows APOBEC3G to act unopposed. Intact cellular APOBEC3G packages with virus particles and is delivered to newly infected cells with viral RNA. Following reverse transcription, APOBEC3G can edit nascent (−)-strand viral cDNA, which is degraded or incorporated into a hypermutated provirus. (**See Color Plate 8.**)

Despite these findings, the significance of cytidine deamination in APOBEC3G antiretroviral activity is not entirely clear. In agreement with overexpression experiments, endogenous APOBEC3G inhibits Vif-deficient HIV infection of primary resting CD4+ T cells, the main physiological target of the virus (Chiu et al., 2005). However, despite potent restriction, retroviral reverse transcripts isolated from these cells contain very few G-to-A mutations. In addition, work by Newman et al. (2005) asserts that APOBEC3G can maintain its antiretroviral capacity in the absence of functional cytidine deaminase activity. As their results conflict with prior findings, the authors note that previous experiments were performed with epitope-tagged APOBEC proteins, which can behave differently than their untagged counterparts. A report from the same group demonstrates that even with functional active sites, the potency of APOBEC3G retroviral restriction does not correlate with deaminase activity (Bishop et al., 2006). Much work remains to be done in defining a complete molecular mechanism for APOBEC3G antiretroviral activity.

HIV Vif protein acts as a viral countermeasure against the APOBEC3G host defense through a variety of mechanisms, all of which prevent the inclusion of APOBEC3G in newly produced virions. Perhaps most importantly, Vif protein binds APOBEC3G and induces its degradation (Conticello et al., 2003; Marin et al., 2003; Sheehy et al., 2003; Stopak et al., 2003; Yu et al., 2003). More specifically, Vif assembles a complex of cellular proteins (including Cul5, elongins B and C, and Rbx1) that participate in the ubiquitination of APOBEC3G, effectively targeting it for proteasomal destruction (Yu et al., 2003). Vif binding can also sequester APOBEC3G and thereby block its packaging into assembling virions (Mariani et al., 2003). Additionally, Vif has been demonstrated to directly inhibit the translation of newly transcribed APOBEC3G mRNA (Stopak et al., 2003).

The high-stakes evolutionary struggle between host and pathogen can lead to extremely specialized defense and counterattack mechanisms. This seems to be true for APOBEC3G and Vif. Although it efficiently controls human APOBEC3G, HIV Vif does not bind or inhibit the mouse homologue APOBEC3 (Mariani et al., 2003). Furthermore, HIV Vif cannot restrain APOBEC3G from closely related primate species such as African green monkey and macaque (Mariani et al., 2003; Zennou and Bieniasz, 2006). The closely related *Simian immunodeficiency virus* (SIV) Vif does not impede the function of human APOBEC3G (Bogerd et al., 2004). Consequently, HIV cannot efficiently replicate in APOBEC3G-expressing simian cells, and SIV is similarly restricted in human cells. Such exquisite specificity suggests relatively recent evolution under strong selective pressures. In fact, the species restriction of Vif interaction is determined by a single amino acid in the APOBEC3G protein (Bogerd et al., 2004; Mangeat et al., 2004; Schrofelbauer et al., 2004; Xu et al., 2004).

The substitution of aspartate 128 in human APOBEC3G with lysine makes APOBEC3G susceptible to SIV Vif but resistant to HIV Vif. The converse substitution in African green monkey APOBEC3G results in the corresponding reversal in susceptibility. It is possible that the species restriction of HIV infection to humans and SIV to other primates is determined at least in part by this divergent amino acid. However, despite the apparent importance of this residue at present, there have likely been multiple rounds of positive selection for substitutions in the coevolution of APOBEC3G and Vif (Zhang and Webb, 2004). Still, it remains interesting to consider the possibility that mutations in the APOBEC3G–Vif interaction played a role in HIV attaining infectious capacity for human cells. Furthermore, as disrupting a single amino acid can eliminate the interaction between Vif and APOBEC3G, this interface presents an intriguing therapeutic target for small molecule inhibitors.

3.2. APOBEC3G Can Act on a Variety of Viruses

3.2.1. Nonprimate Retroviruses

The antiretroviral activity of human APOBEC3G is not limited to HIV. As discussed above, it can act against the closely related primate lentivirus SIV. Additionally, APOBEC3G has demonstrated activity against a wide range of retroviruses that infect various nonprimate species. *Equine infectious anemia virus* (EIAV), a lentivirus lacking a *vif* gene, is sensitive to APOBEC3G hypermutation and can be protected by coexpression of HIV Vif (Mangeat *et al.*, 2003). *Murine leukemia virus* (MLV) is a gammaretrovirus with a simple genome that does not contain a *vif*-like gene. Human APOBEC3G can package with MLV virions and inhibit subsequent productive infection (Bishop *et al.*, 2004; Harris *et al.*, 2003; Kobayashi *et al.*, 2004; Kremer *et al.*, 2005; Mangeat *et al.*, 2003). Although many parameters determine virus tropisms (e.g., surface receptors, intracellular factors, immune response, and so on), these examples suggest that APOBEC3G may protect humans from animal retroviruses.

Interestingly, despite the absence of a *vif* gene, MLV infection is not restricted by the antiviral mouse homologue APOBEC3. This implies that MLV may have evolved novel, Vif-independent processes to escape from the antiviral pressure of mouse cytidine deaminases. Indeed, recent work proposes that MLV protects itself from mouse APOBEC3 via two distinct mechanisms (Abudu *et al.*, 2006). First, MLV viral RNA disrupts the binding of APOBEC3 to Gag, excluding it from assembling virions. Second, the MLV viral protease directly eliminates APOBEC3 by proteolytic cleavage. Neither of these mechanisms is effective at defending MLV from human APOBEC3G, again demonstrating the effects of selective pressures from a specific host–pathogen relationship on adaptive evolution.

3.2.2. Human T-Lymphotropic Virus 1

APOBEC3G may also have antiviral activity against other human retroviruses. Human T-lymphotropic virus 1 (HTLV-1) is one of only four pathogenic human retroviruses. Infection can cause lymphoproliferative disease as well as inflammatory and neurological disorders. The HTLV-1 genome contains basic genetic elements common to HIV and other retroviruses: the *gag-pol-env* genes flanked by long terminal repeat (LTR) motifs. HTLV-1 also contains additional genes involved in pathogenesis and feedback regulation of viral replication (Feuer and Green, 2005). As a retrovirus that shares one of HIV's main target cells (T lymphocytes), HTLV-1 could be a potential target for APOBEC3G. The first studies addressing this issue present somewhat confusing results. Sasada *et al.* (2005) report that in a cell line system, APOBEC3G can package with HTLV-1 virions and potently inhibit viral infection of a T-cell line. This antiviral effect was blocked by the coexpression of HIV Vif in virus producer cells. Of note, APOBEC3G deaminase activity was dispensable for viral restriction, and no hypermutation was detectable in viral genomes. Similar experiments by Navarro *et al.* (2005) also demonstrated the capacity of APOBEC3G to package with HTLV-1, but did not show a noteworthy reduction of infection. Using a different reporter cell line system, Mahieux *et al.* (2005) did not observe significant inhibition of HTLV-1 infection by APOBEC3G. However, molecular analysis revealed that a small percentage (<5%) of viral genomes packaged in the presence of APOBEC3G displayed hypermutation at nearly all cytidine residues. Although when taken together, these initial reports do not establish a cohesive model, they do suggest a possible role of APOBEC3G in HTLV-1 infection.

Some of the difficulties in characterizing the effects of APOBEC3G on HTLV-1 may stem from a currently unidentified viral mechanism to escape the host's defenses. While HTLV-1 apparently lacks a *vif* gene, it preferentially infects and replicates in CD4+ T cells (Richardson *et al.*, 1990), the same cell type in which APOBEC3G expression restricts Vif-deficient HIV. As described above for MLV and murine APOBEC3, HTLV-1 may protect itself via a mechanism distinct from Vif-mediated exclusion and degradation. Additional work is needed to uncover important details on the significance of APOBEC3G in HTLV-1 infection.

3.2.3. Hepatitis B Virus

After it became clear that the antiviral activity of APOBEC3G is not limited to HIV alone, its potential for restricting viruses beyond the Retroviridae family was investigated. *Hepatitis B virus* (HBV) is not a true retrovirus, but it does replicate its genome through reverse transcription of a pregenomic RNA template in virus producer cells (Ganem, 1996). Unlike true retroviruses, HBV virions already contain a partially double-stranded DNA genome upon their infection of naive cells. Thus, the HBV lifecycle includes a reverse transcription step and single-stranded viral genomic DNA, both of which are implicated in APOBEC3G's activity against HIV and other retroviruses. Beginning with these concepts, Trono and colleagues used a hepatoma cell line (Huh7) system to show that APOBEC3G can effectively inhibit HBV infection (Turelli et al., 2004). Furthermore, APOBEC3G cytidine deaminase activity is not necessary for restriction of HBV, which suggests that another, nonediting mechanism is at work. While hypermutation is apparently not the primary means of inhibiting the virus, it can occur both in vitro and in vivo. APOBEC3G editing of minus- and plus-strand HBV DNA is detectable in other hepatoma cell lines (HepG2) and G-to-A hypermutated HBV genomes are present at very low frequencies in the serum of infected patients with high viremia (Suspene et al., 2005).

Further study of the APOBEC3G–HBV interaction revealed additional details of the antiviral mechanisms at work. HBV-infected cells expressing APOBEC3G produce normal levels of viral protein (as measured by HBV surface antigen and core proteins) but have significantly lower levels of viral RNA and DNA for packaging into new virions (Turelli et al., 2004). This may be a consequence of degradation by cellular RNAses, as APOBEC3G can render core-associated viral pregenomic RNA nuclease sensitive, possibly by preventing its encapsidation (Rosler et al., 2005). In contrast to HIV Vif, the HBV X protein, also a viral factor that is necessary for establishing infection, does not inhibit this function of APOBEC3G.

The protective potential of APOBEC3G against HBV infection in vivo remains to be determined. Healthy human liver does not express significant levels of APOBEC3 family mRNA transcripts (Jarmuz et al., 2002). In vitro, primary hepatocytes stimulated with the antiviral cytokine interferon-α rapidly upregulate APOBEC3G expression (Tanaka et al., 2006). Interferon-α also induces the high-level expression of other gene family members including APOBECs 3B, 3C, and 3F, several of which possess anti-HBV activity (Bonvin et al., 2006). As demonstrated in chimpanzees in vivo, acute HBV infection does not trigger an interferon response in the liver (Wieland et al., 2004). However, interferon-α treatment is an effective therapy for chronic HBV infection (Wong et al., 1993). Perhaps hepatic induction of APOBEC3G or its paralogues contributes to the anti-HBV effects of interferon-α. Additional work and clinical studies are required to determine the physiological role of the APOBEC3 deaminases in HBV infection and treatment.

3.3. Antiviral Activities of Other APOBEC3 Family Cytidine Deaminases

As alluded to in the case of HBV above, APOBEC3G is not the only member of the AID/APOBEC gene family with demonstrated antiviral activity. Although HIV is most effectively restricted by APOBEC3G, -3B, -3DE, and -3F can also antagonize the virus (Bishop et al., 2004; Dang et al., 2006; Doehle et al., 2005). Which of the other APOBEC proteins possess antiviral activity? On which viruses can they act?

Although much work remains before a comprehensive list is completed, antiviral actions (and their respective targets) have already been assigned to several APOBEC family members in humans and rodents. Table 1 provides a snapshot of presently characterized antiviral APOBECs and susceptible viruses. This catalog is likely to expand as additional viruses (and their probable

Table 1 AID/APOBEC Cytidine Deaminases and Their Antiviral Activities

Cytidine deaminase	Antiviral activity							
	Retroviridae					Endogenous retroelements		
	HIV	HTLV-1	MLV	Foamy viruses	HBV	ERV (LTR)	LINE-1 (non-LTR)	AAV
Human								
APOBEC1	−	ND	−	ND	ND	ND	ND	ND
APOBEC2	ND	ND	ND	ND	ND	ND	ND	ND
APOBEC3A	−	ND	−	ND	ND	+	+	+
APOBEC3B	+	−	+/−	+	+	+	+	−
APOBEC3C	+	−	−	+	−	+	+	−
APOBEC3D	ND	ND	ND	ND	ND	ND	−	ND
APOBEC3E	ND	ND	ND	ND	ND	ND	ND	ND
APOBEC3DE	+	ND	−	ND	ND	ND	ND	ND
APOBEC3F	+	−	+	+	+	+	+	ND
APOBEC3G	+	+/−	+	+	+	+	−	−
APOBEC3H	−	ND	−	ND	ND	ND	−	−
AID	−	ND	−	ND	ND	ND	ND	ND
Mouse								
APOBEC1	−	ND	ND	ND	ND	ND	ND	ND
APOBEC2	−	ND	ND	ND	ND	ND	ND	ND
APOBEC3	+	ND	−	+	ND	+	−	ND
AID	−	ND	+[a]	ND	ND	ND	ND	ND

[a]Restricts transformation by Ab-MLV. Table format based in part on Turelli and Trono (2005). +/− indicates conflicting reports; ND, not determined.

countermeasures) are studied. Several examples that demonstrate interesting aspects of the cytidine deaminase–virus relationship are discussed below.

3.3.1. APOBEC Proteins Can Inhibit Infection by Foamy Viruses

Foamy viruses (also known as spumaretroviruses) are part of the Retroviridae family. They infect a range of mammalian hosts and demonstrate a particularly high prevalence in nonhuman primate species. The foamy virus life cycle differs considerably from those of the more familiar lentiviruses (Delelis et al., 2004). Notably, most reverse transcription occurs in the virus producer cell, and as such, new virions contain double-stranded viral DNA. In addition, the foamy virus genome contains two accessory genes: *tas*, a transactivator important for replication (Lochelt et al., 1993), and *bet*, a viral factor implicated in latent infection (Meiering and Linial, 2002). Viral packaging and release can proceed via an unusual mechanism, with new virions budding into the endoplasmic reticulum and subsequently leaving the cell by exocytosis (Linial, 1999).

The interplay between foamy viruses and the APOBEC3 proteins provides another example of host–virus coevolution and corresponding species-specific adaptations. Initial reports show that primate foamy viruses are effectively inhibited by APOBECs from human (3G, 3F, and to a lesser extent 3B and 3C), African green monkey (3G), chimpanzee (3G), and mouse (3) (Delebecque et al., 2006; Russell et al., 2005). Much like HIV, the primate foamy virus can escape APOBEC3 restriction through one of its accessory proteins. Although individual groups have demonstrated different results (likely due to dissimilarities in viral vectors), it appears that primate foamy virus Bet protein can abrogate APOBEC3 antiviral function (Russell et al., 2005). This function likely evolved from selective pressures within the specific nonhuman primate host: although primate foamy virus Bet potently inhibits the antiviral effects of chimpanzee APOBEC3G, it only partially inhibits human APOBEC3G and -3F and has no effect on mouse APOBEC3. This paradigm extends beyond primates and their associated foamy viruses. Possessing significant regions of homology to human APOBEC3F, feline APOBEC3 exerts a strong antiviral effect on Bet-deficient feline foamy virus (Lochelt et al., 2005). This restriction is eliminated by Bet expression in wild-type infection.

3.3.2. APOBEC3A Can Inhibit Adeno-Associated Virus Production

All of the APOBEC-susceptible viruses discussed thus far include a reverse transcription step at some point in their life cycle. However, recent work on adeno-associated virus (AAV) suggests that reverse transcription is not a de facto requirement for APOBEC antiviral activity. AAV, a member of the Parvoviridae family, is a small single-stranded DNA virus that infects a wide range of animal hosts, including humans (Berns, 1996). As its name implies, AAV usually requires the action of a helper virus (often an adenovirus) to establish a productive infection. AAV does not encode a polymerase gene; it utilizes the host cell polymerase machinery (Ni et al., 1998) to replicate its genome by leading strand synthesis and double-stranded DNA intermediates (Berns, 1990). There is no reverse transcription apparent in the viral life cycle.

Studies by Weitzman and colleagues demonstrate that AAV production is susceptible to inhibition by human APOBEC3A (Chen et al., 2006). Other APOBEC family members with well-characterized antiviral activities (3C, 3G, and 3F) have no effect. APOBEC3A is expressed in the nucleus, where it interferes with the formation of AAV replication centers in viral producer cells. As a result, viral replication and production are reduced to virtually undetectable levels. Although the specific biochemical mechanism for this disruption remains unclear, it is dependent on an intact zinc-coordination motif in the APOBEC3A active site, perhaps implicating DNA binding or deamination as necessary events.

The susceptibility of AAV to APOBEC3A-mediated restriction independent of any reverse transcription activity suggests that the AID/APOBEC family may possess much broader antiviral potential than initially thought and this possibility raises many new questions. Can APOBEC3A act on other single-stranded DNA viruses? More generally, which other virus types (double-stranded DNA, various RNA varieties, and so on) can be inhibited by which APOBECs? Mounting evidence suggests that particular APOBECs may target certain viruses more effectively than others. Perhaps each family member is specialized to defend against a particular class of viruses: APOBEC3G for retroviruses, APOBEC3A for single-stranded DNA viruses, and so on. Alternatively (or additionally), each family member might possess broad antiviral activity, but attain physiological specialization against particular viruses based on tissue distribution and regulation. Such a scenario could work to the advantage of the host or the pathogen, as may be the case for HIV. Vif-deficient HIV is restricted by both APOBEC3G and APOBEC3B *in vitro*. Yet unlike APOBEC3G, APOBEC3B cannot be restrained by HIV-Vif (Doehle et al., 2005). Thus, APOBEC3B appears to provide an ideal defense against HIV. However, *in vivo*, APOBEC3B is not typically expressed in lymphocytes, important targets of HIV infection in which constitutive production of APOBEC3G is foiled by Vif. The *in vivo* roles of APOBEC3B and other family members in viral defense remain important research problems, as they may lead to new therapeutic strategies. Such considerations are also relevant beyond traditional pathogenic viral infection. For example, recombinant AAV is in development as a promising gene therapy vector due to an attractive list of features: small DNA genome, nonpathogenic infection, preferential targeting of transformed cells, and site-specific genomic integration (Goncalves, 2005). Ultimately, a successful treatment program may need to consider the influence of APOBEC3A activity on the viral vector in producer or target cells.

3.4. Endogenous Retroelements Can Be Suppressed by Many APOBEC3 Deaminases

3.4.1. Endogenous Retroviruses

The above examples clearly demonstrate the capacity of the APOBEC3 proteins to protect against a rapidly expanding list of infectious viruses. In addition to these exogenous threats, most mammals are also impacted by endogenous genetic elements that can alter their genomes. Of these host-encoded elements, the endogenous retroviruses (ERVs) are of note for their high frequency [almost 10% of the human genome (Deininger and Batzer, 2002)] and for their similarities to infectious retroviruses.

ERVs are retroelements that, when active, can replicate and insert elsewhere in the genome. This retrotransposition is achieved via an RNA intermediate, which is reverse transcribed (by the ERV *pol* reverse transcriptase) and integrated into genomic DNA. These insertions have had a major impact on genome evolution (Hughes and Coffin, 2001; Johnson and Coffin, 1999; Kazazian, 2004), but can also be harmful to the host; some evidence suggest an association of ERVs with autoimmune disease (Nakagawa and Harrison, 1996) and oncogenesis (Taruscio and Mantovani, 2004). As genomic remnants of ancient retroviral infections, mobile ERVs share a number of genetic and mechanistic similarities with infectious retroviruses. These include the traditional retroviral *gag-pro-pol* genes, flanking LTRs, reverse transcription-dependent replication, and even the ability (in some cases) to form virus-like particles (VLPs). Likely due to the importance of maintaining genomic integrity, complex organisms have developed mechanisms for restraining mobile ERV activity, including gene methylation (Bourc'his and Bestor, 2004; Walsh *et al.*, 1998), and cosuppression/RNA interference (Ketting and Plasterk, 2000; Sijen and Plasterk, 2003; Tabara *et al.*, 1999). It is now clear that APOBEC3 cytidine deaminases can also inhibit ERVs, further expanding their repertoire of host defense activities.

Human APOBEC3G was the first family member demonstrated to have anti-ERV activity. Using a cell-based retrotransposition assay, Esnault *et al.* (2005) observed that human APOBEC3G or mouse APOBEC3 expression causes a drastic reduction in the retrotransposition of two different murine ERV sequences, intracisternal A-particle (IAP) and MusD. These LTR-containing retroelements, which can undergo reverse transcription and form VLPs, are capable of active retrotransposition in the mouse genome. In this cell-based system, APOBEC inhibition of IAP and MusD is accompanied by a large number of G-to-A mutations in the reduced number of provirus sequences that persist. Sequence analysis of the mouse genome showed that naturally occurring IAP and MusD elements also carry a high rate of G-to-A mutations, particularly in GXA trinucleotide motifs, the target sequence preferred by mouse APOBEC3 (Yu *et al.*, 2004).

Additional APOBEC proteins are also capable of inhibiting retrotransposable elements. Human APOBEC3A and -3B effectively restrict IAP retrotransposition (Bogerd *et al.*, 2006; Chen *et al.*, 2006). APOBEC3B packages with IAP VLPs and hypermutates the reverse transcribed DNA. Interestingly, APOBEC3A does not package or edit, yet it reduces IAP retrotransposition to much lower levels than APOBEC3B or -3G (Bogerd *et al.*, 2006). It remains unclear if APOBEC3A inhibits IAP through a novel mechanism or if a shared process upstream of packaging and editing is sufficient for restricting retrotransposition. Recent work suggests that other APOBEC proteins (human 3G and 3F, mouse 3) suppress ERV retrotransposition in two distinct steps: first by reducing retroelement cDNA levels and then by hyperediting the remaining copies that successfully transpose (Esnault *et al.*, 2006). Perhaps APOBEC3A utilizes only the first of these dual mechanisms to effectively control ERV retrotransposition.

Other types of LTR retrotransposable elements are susceptible to APOBEC inhibition as well. In yeast systems, the Ty1 LTR retrotransposon can be effectively suppressed by ectopic expression of a range of APOBEC proteins including human 3C, -3F, -3G, and mouse 3 (Dutko *et al.*, 2005; Schumacher *et al.*, 2005).

3.4.2. Non-LTR Retroelements

In addition to the LTR retroelements discussed thus far (IAP, MusD, Ty1), mammalian genomes harbor large numbers of non-LTR retrotransposons, of which the long interspersed nuclear element-1 (LINE-1) class is particularly abundant (∼500,000 copies in human) (Lander *et al.*, 2001). Full-length and active LINE-1 elements are detectable in mouse and human genomes (Brouha *et al.*, 2003; Ostertag and Kazazian, 2001; Sassaman *et al.*, 1997). Unlike LTR sequences, LINE-1 reverse transcription occurs in the nucleus and does not involve the formation of VLPs. Despite these considerable differences, LINE-1 elements may be susceptible to APOBEC-mediated inhibition. Although APOBEC3G has no effect on LINE-1 elements (Esnault *et al.*, 2005; Turelli *et al.*, 2004), individual overexpression of several family members (3A, 3B, 3C, 3F) effectively inhibits LINE-1 retrotransposition (Muckenfuss *et al.*, 2006).

Endogenous APOBEC3C can also restrict LINE-1 elements, as demonstrated by cell line RNA interference experiments.

3.4.3. Physiological Role for Suppression of Retroelements by APOBECs

In the mouse, ERV expression is typically suppressed by methylation in somatic cells. As such, the physiological role for APOBEC restriction remains to be determined. ERV sequences are not methylated in germ cells in which several AID/APOBEC family members are expressed at high levels (Turelli and Trono, 2005). Perhaps APOBEC suppression of ERVs protects genomic integrity during the "reprogramming" of methylation sites in gametogenesis or early embryogenesis. However, APOBEC3-deficient mice are fertile and show no evidence of derepression of endogenous retroelements (Mikl et al., 2005). Thus, the function of APOBEC3 in the mouse remains unclear.

In humans, the existence of functionally active ERVs remains uncertain, so a physiological role for retroelement suppression by APOBECs is not obvious. However, proven retroelement inhibition *in vitro* and phylogenetic analysis suggest that APOBEC function may have developed as an ancient system of genome defense. In the human APOBEC3 subfamily, all members with demonstrable *in vivo* expression have the capacity to inhibit at least one type of endogenous retroelement (ERVs, LINE-1, and so on). Furthermore, all but one of these (3A) has undergone many rounds of strong positive selection throughout primate evolution, indicating a likely role in host defense (Sawyer et al., 2004; Zhang and Webb, 2004). Despite the potent activity of some APOBEC3 proteins against exogenous retroviruses such as HIV, the apparent selective pressures driving their adaptive evolution predates the emergence of modern primate lentiviruses by millions of years (Sawyer et al., 2004; Zhang and Webb, 2004). Furthermore, the expansion of the APOBEC3 family directly correlates with a sharp reduction of endogenous retrotransposon activity in primate genomes as compared to rodents (Waterston et al., 2002). These observations support a theory in which the "original" function of the APOBEC3 genes was to protect the genome from actively mobile retroelements or the ancient retroviruses from which they were derived. The ability to inhibit exogenous lentiviruses may simply be a fortuitous extension of this function. Alternatively, with recent evidence for antiviral APOBEC activity beyond retroviruses (HBV, AAV), it is also possible that APOBEC proteins represent an evolutionarily ancient defense system against a broad range of genetic threats, including exogenous DNA or RNA viruses and endogenous retroelements. Efforts to define the antiviral spectrum of AID/APOBEC family members and their physiological role(s) in host defense will likely provide important insights into the selective pressures that shaped their evolution.

4. AID in the Host Response to Viral Infection

AID is one of the key players in the adaptive immune system. In activated B cells, AID is necessary for antibody SHM and CSR. These two AID-dependent processes shape humoral immunity in response to particular threats. SHM allows for increased antibody specificity, while CSR assigns antibodies antigen-appropriate effector function. The dynamic molecular flexibility provided by these AID-mediated processes is in sharp contrast to the fixed molecular machinery of innate immunity.

Nevertheless, a robust innate antiviral defense is provided by APOBEC3 genes very closely related to AID. These very similar genes exert markedly different functions, and yet both participate in host defense. This implies an intriguing evolutionary connection of innate and adaptive immune mechanisms. Phylogenetically, the appearance of AID precedes that of APOBEC1 and APOBEC3, both of which apparently share AID as a common ancestor (Conticello *et al.*, 2005). An AID homologue can be detected as far back as cartilaginous fish, and its evolutionary appearance correlates with hypermutation of immunoglobulin genes (Diaz *et al.*, 1998; Hinds-Frey *et al.*, 1993). However, in light of the antiviral activities of the APOBEC3 subfamily, it is possible that AID also has innate immune functions. This possibility was confirmed by the recent identification of an AID-dependent host response to Abelson (Ab)-MLV.

4.1. AID Is a Host Response Factor Against Ab-MLV

Ab-MLV is a replication-deficient retrovirus that infects murine pre-B cells. The virus is highly oncogenic; infection causes pre-B cell transformation *in vitro* and acute pre-B cell leukemia *in vivo*. Both are dependent on viral transduction of the *v-abl* oncogene (Rosenberg, 1994). Unlike the primate lentiviruses, Ab-MLV does not replicate or form new virus particles in infected cells.

Recent work (Gourzi *et al.*, 2006) has demonstrated that AID protects the host from Ab-MLV oncogenesis and does so independently of its antibody diversification functions. Infected bone marrow cells from $AID^{-/-}$ mice are considerably more susceptible to Ab-MLV transformation than their wild-type counterparts. A similar phenotype is apparent *in vivo* when Ab-MLV-infected bone marrow cells are transferred to wild-type animals. Mice engrafted with infected $AID^{-/-}$ cells die faster and with considerably more aggressive pre-B cell leukemias than those that receive infected wild-type cells. Because all graft recipients were wild-type mice, the benefit provided by AID must be distinct from its function in antibody diversification.

How does AID protect against retroviral transformation? Unlike APOBEC3-mediated antiretroviral activity, it appears that AID targets the host genome rather than the virus. A possible mechanism is diagrammed in Fig. 2. Ab-MLV infection of pre-B cells induces expression of AID, which is typically restricted to germinal center B cells. Induced AID is functionally active and causes somatic mutation of host genes. It appears that AID-mediated damage to host DNA triggers a genotoxic stress response, which in turn restricts the proliferation of Ab-MLV infected cells. This response also causes surface expression of the NK-cell-activating ligand Rae-1. Neither of these events is observed with infection of $AID^{-/-}$ pre-B cells. Thus, it seems that AID counteracts viral oncogenesis by restricting the proliferation of infected cells and flagging them as targets for elimination by NK cells.

The precise molecular mechanism that AID employs to restrict proliferation of infected cells is not understood. AID activity in infected cells leads to Chk-1 phosphorylation and activation of cell cycle damage checkpoints, but whether this host cell restriction is dependent on the ability of AID to catalyze deamination is not known. As is apparent for the antiviral activity of the APOBEC3 deaminases, AID may not need an intact active site to initiate damage repair pathways and restrict host cell proliferation. *In vitro*, both wild-type and catalytically inactive AID can bind RNA (Dickerson *et al.*, 2003), so perhaps AID could restrict host cell proliferation by binding RNA nonspecifically and interfering with translation independent of deaminase activity. A number of other possibilities can be envisioned, but further work is necessary to clarify the mechanism of action of AID in this setting.

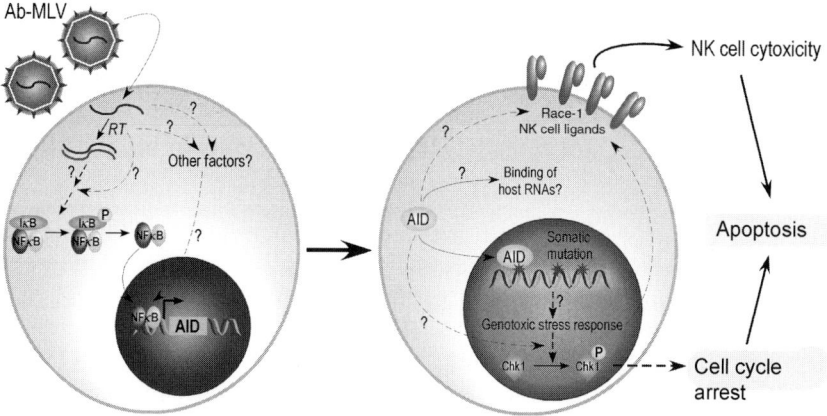

Figure 2 AID and Ab-MLV transformation. Infection of pre-B cells with Ab-MLV triggers the NF-κB-dependent expression of AID. AID mediates somatic mutation of the host genome which is associated with a broad cellular genotoxic stress response. An upregulation of Rae-1 ligands "flags" the infected cell for killing by NK cells and Chk-1 phosphorylation signals for cell cycle arrest. Ultimately, these diverse pathways converge in the elimination of the infected cell by apoptosis. (**See Color Plate 9.**)

The newly discovered role of AID in the host response to an oncogenic retrovirus raises many important questions. Unlike the constitutive expression of some APOBEC3 proteins, AID transcription is tightly regulated. Using a transgenic mouse where endogenous AID transcription effects the expression of a YFP reporter (designated AID-cre-YFP), Casellas and colleagues confirmed that AID is expressed in germinal center B cells and is also induced in bone marrow B cells after infection with Ab-MLV (Li et al., 2007). How does Ab-MLV trigger AID expression in pre-B cells? One possibility is toll-like receptor (TLR) recognition and associated signaling. However, recent data do not favor this hypothesis, as mice deficient in TLR signaling ($myd88^{-/-}$ $trif^{-/-}$) can still induce AID on infection (Gourzi et al., 2007). Additionally, pre-B cells do not express AID in response to Type I interferons, making it unlikely that induction is part of a general antiviral response. Although other signals are probably necessary, the transcription factor NF-κB is required for expression of virus-induced AID. It has previously been shown that NF-κB can bind and activate the AID promoter in response to IL-4 and CD40 ligation (Dedeoglu et al., 2004). Furthermore, many different antiviral pathways depend on distinct signaling components ultimately linked by NF-κB activation (reviewed in Honda et al., 2005). Thus, viral infection could induce AID expression through a number of different pathways that culminate in NF-κB activation, underscoring the potential versatility of this host defense program.

It remains to be seen if this AID-mediated host response extends beyond Ab-MLV to other oncogenic viruses. Also, it is presently not known if this function is restricted to AID or belongs to APOBEC proteins as well. From an evolutionary standpoint, this mechanism raises the possibility that AID's genetic ancestor was a mediator of innate immunity whose function was later co-opted by the adaptive immune system or its predecessors (Pancer and Cooper, 2006).

4.2. AID and Other Viruses

The example of Ab-MLV provides clear evidence of AID function in the host response to an oncogenic virus. Additional work suggests that AID may play a role in other viral infections as well. Two of these, Epstein-Barr virus (EBV) and *Hepatitis C virus* (HCV), are important pathogens with high prevalence in humans.

4.2.1. Epstein-Barr Virus

EBV is a gamma herpesvirus that is extremely prevalent in human populations throughout the world. The virus primarily infects B cells, though less efficient infection of other lymphoid and epithelial cells is also possible. In the vast majority of infected individuals, EBV exists as a lifelong asymptomatic infection that persists in the memory B-lymphocyte pool (Kuppers, 2003). Delayed initial infection in young adulthood can cause infectious mononucleosis (IM): a common, self-limiting lymphoproliferative illness. However, it is widely accepted that EBV also has oncogenic potential and contributes to the development of endemic Burkitt's lymphoma (eBL) and nasopharyngeal carcinoma. Infection is also associated with Hodgkin's lymphomas, AIDS-associated lymphomas, and a variety of other lymphoid malignancies (reviewed in Young and Rickinson, 2004). *In vitro*, EBV infection effectively transforms resting B cells, thus establishing "lymphoblastoid cell lines" (LCLs), which can be continually propagated in culture. Although far from a comprehensive model of physiological EBV oncogenesis, LCLs are extremely useful in studying the mechanisms of establishing latent infection and the related consequences for the host cell.

AID is believed to play a role in the pathogenesis of at least some of the EBV-associated lymphomas. Chromosomal translocations at the immunoglobulin locus, the hallmark of several EBV-associated B-cell lymphomas, are likely caused by aberrant CSR or mistargeted SHM (Kuppers and Dalla-Favera, 2001). In a particularly well-characterized example, eBL cells all harbor a trademark t(8:14) translocation, which juxtaposes the *c-myc* proto-oncogene and the IgH locus. Although the identity of the primary B-cell subset initially infected by EBV *in vivo* remains controversial (and beyond the scope of this chapter), it appears that eBL and several other EBV-associated lymphoma cells are derived from germinal center B cells. Thus, the faulty CSR and oncogenic translocation found in eBL likely occur in a cell type that expresses AID physiologically or driven additionally by EBV infection. However, this may not be the only site where EBV encounters AID.

Several groups reported that EBV infection induces AID expression in non-GC B cells. In one study, peripheral blood resting B cells were infected with EBV and AID transcripts were detectable 10 days later (Epeldegui *et al.*, 2006). Another report describes AID expression in freshly transformed LCLs (He *et al.*, 2003). In such cases, AID expression correlated with detectable SHM (Gil *et al.*, 2007) and CSR (He *et al.*, 2003) events. Somatic mutation at nonimmunoglobulin loci was also detected (Epeldegui *et al.*, 2006).

At first glance, this induction of AID appears analogous to that observed in Ab-MLV infection of mouse pre-B cells. However, the expression observed in EBV-transformed LCLs is more likely caused by a viral gene product, latent membrane protein-1 (LMP-1). LMP-1 is a membrane spanning viral protein expressed during two main phases of EBV infection: the viral "growth" program (Type III latency) and the "survival" program (Type II latency). Although it does not share any sequence similarity, LMP-1 is functionally homologous to CD40 (Gires *et al.*, 1997; Kilger *et al.*, 1998; Mosialos *et al.*, 1995). Both signal through many of the same downstream cellular components and both activate NF-κB. However, unlike CD40, LMP-1 does not contain a significant extracellular domain and constitutively signals in the absence of ligand binding. During normal B-cell activation, AID expression is induced by CD40 ligation (provided by cognate CD4+ T cell "help") and subsequent NF-κB activation. In cell line transfection experiments, EBV-encoded LMP-1 expression is sufficient to induce the NF-κB-dependent expression of AID (He *et al.*, 2003). In EBV infection, the expression of AID correlates with that of LMP-1 and is further upregulated by BAFF and APRIL, two B-cell gene products also induced by LMP-1 signaling. Thus, it appears that AID is induced by EBV infection as part of the virus growth and survival programs.

How do these observations relate to a role for AID in the host response to viral infection? Although EBV can induce its expression, at present it is unclear whether AID is beneficial or harmful to the virus and its efforts to establish latent infection. Similarly to Ab-MLV, EBV-infected B cells accumulate somatic mutations and are susceptible to NK-cell cytotoxicity (Moretta *et al.*, 1997; Wilson and Morgan, 2002). Survival in light of such cellular stresses could be explained by the anti-apoptotic signals also provided by LMP-1 and at this point any role of AID in restricting EBV transformation or latency remains speculative. However, new evidence that EBV can also inhibit AID expression in certain situations suggests that decreased AID activity could be advantageous to the virus. A study shows that, in contrast to LMP-1, EBV-encoded nuclear antigen-2 (EBNA-2) downregulates AID expression (Tobollik *et al.*, 2006). EBNA-2 is a transcription factor that acts on many EBV as well as host cell loci (Zimber-Strobl *et al.*, 1994). Much like the LMP-1/CD40-signaling similarities, EBNA-2 is a functional analogue of the cellular transcription factor Notch in its active form. Using a variety of cell line expression systems, Tobollik *et al.* (2006) demonstrated that EBNA-2 inhibits AID transcription, even in conjunction with LMP-1 expression. In the EBV growth program (Type III latency) of gene expression, EBNA-2 and LMP-1 are simultaneously expressed. This genetic program is utilized by EBV in LCLs *in vitro* and acute IM *in vivo*. Although LCLs express AID as described above, immunohistochemical staining of IM patient tonsils revealed a different expression pattern. EBV-infected, proliferating B cells were predominantly AID-negative. Furthermore, most (>90%) EBNA-2-positive cells were also AID-negative. In contrast to LCLs *in vitro*, very few (<10%) of LMP-positive cells expressed detectable amounts of AID. Contrary to the growth program, the survival program found in GC B-cells allows LMP-1 expression in the absence of EBNA-2. Therefore, EBV could augment AID expression in the GC, posing an additional risk of oncogenic mutations.

These results indicate that the regulation of AID expression in EBV infection is a complex process. EBV has apparently evolved dual mechanisms that can initiate or inhibit AID expression, which is typically under very tight cellular control. In the EBV growth program, these mechanisms are in apparent opposition with regard to AID. Perhaps AID induction is an indirect consequence of pro-survival LMP-1 signaling. EBNA-2 may then repress AID to minimize genetic damage to the host and viral genomes. In contrast, AID expression, further enhanced via LMP-1 during the GC reaction, might allow the infected cell to proceed with the B cell differentiation program. This could facilitate incorporation into the memory B cell compartment, the site of long-term EBV persistence. Many other possible scenarios can be envisioned. Ultimately, additional experiments that examine the actions of AID in the context of EBV infection, particularly *in vivo*, are needed to explain this intriguing host–pathogen genetic relationship.

4.2.2. Hepatitis C Virus

HCV is a significant global health problem, with more than 170 million people infected worldwide (Lauer and Walker, 2001). HCV is a small, single-stranded RNA virus of the Flaviviridae family. On infection with HCV, a limited number of people successfully clear the virus. Most ($\sim$70%), however, progress to chronic infection in which the virus persists despite an adaptive immune response (Alter *et al.*, 1999). The liver is the major target organ for HCV, and chronic infection is associated with hepatitis, cirrhosis, and hepatocellular carcinoma. In addition, HCV is associated with several B-cell abnormalities, including mixed cryoglobulinemia and B-cell non-Hodgkin's lymphoma (NHL).

Several lines of evidence suggest that B cells can be infected with HCV under certain conditions, but a definitive role for direct B-cell infection in the disease remains elusive. HCV RNA has been detected in NHL B cells isolated from an HCV-infected patient (Sung *et al.*, 2003). One cell line derived from this lymphoma can also release infectious particles in culture ("SB HCV"). However, B-cell infection is not a requirement for oncogenesis, as a survey of HCV-associated NHLs found detectable viral RNA in lymphoma cells from only a fraction of patients (De Vita *et al.*, 2002). Progress on this problem has been delayed in part because until very recently, HCV has been notoriously difficult to propagate and work with *in vitro*. It was reported that normal peripheral B cells can be infected with the *in vitro* derived SB HCV, but this system requires EBV transformation for survival and subsequent detection of HCV RNA (Sung *et al.*, 2003). In contrast, virus produced from a recently developed HCV cell culture (HCVcc) system (Lindenbach *et al.*, 2005, 2006) cannot infect normal peripheral B cells *in vitro* (Dustin and Rice, 2006).

Although the physiological mechanism remains uncertain, it is clear that B cells can play a role in HCV pathogenesis. Some evidence suggests that B-cell abnormalities associated with HCV infection may be related to the action of

AID. Using lymphoma cell lines and SB HCV, Machida *et al.* (2004) report that HCV infection of B cells induces the expression of AID and several error-prone DNA polymerases. This induction correlates with an increase in somatic mutation and DNA double-stranded breaks. The frequency of mutations was diminished by RNA interference directed against AID. Given that AID-dependent mutations were detected in both V_H regions and cellular proto-oncogenes, the authors propose an oncogenic role for AID in HCV-associated malignancies.

Additional work from the same group suggests that direct HCV infection of B cells may not be necessary for the observed induction of AID and corresponding mutations. High-concentration binding of HCV E2 glycoprotein to B-cell surface CD81 is sufficient to initiate AID expression (Machida *et al.*, 2005). CD81, a broadly expressed tetraspanin transmembrane protein, is a necessary receptor for HCV entry (Cormier *et al.*, 2004; Lindenbach *et al.*, 2005; Zhang *et al.*, 2004). However, it is not sufficient for infection, which apparently requires additional and as yet unidentified coreceptors. In B cells, CD81 exists as part of a surface signaling complex that also includes CD19, CD21, and CD225 (reviewed in Fearon and Carter, 1995; Levy *et al.*, 1998). Other cell types (such as hepatoma cell lines) in which CD81 is not part of such a signaling complex do not express AID in response to HCV-E2 binding. This suggests a unique role for the E2–CD81 interaction in B cells.

These initial reports provide another example of virally induced AID activity in B cells outside of the germinal center. Unlike Ab-MLV and EBV, HCV is not a transforming virus, despite its association with various malignancies. It remains to be determined if HCV-triggered AID activity is beneficial or harmful to the virus and/or the host. AID-associated mutations triggered by HCV infection could certainly impact the development of B-cell NHL. Alternatively, similar to the proposed mechanism in Ab-MLV transformation, AID activity could be advantageous to the host in providing an inhospitable cellular setting for infection. As the interaction of HCV and B cells *in vivo* is further characterized, the functional impact of AID activity may become more apparent.

5. Concluding Remarks

The discovery of APOBEC3G antiretroviral activity revealed a novel mechanism of antiviral innate immunity. Evolutionary considerations and genetic similarities between AID and the APOBEC3 subfamily prompted an investigation into whether AID also participates in the innate defense against viral infection. The recent finding that AID protects the host from Ab-MLV oncogenesis and does so independently of its antibody diversification functions confirms this hypothesis and raises a number of important questions. Is AID activity in response to viral infection restricted to B cells? By what molecular mechanism does AID restrict the proliferation of infected cells? For what viruses does AID contribute to host defense and in particular, what is the role of AID in the response to EBV and HCV infection? Is AID induction a feature of transforming or persistent infections in general? The newly generated AID-cre-YFP reporter mouse (Li et al., 2007) should greatly facilitate the search for answers to some of these questions. Furthermore, as the probable founding member of the APOBEC family of polynucleotide deaminases, AID harbors an antiviral mechanism that may precede that of the phylogenetically most recent APOBEC3 proteins. This raises the question of whether APOBEC1 and APOBEC2 also possess antiviral activity. Both of these enzymes will undoubtedly be the focus of future work in the field.

In their initial characterization, the APOBEC3 genes were attributed putative cytidine deaminase activity primarily on account of their sequence homology to APOBEC1 and AID (Jarmuz et al., 2002). With the subsequent identification of APOBEC3G antiretroviral activity and its association with G-to-A mutations in the viral genome (Harris et al., 2003), a model for retroviral restriction began to take shape. Briefly, APOBEC3G in infected cells (in the absence of Vif) is packaged with newly assembled virions. On subsequent infection of naive cells, APOBEC3G deaminates cytidines throughout the newly reverse transcribed viral (–)-strand cDNA, hypermutating, and effectively crippling the retroviral genome. This model was bolstered by additional work showing that APOBEC3G does, in fact, deaminate retroviral cDNA and catalytically inert APOBEC3G mutants are unable to inhibit retroviral infection (Mangeat et al., 2003; Zhang et al., 2003).

But is hypermutation a primary (or necessary) mechanism of APOBEC-mediated retroviral restriction? In light of recent data (Chiu et al., 2005; Newman et al., 2005), a definitive answer remains elusive. It is possible that the G-to-A mutations observed in reverse transcripts are coincidental side effects of a yet to be determined APOBEC3 mechanism upstream of DNA deamination. APOBEC3G strongly binds single-stranded cDNA (Chelico et al., 2006) and can effectively package into retrovirus particles without a functional deaminase active site (Kremer et al., 2005). Perhaps packaged APOBEC3 protein binds nascent viral cDNA, promoting its degradation and/or blocking access for other proviral factors while coincidentally deaminating the bound substrate. In this scheme, G-to-A mutations could simply represent a readily detectable feature linked to APOBEC function—a molecular "footprint in the sand." Although such a scenario for retroviral restriction remains purely speculative, APOBEC suppression of HBV appears to follow a similar model. As an important scientific question and therapeutic target, the mechanism of APOBEC antiretroviral activity demands additional investigation.

Although cytidine deaminase activity may be dispensable for inhibiting infection, some degree of mutation could be advantageous to viruses. A relatively low level of mutation could increase viral genetic diversity without completely crippling infectivity. In the case of HIV, though Vif acts an effective countermeasure against APOBEC3G and APOBEC3F, inhibition is incomplete and may allow for some deaminase activity. Furthermore, defective *vif* alleles can readily be found in infected patients and can result in incomplete neutralization of APOBEC3G or -3F (Simon *et al.*, 2005). Indeed, patient-derived viral sequences display G-to-A mutations characteristic of APOBEC3G- and -3F-targeted editing (Liddament *et al.*, 2004; Simon *et al.*, 2005). Although the rapid adaptation of HIV *in vivo* is likely propelled primarily by error-prone reverse transcriptase, a contribution from cytidine deaminases is also likely. Perhaps HIV or other viruses can draw on the editing capacity of these antiviral factors to develop drug resistance or escape the adaptive immune response. The impact of such mutations in the generation and selection of virus variants remains to be determined, but may reveal another evolutionary battlefield in host–pathogen conflicts.

Notes Added in Proof

Chiba and colleagues recently reported significant AID expression in human liver in the context of viral hepatitis (HBV and HCV) and cirrhosis Kou *et al.*, 2007. Though AID was not detectable in normal liver, expression was upregulated in hepatocellular carcinoma and surrounding noncancerous tissue with underlying inflammation. These findings further support a role for AID in the host response to viral infection and/or oncogenesis.

Acknowledgments

We wish to thank Dr. Charles Rice, Dr. Christian Munz, and Dr. Lynn Dustin for critical review of the chapter and helpful advice. We also thank Joanna Spencer and Robert McGinty for additional editorial assistance. BRR is supported by NIH MSTP grant GM07739. NPP is supported in part by NIH/NIAID grant AI071029.

References

Abudu, A., Takaori-Kondo, A., Izumi, T., Shirakawa, K., Kobayashi, M., Sasada, A., Fukunaga, K., and Uchiyama, T. (2006). Murine retrovirus escapes from murine APOBEC3 via two distinct novel mechanisms. *Curr. Biol.* **16,** 1565–1570.

Alter, M. J., Kruszon-Moran, D., Nainan, O. V., McQuillan, G. M., Gao, F., Moyer, L. A., Kaslow, R. A., and Margolis, H. S. (1999). The prevalence of hepatitis C virus infection in the United States, 1988 through 1994. *N. Engl. J. Med.* **341,** 556–562.

Berns, K. I. (1990). Parvovirus replication. *Microbiol. Rev.* **54**, 316–329.
Berns, K. I. (1996). *In* "Fields Virology" (B. N. Fields, D. M. Knipe, and P. M. Howley, Eds.), p. 2173. Lipincott-Raven, Philadelphia.
Bishop, K. N., Holmes, R. K., Sheehy, A. M., Davidson, N. O., Cho, S. J., and Malim, M. H. (2004). Cytidine deamination of retroviral DNA by diverse APOBEC proteins. *Curr. Biol.* **14**, 1392–1396.
Bishop, K. N., Holmes, R. K., and Malim, M. H. (2006). Antiviral potency of APOBEC proteins does not correlate with cytidine deamination. *J. Virol.* **80**, 8450–8458.
Bogerd, H. P., Doehle, B. P., Wiegand, H. L., and Cullen, B. R. (2004). A single amino acid difference in the host APOBEC3G protein controls the primate species specificity of HIV type 1 virion infectivity factor. *Proc. Natl. Acad. Sci. USA* **101**, 3770–3774.
Bogerd, H. P., Wiegand, H. L., Doehle, B. P., Lueders, K. K., and Cullen, B. R. (2006). APOBEC3A and APOBEC3B are potent inhibitors of LTR-retrotransposon function in human cells. *Nucleic Acids Res.* **34**, 89–95.
Bonvin, M., Achermann, F., Greeve, I., Stroka, D., Keogh, A., Inderbitzin, D., Candinas, D., Sommer, P., Wain-Hobson, S., Vartanian, J. P., and Greeve, J. (2006). Interferon-inducible expression of APOBEC3 editing enzymes in human hepatocytes and inhibition of hepatitis B virus replication. *Hepatology* **43**, 1364–1374.
Bourc'his, D., and Bestor, T. H. (2004). Meiotic catastrophe and retrotransposon reactivation in male germ cells lacking Dnmt3L. *Nature* **431**, 96–99.
Brouha, B., Schustak, J., Badge, R. M., Lutz-Prigge, S., Farley, A. H., Moran, J. V., and Kazazian, H. H., Jr. (2003). Hot L1s account for the bulk of retrotransposition in the human population. *Proc. Natl. Acad. Sci. USA* **100**, 5280–5285.
Chelico, L., Pham, P., Calabrese, P., and Goodman, M. F. (2006). APOBEC3G DNA deaminase acts processively $3' \rightarrow 5'$ on single-stranded DNA. *Nat. Struct. Mol. Biol.* **13**, 392–399.
Chen, H., Lilley, C. E., Yu, Q., Lee, D. V., Chou, J., Narvaiza, I., Landau, N. R., and Weitzman, M. D. (2006). APOBEC3A is a potent inhibitor of adeno-associated virus and retrotransposons. *Curr. Biol.* **16**, 480–485.
Chiu, Y. L., Soros, V. B., Kreisberg, J. F., Stopak, K., Yonemoto, W., and Greene, W. C. (2005). Cellular APOBEC3G restricts HIV-1 infection in resting CD4+ T cells. *Nature* **435**, 108–114.
Conticello, S. G., Harris, R. S., and Neuberger, M. S. (2003). The Vif protein of HIV triggers degradation of the human antiretroviral DNA deaminase APOBEC3G. *Curr. Biol.* **13**, 2009–2013.
Conticello, S. G., Thomas, C. J., Petersen-Mahrt, S. K., and Neuberger, M. S. (2005). Evolution of the AID/APOBEC family of polynucleotide (deoxy)cytidine deaminases. *Mol. Biol. Evol.* **22**, 367–377.
Cormier, E. G., Tsamis, F., Kajumo, F., Durso, R. J., Gardner, J. P., and Dragic, T. (2004). CD81 is an entry coreceptor for hepatitis C virus. *Proc. Natl. Acad. Sci. USA* **101**, 7270–7274.
Cullen, B. R. (2003). HIV-1 Vif: Counteracting innate antiretroviral defenses. *Mol. Ther.* **8**, 525–527.
Dang, Y., Wang, X., Esselman, W. J., and Zheng, Y. H. (2006). Identification of APOBEC3DE as another antiretroviral factor from the human APOBEC family. *J. Virol.* **80**, 10522–10533.
De Vita, S., De Re, V., Sansonno, D., Gloghini, A., Gasparotto, D., Libra, M., Sacco, S., Carbone, A., Ferraccioli, G., and Boiocchi, M. (2002). Lack of HCV infection in malignant cells refutes the hypothesis of a direct transforming action of the virus in the pathogenesis of HCV-associated B-cell NHLs. *Tumori* **88**, 400–407.
Dedeoglu, F., Horwitz, B., Chaudhuri, J., Alt, F. W., and Geha, R. S. (2004). Induction of activation-induced cytidine deaminase gene expression by IL-4 and CD40 ligation is dependent on STAT6 and NFkappaB. *Int. Immunol.* **16**, 395–404.

Deininger, P. L., and Batzer, M. A. (2002). Mammalian retroelements. *Genome Res.* **12**, 1455–1465.
Delebecque, F., Suspene, R., Calattini, S., Casartelli, N., Saib, A., Froment, A., Wain-Hobson, S., Gessain, A., Vartanian, J. P., and Schwartz, O. (2006). Restriction of foamy viruses by APOBEC cytidine deaminases. *J. Virol.* **80**, 605–614.
Delelis, O., Lehmann-Che, J., and Saib, A. (2004). Foamy viruses—a world apart. *Curr. Opin. Microbiol.* **7**, 400–406.
Diaz, M., Greenberg, A. S., and Flajnik, M. F. (1998). Somatic hypermutation of the new antigen receptor gene (NAR) in the nurse shark does not generate the repertoire: Possible role in antigen-driven reactions in the absence of germinal centers. *Proc. Natl. Acad. Sci. USA* **95**, 14343–14348.
Dickerson, S. K., Market, E., Besmer, E., and Papavasiliou, F. N. (2003). AID mediates hypermutation by deaminating single stranded DNA. *J. Exp. Med.* **197**, 1291–1296.
Doehle, B. P., Schafer, A., and Cullen, B. R. (2005). Human APOBEC3B is a potent inhibitor of HIV-1 infectivity and is resistant to HIV-1 Vif. *Virology* **339**, 281–288.
Dustin, L. B., and Rice, C. M. (2006). Personal communication.
Dutko, J. A., Schafer, A., Kenny, A. E., Cullen, B. R., and Curcio, M. J. (2005). Inhibition of a yeast LTR retrotransposon by human APOBEC3 cytidine deaminases. *Curr. Biol.* **15**, 661–666.
Epeldegui, M., Hung, Y. P., McQuay, A., Ambinder, R. F., and Martinez-Maza, O. (2006). Infection of human B cells with Epstein-Barr virus results in the expression of somatic hypermutation-inducing molecules and in the accrual of oncogene mutations. *Mol. Immunol.* **44**, 934–942.
Esnault, C., Heidmann, O., Delebecque, F., Dewannieux, M., Ribet, D., Hance, A. J., Heidmann, T., and Schwartz, O. (2005). APOBEC3G cytidine deaminase inhibits retrotransposition of endogenous retroviruses. *Nature* **433**, 430–433.
Esnault, C., Millet, J., Schwartz, O., and Heidmann, T. (2006). Dual inhibitory effects of APOBEC family proteins on retrotransposition of mammalian endogenous retroviruses. *Nucleic Acids Res.* **34**, 1522–1531.
Fearon, D. T., and Carter, R. H. (1995). The CD19/CR2/TAPA-1 complex of B lymphocytes: Linking natural to acquired immunity. *Annu. Rev. Immunol.* **13**, 127–149.
Feuer, G., and Green, P. L. (2005). Comparative biology of human T-cell lymphotropic virus type 1 (HTLV-1) and HTLV-2. *Oncogene* **24**, 5996–6004.
Ganem, D. (1996). *In* "Fields Virology" (B. N. Fields, D. M. Knipe, and P. M. Howley, Eds.), p. 2703. Lipincott-Raven, Philadelphia.
Gil, Y., Levy-Nabot, S., Steinitz, M., and Laskov, R. (2007). Somatic mutations and activation-induced cytidine deaminase (AID) expression in established rheumatoid factor-producing lymphoblastoid cell line. *Mol. Immunol.* **44**, 494–505.
Gires, O., Zimber-Strobl, U., Gonnella, R., Ueffing, M., Marschall, G., Zeidler, R., Pich, D., and Hammerschmidt, W. (1997). Latent membrane protein 1 of Epstein-Barr virus mimics a constitutively active receptor molecule. *EMBO J.* **16**, 6131–6140.
Goncalves, M. A. (2005). Adeno-associated virus: From defective virus to effective vector. *Virol. J.* **2**, 43.
Gourzi, P., Leonova, T., and Papavasiliou, F. N. (2007). Viral induction of AID is independent of the interferon and the Toll-like receptor signaling pathways but requires NFκB. *J. Exp. Med.* **204**(2), 259–265.
Gourzi, P., Leonova, T., and Papavasiliou, F. N. (2006). A role for activation-induced cytidine deaminase in the host response against a transforming retrovirus. *Immunity* **24**, 779–786.

Gu, Y., and Sundquist, W. I. (2003). Good to CU. *Nature* **424,** 21–22.
Harris, R. S., Bishop, K. N., Sheehy, A. M., Craig, H. M., Petersen-Mahrt, S. K., Watt, I. N., Neuberger, M. S., and Malim, M. H. (2003). DNA deamination mediates innate immunity to retroviral infection. *Cell* **113,** 803–809.
He, B., Raab-Traub, N., Casali, P., and Cerutti, A. (2003). EBV-encoded latent membrane protein 1 cooperates with BAFF/BLyS and APRIL to induce T cell-independent Ig heavy chain class switching. *J. Immunol.* **171,** 5215–5224.
Hinds-Frey, K. R., Nishikata, H., Litman, R. T., and Litman, G. W. (1993). Somatic variation precedes extensive diversification of germline sequences and combinatorial joining in the evolution of immunoglobulin heavy chain diversity. *J. Exp. Med.* **178,** 815–824.
Honda, K., Yanai, H., Takaoka, A., and Taniguchi, T. (2005). Regulation of the type I IFN induction: A current view. *Int. Immunol.* **17,** 1367–1378.
Hughes, J. F., and Coffin, J. M. (2001). Evidence for genomic rearrangements mediated by human endogenous retroviruses during primate evolution. *Nat. Genet.* **29,** 487–489.
Jarmuz, A., Chester, A., Bayliss, J., Gisbourne, J., Dunham, I., Scott, J., and Navaratnam, N. (2002). An anthropoid-specific locus of orphan C to U RNA-editing enzymes on chromosome 22. *Genomics* **79,** 285–296.
Johnson, W. E., and Coffin, J. M. (1999). Constructing primate phylogenies from ancient retrovirus sequences. *Proc. Natl. Acad. Sci. USA* **96,** 10254–10260.
Kazazian, H. H., Jr. (2004). Mobile elements: Drivers of genome evolution. *Science* **303,** 1626–1632.
Ketting, R. F., and Plasterk, R. H. (2000). A genetic link between co-suppression and RNA interference in *C. elegans*. *Nature* **404,** 296–298.
Kilger, E., Kieser, A., Baumann, M., and Hammerschmidt, W. (1998). Epstein-Barr virus-mediated B-cell proliferation is dependent upon latent membrane protein 1, which simulates an activated CD40 receptor. *EMBO J.* **17,** 1700–1709.
Kobayashi, M., Takaori-Kondo, A., Shindo, K., Abudu, A., Fukunaga, K., and Uchiyama, T. (2004). APOBEC3G targets specific virus species. *J. Virol.* **78,** 8238–8244.
Kou, T., Marusawa, H., Kinoshita, K., Endo, Y., Okazaki, I. M., Ueda, Y., Kodama, Y., Haga, H., Ikai, I., and Chiba, T. (2007). Expression of activation-induced cytidine deaminase in human hepatocytes during hepatocarcinogenesis. *Int. J. Cancer.* **120**(3), 469–476.
Kremer, M., Bittner, A., and Schnierle, B. S. (2005). Human APOBEC3G incorporation into murine leukemia virus particles. *Virology* **337,** 175–182.
Kuppers, R. (2003). B cells under influence: Transformation of B cells by Epstein-Barr virus. *Nat. Rev. Immunol.* **3,** 801–812.
Kuppers, R., and Dalla-Favera, R. (2001). Mechanisms of chromosomal translocations in B cell lymphomas. *Oncogene* **20,** 5580–5594.
Lander, E. S., Linton, L. M., Birren, B., Nusbaum, C., Zody, M. C., Baldwin, J., Devon, K., Dewar, K., Doyle, M., FitzHugh, W., Funke, R., Gage, D., *et al.* (2001). Initial sequencing and analysis of the human genome. *Nature* **409,** 860–921.
Lauer, G. M., and Walker, B. D. (2001). Hepatitis C virus infection. *N. Engl. J. Med.* **345,** 41–52.
Lecossier, D., Bouchonnet, F., Clavel, F., and Hance, A. J. (2003). Hypermutation of HIV-1 DNA in the absence of the Vif protein. *Science* **300,** 1112.
Levy, S., Todd, S. C., and Maecker, H. T. (1998). CD81 (TAPA-1): A molecule involved in signal transduction and cell adhesion in the immune system. *Annu. Rev. Immunol.* **16,** 89–109.
Li, Z., Crouch, E., Takizawa, M., Gourzi, P., Feigenbaum, L., Papavasiliou, F. N., Janz, S., and Casselas, R. (2007). Regulation of AID in the immune response. *J. Exp. Med.* in press.

Liddament, M. T., Brown, W. L., Schumacher, A. J., and Harris, R. S. (2004). APOBEC3F properties and hypermutation preferences indicate activity against HIV-1 *in vivo*. *Curr. Biol.* **14,** 1385–1391.

Lindenbach, B. D., Evans, M. J., Syder, A. J., Wolk, B., Tellinghuisen, T. L., Liu, C. C., Maruyama, T., Hynes, R. O., Burton, D. R., McKeating, J. A., and Rice, C. M. (2005). Complete replication of hepatitis C virus in cell culture. *Science* **309,** 623–626.

Lindenbach, B. D., Meuleman, P., Ploss, A., Vanwolleghem, T., Syder, A. J., McKeating, J. A., Lanford, R. E., Feinstone, S. M., Major, M. E., Leroux-Roels, G., and Rice, C. M. (2006). Cell culture-grown hepatitis C virus is infectious *in vivo* and can be recultured *in vitro*. *Proc. Natl. Acad. Sci. USA* **103,** 3805–3809.

Linial, M. L. (1999). Foamy viruses are unconventional retroviruses. *J. Virol.* **73,** 1747–1755.

Lochelt, M., Muranyi, W., and Flugel, R. M. (1993). Human foamy virus genome possesses an internal, Bel-1-dependent and functional promoter. *Proc. Natl. Acad. Sci. USA* **90,** 7317–7321.

Lochelt, M., Romen, F., Bastone, P., Muckenfuss, H., Kirchner, N., Kim, Y. B., Truyen, U., Rosler, U., Battenberg, M., Saib, A., Flory, E., Cichutek, K., and Munk, C. (2005). The antiretroviral activity of APOBEC3 is inhibited by the foamy virus accessory Bet protein. *Proc. Natl. Acad. Sci. USA* **102,** 7982–7987.

Machida, K., Cheng, K. T., Sung, V. M., Shimodaira, S., Lindsay, K. L., Levine, A. M., Lai, M. Y., and Lai, M. M. (2004). Hepatitis C virus induces a mutator phenotype: Enhanced mutations of immunoglobulin and protooncogenes. *Proc. Natl. Acad. Sci. USA* **101,** 4262–4267.

Machida, K., Cheng, K. T., Pavio, N., Sung, V. M., and Lai, M. M. (2005). Hepatitis C virus E2-CD81 interaction induces hypermutation of the immunoglobulin gene in B cells. *J. Virol.* **79,** 8079–8089.

Madani, N., and Kabat, D. (1998). An endogenous inhibitor of human immunodeficiency virus in human lymphocytes is overcome by the viral Vif protein. *J. Virol.* **72,** 10251–10255.

Mahieux, R., Suspene, R., Delebecque, F., Henry, M., Schwartz, O., Wain-Hobson, S., and Vartanian, J. P. (2005). Extensive editing of a small fraction of human T-cell leukemia virus type 1 genomes by four APOBEC3 cytidine deaminases. *J. Gen. Virol.* **86,** 2489–2494.

Mangeat, B., Turelli, P., Caron, G., Friedli, M., Perrin, L., and Trono, D. (2003). Broad antiretroviral defence by human APOBEC3G through lethal editing of nascent reverse transcripts. *Nature* **424,** 99–103.

Mangeat, B., Turelli, P., Liao, S., and Trono, D. (2004). A single amino acid determinant governs the species-specific sensitivity of APOBEC3G to Vif action. *J. Biol. Chem.* **279,** 14481–14483.

Mariani, R., Chen, D., Schrofelbauer, B., Navarro, F., Konig, R., Bollman, B., Munk, C., Nymark-McMahon, H., and Landau, N. R. (2003). Species-specific exclusion of APOBEC3G from HIV-1 virions by Vif. *Cell* **114,** 21–31.

Marin, M., Rose, K. M., Kozak, S. L., and Kabat, D. (2003). HIV-1 Vif protein binds the editing enzyme APOBEC3G and induces its degradation. *Nat. Med.* **9,** 1398–1403.

Meiering, C. D., and Linial, M. L. (2002). Reactivation of a complex retrovirus is controlled by a molecular switch and is inhibited by a viral protein. *Proc. Natl. Acad. Sci. USA* **99,** 15130–15135.

Mikl, M. C., Watt, I. N., Lu, M., Reik, W., Davies, S. L., Neuberger, M. S., and Rada, C. (2005). Mice deficient in APOBEC2 and APOBEC3. *Mol. Cell. Biol.* **25,** 7270–7277.

Moretta, A., Comoli, P., Montagna, D., Gasparoni, A., Percivalle, E., Carena, I., Revello, M. G., Gerna, G., Mingrat, G., Locatelli, F., Rondini, G., and Maccario, R. (1997). High frequency of Epstein-Barr virus (EBV) lymphoblastoid cell line-reactive lymphocytes in cord blood: Evaluation of cytolytic activity and IL-2 production. *Clin. Exp. Immunol.* **107,** 312–320.

Mosialos, G., Birkenbach, M., Yalamanchili, R., VanArsdale, T., Ware, C., and Kieff, E. (1995). The Epstein-Barr virus transforming protein LMP1 engages signaling proteins for the tumor necrosis factor receptor family. *Cell* **80,** 389.

Muckenfuss, H., Hamdorf, M., Held, U., Perkovic, M., Lower, J., Cichutek, K., Flory, E., Schumann, G. G., and Munk, C. (2006). APOBEC3 proteins inhibit human LINE-1 retrotransposition. *J. Biol. Chem.* **281,** 22161–22172.

Muramatsu, M., Sankaranand, V. S., Anant, S., Sugai, M., Kinoshita, K., Davidson, N. O., and Honjo, T. (1999). Specific expression of activation-induced cytidine deaminase (AID), a novel member of the RNA-editing deaminase family in germinal center B cells. *J. Biol. Chem.* **274,** 18470–18476.

Nakagawa, K., and Harrison, L. C. (1996). The potential roles of endogenous retroviruses in autoimmunity. *Immunol. Rev.* **152,** 193–236.

Navaratnam, N., Morrison, J. R., Bhattacharya, S., Patel, D., Funahashi, T., Giannoni, F., Teng, B. B., Davidson, N. O., and Scott, J. (1993). The p27 catalytic subunit of the apolipoprotein B mRNA editing enzyme is a cytidine deaminase. *J. Biol. Chem.* **268,** 20709–20712.

Navarro, F., Bollman, B., Chen, H., Konig, R., Yu, Q., Chiles, K., and Landau, N. R. (2005). Complementary function of the two catalytic domains of APOBEC3G. *Virology* **333,** 374–386.

Neuberger, M. S., and Scott, J. (2000). Immunology: RNA editing AIDs antibody diversification? *Science* **289,** 1705–1706.

Newman, E. N., Holmes, R. K., Craig, H. M., Klein, K. C., Lingappa, J. R., Malim, M. H., and Sheehy, A. M. (2005). Antiviral function of APOBEC3G can be dissociated from cytidine deaminase activity. *Curr. Biol.* **15,** 166–170.

Ni, T. H., McDonald, W. F., Zolotukhin, I., Melendy, T., Waga, S., Stillman, B., and Muzyczka, N. (1998). Cellular proteins required for adeno-associated virus DNA replication in the absence of adenovirus coinfection. *J. Virol.* **72,** 2777–2787.

Ostertag, E. M., and Kazazian, H. H., Jr. (2001). Biology of mammalian L1 retrotransposons. *Annu. Rev. Genet.* **35,** 501–538.

Pancer, Z., and Cooper, M. D. (2006). The evolution of adaptive immunity. *Annu. Rev. Immunol.* **24,** 497–518.

Richardson, J. H., Edwards, A. J., Cruickshank, J. K., Rudge, P., and Dalgleish, A. G. (1990). In vivo cellular tropism of human T-cell leukemia virus type 1. *J. Virol.* **64,** 5682–5687.

Rosenberg, N. (1994). Abl-mediated transformation, immunoglobulin gene rearrangements and arrest of B lymphocyte differentiation. *Semin. Cancer Biol.* **5,** 95–102.

Rosler, C., Kock, J., Kann, M., Malim, M. H., Blum, H. E., Baumert, T. F., and von Weizsacker, F. (2005). APOBEC-mediated interference with hepadnavirus production. *Hepatology* **42,** 301–309.

Russell, R. A., Wiegand, H. L., Moore, M. D., Schafer, A., McClure, M. O., and Cullen, B. R. (2005). Foamy virus Bet proteins function as novel inhibitors of the APOBEC3 family of innate antiretroviral defense factors. *J. Virol.* **79,** 8724–8731.

Sasada, A., Takaori-Kondo, A., Shirakawa, K., Kobayashi, M., Abudu, A., Hishizawa, M., Imada, K., Tanaka, Y., and Uchiyama, T. (2005). APOBEC3G targets human T-cell leukemia virus type 1. *Retrovirology* **2,** 32.

Sassaman, D. M., Dombroski, B. A., Moran, J. V., Kimberland, M. L., Naas, T. P., DeBerardinis, R. J., Gabriel, A., Swergold, G. D., and Kazazian, H. H., Jr. (1997). Many human L1 elements are capable of retrotransposition. *Nat. Genet.* **16,** 37–43.

Sawyer, S. L., Emerman, M., and Malik, H. S. (2004). Ancient adaptive evolution of the primate antiviral DNA-editing enzyme APOBEC3G. *PLoS Biol.* **2,** E275.

Schrofelbauer, B., Chen, D., and Landau, N. R. (2004). A single amino acid of APOBEC3G controls its species-specific interaction with virion infectivity factor (Vif). *Proc. Natl. Acad. Sci. USA* **101,** 3927–3932.

Schumacher, A. J., Nissley, D. V., and Harris, R. S. (2005). APOBEC3G hypermutates genomic DNA and inhibits Ty1 retrotransposition in yeast. *Proc. Natl. Acad. Sci. USA* **102,** 9854–9859.

Sheehy, A. M., Gaddis, N. C., Choi, J. D., and Malim, M. H. (2002). Isolation of a human gene that inhibits HIV-1 infection and is suppressed by the viral Vif protein. *Nature* **418,** 646–650.

Sheehy, A. M., Gaddis, N. C., and Malim, M. H. (2003). The antiretroviral enzyme APOBEC3G is degraded by the proteasome in response to HIV-1 Vif. *Nat. Med.* **9,** 1404–1407.

Sijen, T., and Plasterk, R. H. (2003). Transposon silencing in the *Caenorhabditis elegans* germ line by natural RNAi. *Nature* **426,** 310–314.

Simon, J. H., Gaddis, N. C., Fouchier, R. A., and Malim, M. H. (1998). Evidence for a newly discovered cellular anti-HIV-1 phenotype. *Nat. Med.* **4,** 1397–1400.

Simon, V., Zennou, V., Murray, D., Huang, Y., Ho, D. D., and Bieniasz, P. D. (2005). Natural variation in Vif: Differential impact on APOBEC3G/3F and a potential role in HIV-1 diversification. *PLoS Pathog.* **1,** e6.

Stopak, K., de Noronha, C., Yonemoto, W., and Greene, W. C. (2003). HIV-1 Vif blocks the antiviral activity of APOBEC3G by impairing both its translation and intracellular stability. *Mol. Cell* **12,** 591–601.

Sung, V. M., Shimodaira, S., Doughty, A. L., Picchio, G. R., Can, H., Yen, T. S., Lindsay, K. L., Levine, A. M., and Lai, M. M. (2003). Establishment of B-cell lymphoma cell lines persistently infected with hepatitis C virus *in vivo* and *in vitro*: The apoptotic effects of virus infection. *J. Virol.* **77,** 2134–2146.

Suspene, R., Guetard, D., Henry, M., Sommer, P., Wain-Hobson, S., and Vartanian, J. P. (2005). Extensive editing of both hepatitis B virus DNA strands by APOBEC3 cytidine deaminases *in vitro* and *in vivo*. *Proc. Natl. Acad. Sci. USA* **102,** 8321–8326.

Tabara, H., Sarkissian, M., Kelly, W. G., Fleenor, J., Grishok, A., Timmons, L., Fire, A., and Mello, C. C. (1999). The rde-1 gene, RNA interference, and transposon silencing in *C. elegans*. *Cell* **99,** 123–132.

Tanaka, Y., Marusawa, H., Seno, H., Matsumoto, Y., Ueda, Y., Kodama, Y., Endo, Y., Yamauchi, J., Matsumoto, T., Takaori-Kondo, A., Ikai, I., and Chiba, T. (2006). Anti-viral protein APOBEC3G is induced by interferon-alpha stimulation in human hepatocytes. *Biochem. Biophys. Res. Commun.* **341,** 314–319.

Taruscio, D., and Mantovani, A. (2004). Factors regulating endogenous retroviral sequences in human and mouse. *Cytogenet Genome Res.* **105,** 351–362.

Teng, B., Burant, C. F., and Davidson, N. O. (1993). Molecular cloning of an apolipoprotein B messenger RNA editing protein. *Science* **260,** 1816–1819.

Tobollik, S., Meyer, L., Buettner, M., Klemmer, S., Kempkes, B., Kremmer, E., Niedobitek, G., and Jungnickel, B. (2006). Epstein-Barr-virus nuclear antigen 2 inhibits AID expression during EBV-driven B cell growth. *Blood* **108**(12), 3859–3864.

Turelli, P., and Trono, D. (2005). Editing at the crossroad of innate and adaptive immunity. *Science* **307,** 1061–1065.

Turelli, P., Mangeat, B., Jost, S., Vianin, S., and Trono, D. (2004). Inhibition of hepatitis B virus replication by APOBEC3G. *Science* **303,** 1829.

Turelli, P., Vianin, S., and Trono, D. (2004). The innate antiretroviral factor APOBEC3G does not affect human LINE-1 retrotransposition in a cell culture assay. *J. Biol. Chem.* **279,** 43371–43373.

Walsh, C. P., Chaillet, J. R., and Bestor, T. H. (1998). Transcription of IAP endogenous retroviruses is constrained by cytosine methylation. *Nat. Genet.* **20**, 116–117.
Waterston, R. H., Lindblad-Toh, K., Birney, E., Rogers, J., Abril, J. F., Agarwal, P., Agarwala, R., Ainscough, R., Alexandersson, M., An, P., Antonarakis, S. E., Attwood, J., *et al.* (2002). Initial sequencing and comparative analysis of the mouse genome. *Nature* **420**, 520–562.
Wieland, S., Thimme, R., Purcell, R. H., and Chisari, F. V. (2004). Genomic analysis of the host response to hepatitis B virus infection. *Proc. Natl. Acad. Sci. USA* **101**, 6669–6674.
Wilson, A. D., and Morgan, A. J. (2002). Primary immune responses by cord blood CD4(+) T cells and NK cells inhibit Epstein-Barr virus B-cell transformation *in vitro*. *J. Virol.* **76**, 5071–5081.
Wong, D. K., Cheung, A. M., O'Rourke, K., Naylor, C. D., Detsky, A. S., and Heathcote, J. (1993). Effect of alpha-interferon treatment in patients with hepatitis B e antigen-positive chronic hepatitis B. A meta-analysis. *Ann. Intern. Med.* **119**, 312–323.
Xu, H., Svarovskaia, E. S., Barr, R., Zhang, Y., Khan, M. A., Strebel, K., and Pathak, V. K. (2004). A single amino acid substitution in human APOBEC3G antiretroviral enzyme confers resistance to HIV-1 virion infectivity factor-induced depletion. *Proc. Natl. Acad. Sci. USA* **101**, 5652–5657.
Young, L. S., and Rickinson, A. B. (2004). Epstein-Barr virus: 40 years on. *Nat. Rev. Cancer* **4**, 757–768.
Yu, Q., Konig, R., Pillai, S., Chiles, K., Kearney, M., Palmer, S., Richman, D., Coffin, J. M., and Landau, N. R. (2004). Single-strand specificity of APOBEC3G accounts for minus-strand deamination of the HIV genome. *Nat. Struct. Mol. Biol.* **11**, 435–442.
Yu, X., Yu, Y., Liu, B., Luo, K., Kong, W., Mao, P., and Yu, X. F. (2003). Induction of APOBEC3G ubiquitination and degradation by an HIV-1 Vif-Cul5-SCF complex. *Science* **302**, 1056–1060.
Zennou, V., and Bieniasz, P. D. (2006). Comparative analysis of the antiretroviral activity of APOBEC3G and APOBEC3F from primates. *Virology* **349**, 31–40.
Zhang, H., Yang, B., Pomerantz, R. J., Zhang, C., Arunachalam, S. C., and Gao, L. (2003). The cytidine deaminase CEM15 induces hypermutation in newly synthesized HIV-1 DNA. *Nature* **424**, 94–98.
Zhang, J., and Webb, D. M. (2004). Rapid evolution of primate antiviral enzyme APOBEC3G. *Hum. Mol. Genet.* **13**, 1785–1791.
Zhang, J., Randall, G., Higginbottom, A., Monk, P., Rice, C. M., and McKeating, J. A. (2004). CD81 is required for hepatitis C virus glycoprotein-mediated viral infection. *J. Virol.* **78**, 1448–1455.
Zimber-Strobl, U., Strobl, L. J., Meitinger, C., Hinrichs, R., Sakai, T., Furukawa, T., Honjo, T., and Bornkamm, G. W. (1994). Epstein-Barr virus nuclear antigen 2 exerts its transactivating function through interaction with recombination signal binding protein RBP-J kappa, the homologue of Drosophila Suppressor of Hairless. *EMBO J.* **13**, 4973–4982.

Role of AID in Tumorigenesis

Il-mi Okazaki, Ai Kotani,[1] and Tasuku Honjo

Department of Immunology and Genomic Medicine, Graduate School of Medicine, Kyoto University, Kyoto, Japan

Abstract 245
1. Introduction 246
2. AID Transgenic Mouse Models 247
3. Role of AID in Chromosomal Translocation and Subsequent Lymphomagenesis 249
4. AID Expression in Human B-Cell Malignancies 252
5. Mechanism of AID Expression in Normal and Malignant B Cells 259
6. AID Expression in Normal and Malignant Nonlymphoid Cells 263
7. Concluding Remarks 265
   References 265

Abstract

A hallmark of mature B-cell lymphomas is reciprocal chromosomal translocations involving the Ig locus and a proto-oncogene, which usually result in the deregulated, constitutive expression of the translocated gene. In addition to such translocations, proto-oncogenes are frequently hypermutated in germinal center (GC)-derived B-cell lymphomas. Although aberrant, mistargeted class switch recombination (CSR) and somatic hypermutation (SHM) events have long been suspected of causing chromosomal translocations and mutations in oncogenes, and thus of playing a critical role in the pathogenesis of most B-cell lymphomas, the molecular basis for such deregulation of CSR and SHM is only beginning to be elucidated by recent genetic approaches. The tumorigenic ability of activation-induced cytidine deaminase (AID), a key enzyme that initiates CSR and SHM, was revealed in studies on AID transgenic mice. In addition, experiments with AID-deficient mice clearly showed that AID is required not only for the c-myc/IgH translocation but also for the malignant progression of translocation-bearing lymphoma precursor cells, probably by introducing additional genetic hits. Normally, AID expression is only transiently and specifically induced in activated B cells in GCs. However, recent studies indicate that AID can be induced directly in B cells outside the GCs by various pathogens, including transforming viruses associated with human malignancies. Indeed, AID expression is not restricted to GC-derived B-cell lymphomas, but is also found in other types of B-cell lymphoma and even in nonlymphoid

---

[1]Present address: Whitehead Institute for Biomedical Research, Nine Cambridge Center, Cambridge, Massachusetts 02142.

tumors, suggesting that ectopically expressed AID is involved in tumorigenesis and disease progression in a wide variety of cell types.

1. Introduction

Lymphomas diagnosed in the Western world are mostly of B-cell origin, and most of these are derived from germinal-center (GC) or post-GC B cells (Kuppers, 2005), suggesting that events occurring in the GC environment contribute to the pathogenesis of B-cell lymphomas. In the GC, antigen-stimulated mature B cells proliferate extensively and undergo two distinct genetic alterations in the immunoglobulin (Ig) genes, namely somatic hypermutation (SHM) and class switch recombination (CSR), both of which involve DNA strand breaks (Honjo et al., 2002; Neuberger and Milstein, 1995). SHM causes accumulated point mutations in the rearranged variable (V) region genes, which result in the generation of antibodies with a potentially higher affinity for their antigen (Neuberger and Milstein, 1995). CSR changes the Ig heavy-chain constant region (C_H) gene from $C\mu$ to another C_H gene, by recombination between the μ switch ($S\mu$) region and one of the downstream switch (S) regions, located 5' to each C_H gene. This results in the generation of antibodies with different effector functions but the same antigen specificity (Honjo et al., 2002). These frequent genetic alterations in the Ig loci have long been suspected to contribute to lymphoma pathogenesis.

A hallmark of mature B-cell lymphomas is reciprocal chromosomal translocations involving the Ig locus and a proto-oncogene such as the c-myc/IgH translocations in Burkitt's lymphoma (BL) (Kuppers, 2005; Kuppers and Dalla-Favera, 2001). As a result of such translocations, the oncogene is brought under the control of the active Ig locus, leading to deregulated, constitutive expression of the translocated gene. In most cases, the breakpoints are found either in rearranged V region genes or in S regions of the Ig loci, suggesting that these chromosomal translocations are mediated by aberrant SHM and CSR activity (Kuppers and Dalla-Favera, 2001). In addition to such chromosomal translocations, an aberrant SHM process also seems to contribute to lymphoma pathogenesis by mutating non-Ig genes. Multiple proto-oncogenes are hypermutated in GC-derived B-cell lymphomas, such as diffuse large B-cell lymphoma (DLBCL) and BL, in a way that is similar to the normal SHM of Ig genes (Pasqualucci et al., 2001). Some of these genes, such as Bcl-6 and c-myc, accumulate mutations in the same regions as the translocation breakpoint clusters (Pasqualucci et al., 2001). Collectively, aberrant, mistargeted CSR and SHM activity is thought to play critical roles in the pathogenesis of the majority of B-cell lymphomas by causing chromosomal translocations and mutations in oncogenes. However, the molecular basis for CSR and SHM deregulation was not clearly described until activation-induced cytidine deaminase (AID), a key enzyme that initiates CSR and SHM, was described (Muramatsu et al., 2000; Revy et al., 2000).

AID is specifically expressed in GC B cells (Muramatsu et al., 1999) and is required for both SHM and CSR (Muramatsu et al., 2000; Revy et al., 2000). Furthermore, the expression of AID alone is sufficient to induce CSR and SHM in transcribed artificial substrates in fibroblasts as well as B cells (Martin and Scharff, 2002; Martin et al., 2002; Okazaki et al., 2002; Yoshikawa et al., 2002), indicating that AID triggers these two events. Importantly, targets of AID activity are not restricted to the Ig genes but include non-Ig genes, as evidenced by the mutations induced in non-Ig genes by AID expression (Martin and Scharff, 2002; Yoshikawa et al., 2002). Therefore, it is reasonable to speculate that the deregulation of AID could lead to aberrant CSR and SHM activity and play a critical role in lymphoma pathogenesis. This chapter discusses both the known contributions of AID to the pathogenesis of B-cell lymphomas and the possible contributions that ectopically expressed AID may make to promote non-B-cell tumorigenesis and disease progression.

2. AID Transgenic Mouse Models

One possible molecular mechanism for aberrant CSR and SHM activity is deregulated AID expression. However, the presence of AID expression in developed lymphomas does not always imply that AID expression is responsible for the lymphomagenesis. Conversely, the absence of AID expression does not mean it has no role in lymphomagenesis; for example, its expression might be terminated after the cell is transformed. A direct correlation between deregulated AID expression and tumorigenesis was tested using AID transgenic mice in which AID was expressed under control of a promoter that drives ubiquitous and constitutive expression (Okazaki et al., 2003). The AID transgenic mice spontaneously and frequently developed T-cell lymphomas. The genes for T-cell receptor (TCR), c-myc, Pim1, CD4, and CD5 were extensively mutated in these T-cell lymphomas; however, no clonal chromosomal translocations were found by spectral karyotyping (Kotani et al., 2005; Okazaki et al., 2003), suggesting that in the AID transgenic mice, the deregulated expression of AID contributes to T-cell lymphomagenesis by introducing mutations in non-Ig genes, including oncogenes, rather than by generating chromosomal translocations. Nonetheless, the existence of nonclonal translocations cannot be excluded because the overexpression of AID quickly induces the generation of c-myc/IgH translocations in activated B cells *in vitro* (Ramiro et al., 2006). Downregulation of tumor suppressor genes, such as those in the p53 pathway, might also be required for nonclonal translocations, if any, to become clonal translocations in the T-cell lymphomas of the AID transgenic mice.

Interestingly, these mice frequently developed multiple lung microadenomas and occasionally adenocarcinomas (Okazaki et al., 2003). Although much less frequent than the T-cell lymphomas and lung microadenomas, other types of tumor such as hepatocellular carcinomas (HCCs), melanomas, and sarcomas were found in the AID transgenic mice (Okazaki et al., 2003; I.M.O., unpublished data). In contrast, no B-cell lymphomas were observed in the AID transgenic mice (Okazaki et al., 2003). These observations may indicate that the sensitivity to AID activity is variable among different types of cells, although many tissues are potentially affected by the tumorigenic activity of AID in these mice. Alternatively, T-cell lymphomas may simply expand well in advance of the tumor generation in other cells.

Tissue-specific sensitivity to AID expression was tested by comparing three sets of transgenic mice in which AID expression was under the control of the lck, HTLV-1, or MMTV promoters (Rucci et al., 2006). Most of the lck-AID transgenic mice died with thymic lymphomas, in accordance with the lck promoter's high activity in double-positive thymocytes. In contrast, none of the HTLV-1-AID or MMTV-AID transgenic mice developed tumors of T-cell- or mammary gland-origin, although the HTLV-1 and MMTV promoters are, respectively, active in single-positive thymocytes as well as in mature T cells and exocrine glands, including the mammary gland. From these observations, it was concluded that lck-expressing thymocytes are sensitive to the transforming activity of AID, while more mature T cells and mammary gland tissues are resistant to it (Rucci et al., 2006). However, further examination is required to support the above conclusion because (1) only for mice each were analyzed for the HTLV-1- and MMTV-AID transgenic mice (Rucci et al., 2006), (2) the breast of one MMTV-AID transgenic mouse developed glandular hyperplasia, if not a mammary tumor (Rucci et al., 2006), and (3) not only CD4/CD8 double-positive thymocytes but also CD4 single-positive T cells were affected in the transgenic mice expressing AID ubiquitously (Okazaki et al., 2003).

Currently, the reason no B-cell lymphomas developed in the AID transgenic mice is unclear. Because B cells, but not T cells, express AID physiologically, it was tempting to speculate that B cells have a protective system to prevent excessive AID activity by inactivating the transgenic AID, at least in part. This possibility was tested using conditional AID transgenic mice that specifically and constitutively express AID in B cells that have once expressed CD19 (Muto et al., 2006). The activity of the transgenic AID was assessed in the absence of endogenous AID by crossing the conditional AID transgenic mice with the AID-deficient mice. Although the transgenic AID protein was expressed far more abundantly than the endogenous AID, the efficiencies of CSR and SHM in B cells expressing transgenic AID alone were only 30–40% of those in B cells expressing endogenous AID alone (Muto et al., 2006). This could be either because the function of the transgenic AID was inactivated and thus it was less effective than the endogenous AID or because other factors required for CSR and SHM were downregulated in the B cells that constitutively expressed AID. However, additional AID expression by retrovirus infection augmented the CSR in B cells expressing transgenic AID alone to a level similar to or greater than that of wild-type B cells (Muto et al., 2006), indicating that other factors required for CSR were not limiting and that transgenic AID, in spite of its abundance, is much less efficient than the endogenous protein.

Taken together, these results support the idea that most of the constitutively expressed AID was somehow modified to downregulate its CSR- and SHM-initiating activity, by as yet unknown mechanisms. There are several ways AID might be inactivated in B cells. The accumulated AID in transgenic B cells is likely to be inactivated by protein modifications or by interactions with other molecules. Because the AID function seems to be regulated by its subcellular localization (Ito et al., 2004; McBride et al., 2004), it is also possible that protein–protein interactions cause a change in AID's subcellular localization, reducing its activity. It still needs to be clarified if the inactivation of constitutively expressed AID in B cells can explain the absence of B-cell lymphomas in the AID transgenic mice.

In summary, the constitutive expression of AID is potentially deleterious to B cells as well as non-B cells, because AID may introduce DNA strand breaks not only in the IgV or S region genes but also in other genes, including oncogenes, which further induce chromosomal translocations and mutations. Therefore, AID expression has to be tightly regulated and limited to activated B cells. In addition, B cells seem to have acquired an as yet unknown strategy to limit AID function. B cells probably have multiple regulators for AID function, and elucidating these mechanisms will contribute to our understanding of the pathogenesis of B-cell lymphomas.

3. Role of AID in Chromosomal Translocation and Subsequent Lymphomagenesis

Chromosomal translocations are a hallmark of human hematological malignancies and are involved in the etiologies of many of them. In human B-cell lymphomas and leukemias, chromosomal translocations between IgH and various oncogenes, such as c-myc (BL), Bcl-2 (follicular B-cell lymphoma, FL), Bcl-6 (DLBCL), cyclin D (mantle cell lymphoma, MCL), and FGFR (multiple myeloma, MM), are frequently found (Mitelman, 2000; Willis and Dyer, 2000). These translocations are believed to result from frequent genetic alterations associated with DNA strand breaks that occur during B-cell development, namely V(D)J recombination, SHM, and CSR. Analyses of the DNA breakpoints of these chromosomal translocations suggested that most of the ones found in B-cell lymphomas are caused by aberrations in either V(D)J recombination (Bcl-2/IgH in FL and Bcl-1/IgH MCL), SHM (c-myc/IgH and c-myc/IgL in endemic BL), or CSR (c-myc/IgH in sporadic BL, Bcl-6/IgH in DLBCL, and FGFR/IgH in MM) (Kuppers and Dalla-Favera, 2001; Willis and Dyer, 2000). Indeed, RAG1 and RAG2, key DNA-cleaving enzymes required for V(D)J recombination, have been reported to be essential for chromosomal translocations in several murine lymphoma models (Difilippantonio et al., 2002; Gladdy et al., 2003; Petiniot et al., 2000; Vanasse et al., 1999; Zhu et al., 2002). Similarly, the role of aberrant CSR in chromosomal translocations has been directly tested in mouse models for c-myc/IgH translocation by taking advantage of the absolute requirement for AID in the initiating step of CSR (Ramiro et al., 2004, 2006; Unniraman et al., 2004).

Reciprocal chromosomal translocations between the c-myc gene on chromosome 8 and the IgH or IgL genes on chromosomes 14, 22, or 2, which result in constitutive, deregulated expression of c-myc, are characteristic of human BL and are usually considered to be the initiating oncogenic events (Janz, 2006). The most common translocation, representing 80% of the total c-myc/Ig translocations in BL, is the t(8;14) translocation, in which the majority of breakpoints are in the J_H region, for endemic BL, or the S regions, for the sporadic BL (Neri et al., 1988; Shiramizu et al., 1991), suggesting that SHM and CSR, respectively, are involved in the c-myc/IgH translocations in endemic and sporadic BL. The mouse T(12;15)(IgH/c-myc) translocation, which is characteristic of plasmacytomas and is induced in pristane-injected or IL-6-transgenic BALB/c mice, is widely accepted as the direct counterpart of the human t(8;14) translocation, both structurally and functionally (Janz, 2006; Potter, 2003). Therefore, these two mouse models are useful for dissecting the molecular mechanisms of the c-myc/IgH translocation found in human BL.

The assumption that AID is required for plasmacytoma-associated T(12;15) translocations was tested for the first time using AID-deficient BALB/c-IL-6 transgenic mice (Ramiro et al., 2004). BALB/c-IL-6 transgenic mice develop lymphatic hyperplasia associated with the polyclonal expansion of plasma cells that frequently carry T(12;15) translocations (Kovalchuk et al., 2002; Suematsu et al., 1992). These hyperplastic transgenic B cells are preneoplastic because they can develop into monoclonal plasmacytomas when they are transferred into BALB/c or nude mice (Kovalchuk et al., 2002). Although the AID-deficient IL-6 transgenic mice also developed lymphatic hyperplasia, with a slight delay compared with control mice, the T(12;15)(IgH/c-myc) translocations were absent from the AID-deficient hyperplastic lymph nodes, suggesting that AID is required for these translocations (Ramiro et al., 2004). The breakpoints for the T(12;15) translocations in the IL-6 transgenic mice were mainly in the S regions (Kovalchuk et al., 2002; Ramiro et al., 2004; Suematsu et al., 1992), indicating a major role for aberrant CSR rather than for SHM.

The direct involvement of AID in translocations was further confirmed using primary B cells stimulated in vitro to undergo CSR (Franco et al., 2006; Ramiro et al., 2006). AID overexpression in AID-deficient B cells was sufficient to induce T(12;15)(IgH/c-myc) translocations within hours. In addition, chromosomal translocations involving the IgH locus that were induced in histone H2AX-deficient B cells in vitro were also dependent on AID (Franco et al., 2006). Like the normal CSR (Imai et al., 2003; Rada et al., 2002), the T(12;15) translocations require uracil DNA glycosylase in addition to AID (Ramiro et al., 2006). In contrast, the aberrant joining of c-myc and IgH does not require histone H2AX, p53-binding protein 1, or the nonhomologous end-joining protein Ku80 (Ramiro et al., 2006), all of which are known to be essential for the intrachromosomal repair process during normal CSR (Dudley et al., 2005), indicating that the repair pathways for the DSBs in CSR are distinct from those in AID-dependent chromosomal translocations. Interestingly, translocations seem to be suppressed under normal circumstances by the tumor suppressors ATM, Nbs1, p19 (Arf), and p53, which emphasizes their protective roles against chromosomal translocations (Ramiro et al., 2006).

The requirement for AID in T(12;15)(IgH/c-myc) translocations is now certain. This translocation itself, however, is not sufficient to induce lymphoma, because the lymphomas that develop in transgenic mice bearing the c-myc gene coupled to the IgH enhancer (Eμ), which mimics T(12;15) translocations, are monoclonal, even though the Eμ enhancer is presumably activated in all B-lineage cells (Adams et al., 1985; Harris et al., 1988). Therefore, it is likely that translocation-bearing B cells require additional genetic hits to progress to fully malignant lymphomas. The possibility that AID promotes the outgrowth of translocation-bearing clones (tumor progression) was raised from experiments using the pristane-induced plasmacytoma model (Unniraman et al., 2004). Repeated injections of pristane into BALB/c mice are known to induce T(12;15)(IgH/c-myc) translocation-positive B cells and finally lead to the outgrowth of plasmacytomas (Potter and Wiener, 1992). After repeated injections of pristane, translocation-positive cells greatly increased in AID-sufficient mice but not in AID-deficient ones (Unniraman et al., 2004). From this observation, the authors concluded that AID does not contribute to c-myc/IgH chromosomal translocations but plays critical roles in the outgrowth of cells bearing this translocation (Unniraman et al., 2004). However, this interpretation remains inconclusive because tumor formation was not assessed explicitly, so tumor initiation and progression cannot be distinguished by these experiments.

A direct mechanistic link between AID and the ongoing neoplastic progression of translocation-bearing tumor precursors was demonstrated using

AID-deficient Eμ-cmyc transgenic mice (Kotani et al., 2007). These mice can develop both pre-B- and mature B-cell lymphomas (Adams et al., 1985; Harris et al., 1988). Although the survival curves for these mice showed no significant differences among $AID^{-/-}$, $AID^{+/-}$, and $AID^{+/+}$ Eμ-cmyc transgenic mice, the proportions of lymphoma types were strikingly different among the three groups. Almost all the lymphomas that developed in the $AID^{-/-}$ Eμ-cmyc transgenic mice were pre-B-cell lymphomas, whereas the $AID^{+/+}$ Eμ-cmyc transgenic mice predominantly developed mature B-cell lymphomas. Interestingly, the $AID^{+/-}$ Eμ-cmyc transgenic mice developed both pre-B- and mature B-cell lymphomas at a 1:1 ratio. These results suggest that AID plays a critical and dose-dependent role in the induction of the secondary genetic hits required for the development of mature B- but not pre-B-cell lymphomas from c-myc-overexpressing tumor progenitors.

Currently, it is completely unclear what secondary genetic hits are introduced by AID. AID could cause additional genetic hits in tumor progenitor cells through its mutagenic activity. Indeed, many of the B-cell lymphomas generated in the Eμ-cmyc transgenic mice had an unmutated IgV but a mutated Pim1 gene, while none of the pre-B-cell lymphomas showed mutations in the Pim1 gene (Kotani et al., 2007). Considering that Pim1 is a target gene for aberrant SHM in human DLBCL (Pasqualucci et al., 2001) and that it acts synergistically with c-myc in lymphomagenesis (Shirogane et al., 1999), Pim1 is a candidate target gene for secondary genetic hits leading to the transformation of tumor progenitor cells. In summary, AID has dual functions in B-cell lymphoma development: tumor initiation by causing chromosomal translocations and tumor progression, possibly through its mutagenic activity (Fig. 1). Further investigation will establish the function of AID in the tumor biology of human B-lineage malignancies.

4. AID Expression in Human B-Cell Malignancies

4.1. AID Expression in GC-Derived B-Cell Lymphomas

AID is expressed physiologically in GC B cells (Muramatsu et al., 2000; Yang et al., 2005). Thus, after the discovery of AID, the initial studies on its expression in human hematological malignancy were performed in GC-derived human B-cell lymphomas such as DLBCL, FL, and BL (Table 1). The majority, but not all, of these lymphoma cases express AID constitutively (Faili et al., 2002; Greeve et al., 2003; Hardianti et al., 2004a,b; Muto et al., 2000; Pasqualucci et al., 2001; Smit et al., 2003). These GC-derived B-cell lymphomas frequently carry chromosomal translocations involving IgH, such as Bcl-6/IgH, IgH/Bcl-2, and c-myc/IgH, some of which are thought to stem from

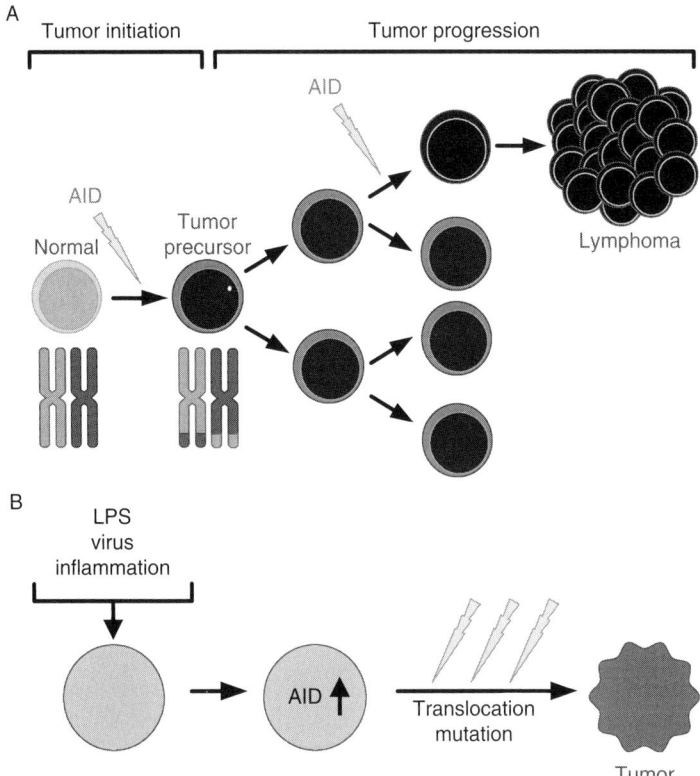

Figure 1 General model of the role of AID in tumor biology. (A) The dual functions of AID in tumorigenesis: initiation and progression. AID is required for chromosomal translocation at the IgH locus during CSR and SHM. Chromosomal translocation-bearing tumor precursors acquire secondary genetic hits and survive to develop into lymphoma, possibly through the mutagenic activity of AID. (B) AID can be induced directly in B cells outside of the GCs, and possibly in non-B cells, by various pathogens including transforming viruses. AID can also be induced under inflammatory conditions and may contribute to tumorigenesis and/or tumor evolution. (**See Color Plate 10.**)

illegitimate CSR (Kuppers and Dalla-Favera, 2001). Moreover, they frequently display hypermutations in oncogenes such as Bcl-6, c-myc, Pim1, RhoH/TTF1, and Pax5 that are similar to the SHM of Ig genes (Gordon *et al.*, 2003; Migliazza *et al.*, 1995; Pasqualucci *et al.*, 2001; Shen *et al.*, 1998). Some of these mutations create amino acid substitutions with potential functional consequences. These findings suggest that the AID expressed in GC-derived B-cell lymphomas is likely to be involved in lymphomagenesis through aberrant CSR and SHM.

Table 1 AID Expression in Human Malignancies of B-Cell Origin[a]

Lymphoma/leukemia	Subtype	Origin	AID expression	Correlation with clinical course	Possible mechanism	References
GC B-cell lymphomas						
DLBCL	ABC-type	GC B-cell expressing markers of plasmacytic differentiation	+/Higher than GCB type and type III	Poorer than GCB-type and type III	Blimp-1 inactivation	Lossos et al., 2004; Pasqualucci et al., 2004
	GCB-type	GC B cell	+			
	Type III	Heterogeneous GC B cell	+			
PCLBCL	PCLBCL-leg	GC B cell	+/Higher than PCFCL	Poorer than PCFCL		Dijkman et al., 2006
	PCFCL	GC B cell	+			
BL		GC B cell	+		EBV?	Faili et al., 2002; Greeve et al., 2003; Hardianti et al., 2004a,b; Muto et al., 2000; Pasqualucci et al., 2001; Smit et al., 2003
FL		GC B cell	+	Elevation of AID expression during transformation into DLBCL		Faili et al., 2002; Greeve et al., 2003; Hardianti et al., 2004a,b; Muto et al., 2000; Pasqualucci et al., 2001; Smit et al., 2003
HL	LPHL	GC B cell	+	Transformation into DLBCL?	EBV? Downregulation of B-cell-specific gene expression	Braeuninger et al., 1997
	cHL	Preapoptotic GC B cell	−			

Non-GC B-cell lymphoma/leukemia				
B-CLL	IgV$_H$ unmutated	Memory B cell	+	Albesiano et al., 2003; Cerutti et al., 2002; Heintel et al., 2004; McCarthy et al., 2003; Oppezzo et al., 2003; Reiniger et al., 2006
	IgV$_H$ mutated	Memory B cell	−	Poorer than M B-CLL
MALT lymphoma		Marginal zone B cell	+	Greeve et al., 2003; Forconi et al., 2004 Smit et al., 2003;
IC		Plasma cell	+	
MM		Plasma cell	−	
HCL		Memory B cell	+	Babbage et al., 2004; Greeve et al., 2003; Klapper et al., 2006; Smit et al., 2003
MCL		Naïve B cell or intermediate between naïve and GC B cells	?	
Pre-B ALL	t(14;18)	Pre-B cell	+	Greeve et al., 2003; Hardianti et al., 2005; Smit et al., 2003
	Others	Pre-B cell	−	

*a*DLBCL, diffuse large B-cell lymphoma; PCLBCL; primary cutaneous large B-cell lymphoma; PCFCL, primary cutaneous follicle center lymphoma; BL, Burkitt's lymphoma; FL, follicular B-cell lymphoma; HL, Hodgkin's lymphoma; LPHL, nodular lymphocyte-predominant HL; cHL, classical HL; B-CLL, B-cell chronic lymphocytic leukemia; M B-CLL, IgV$_H$ mutated B-CLL; IC, immunocytoma; MM, multiple myeloma; HCL, Hairy cell leukemia; MCL, mantle cell lymphoma; ALL, acute lymphocytic leukemia.

Additionally, AID was reported to be consistently expressed in the neoplastic cells of nodular lymphocyte-predominant Hodgkin's lymphoma (LPHL), but infrequently in those of classical Hodgkin's lymphoma (CHL) (Greiner et al., 2005; Mottok et al., 2005). This finding is consistent with our current idea that lymphocytic and histiocytic (L&H) cells, the neoplastic cells in LPHL, carry highly mutated Ig genes and have ongoing SHM and therefore are probably derived from GC B cells (Braeuninger et al., 1997). In contrast, Hodgkin and Reed-Sternberg cells, the neoplastic cells in CHL, carry highly mutated Ig genes without ongoing SHM and are probably derived from preapoptotic GC B cells, which have downregulated B-cell-specific gene expression (Kanzler et al., 1996; Kuppers et al., 2002; Marafioti et al., 2000). An intriguing possibility is that the AID expressed in L&H cells plays a role in the transformation of LPHL, an indolent subtype of Hodgkin's lymphoma, into aggressive DLBCL by introducing additional transforming mutations (Mottok et al., 2005).

4.2. AID Expression in Non-GC-Derived B-Cell Lymphomas

AID expression has also been extensively studied in human B-cell chronic lymphocytic leukemia (B-CLL), which is a non-GC-derived B-cell lymphoma and the most common leukemia in the Western world (Albesiano et al., 2003; Cerutti et al., 2002; Heintel et al., 2004; McCarthy et al., 2003; Oppezzo et al., 2003) (Table 1). B-CLL cells were originally considered to be the neoplastic counterpart of naive B cells, which do not undergo SHM (Hamblin, 2002). However, the demonstration that approximately 50% of B-CLL cases express mutated IgV_H genes (Schroeder and Dighiero, 1994) changed this view. Currently, it is well accepted that there are at least two distinct B-CLL subsets, one with unmutated IgV_H genes (UM B-CLL) and the other with mutated IgV_H genes (M B-CLL); importantly, M B-CLL cases have a better prognosis than UM B-CLL cases (Damle et al., 1999). Gene expression profiles suggest that both subtypes of B-CLL resemble memory B cells but not naive B cells (Klein et al., 2001; Rosenwald et al., 2001). Surprisingly, AID is constitutively expressed in UM B-CLL cells but not in M B-CLL cells (Albesiano et al., 2003; Cerutti et al., 2002; Heintel et al., 2004; McCarthy et al., 2003; Oppezzo et al., 2003), suggesting that the SHM machinery in the UM B-CLL cells is defective or inactivated. In contrast, the B-CLL cells with constitutive expression of AID undergo active CSR without any stimulation (Cerutti et al., 2002; Oppezzo et al., 2003), indicating a dissociation between SHM and CSR in CLL cells. Because AID is differentially expressed in the two subsets of CLL, although the gene expression profile of these two subsets is almost identical

(Klein et al., 2001; Rosenwald et al., 2001), it is tempting to think that AID is involved in poor prognosis of UM B-CLL. In addition, several AID splicing variants are expressed in UM B-CLL cells (McCarthy et al., 2003; Oppezzo et al., 2003). Therefore, it will be interesting to learn whether the splicing variants are involved in the pathogenesis of UM B-CLL.

Recently, studies on AID expression in human B-cell leukemia/lymphoma have been extended from GC-derived B-cell lymphomas and CLL to other kinds of human B-lineage leukemias/lymphomas (Table 1). Several studies show constitutive AID expression in many cases of MALT lymphoma (derived from marginal zone B cells of MALT), immunocytoma (from plasma cells), and Hairy cell leukemia (from memory B cells), but not in any cases of multiple myeloma (from plasma cells) (Forconi et al., 2004; Greeve et al., 2003; Smit et al., 2003). At present, AID expression in mantle cell lymphoma [from naive B cells or an intermediate cell type between naive and GC cells (Kolar et al., 2006)] is controversial (Babbage et al., 2004; Greeve et al., 2003; Klapper et al., 2006; Smit et al., 2003). Of note, constitutive expression of AID was found in a rare subset of pre-B acute lymphoblastic leukemia (pre-B ALL) carrying the t(14;18) translocation (Hardianti et al., 2005), but not in pre-B ALL without the translocation (Greeve et al., 2003; Hardianti et al., 2005; Smit et al., 2003), although the translocation itself is presumed to result from mistakes in V(D)J recombination. These studies indicate that AID can be expressed not only in GC-derived B-cell lymphomas but also in leukemias/lymphomas derived from B cells at various stages of differentiation (Table 1). Because AID expression was detected in a limited number of cases, further studies with more cases are required to clarify whether AID expression in these non-GC-derived leukemias/lymphomas has any clinical implications.

4.3. Potential Importance of AID Expression in Human B-Cell Malignancies

The presence of AID expression in a variety of human B-cell malignancies supports the assumption that AID plays a critical role in their initiation and/or progression. However, the level of AID expression in these malignancies does not always correlate with the level of SHM in the IgV gene or in oncogenes (Heintel et al., 2004; McCarthy et al., 2003; Pasqualucci et al., 2004; Smit et al., 2003). Moreover, AID expression is not always associated with ongoing mutations (Hardianti et al., 2004b; Lossos et al., 2004; Pasqualucci et al., 2001, 2004; Smit et al., 2003), although a clear association is observed in LPHL (Greiner et al., 2005; Mottok et al., 2005). The dissociation between AID expression and SHM activity can be explained at least in part by two possibilities: (1) the SHM machinery or AID itself is functionally impaired in tumor cells; or (2) AID may introduce mutations at earlier stages of the disease, but in later stages, the AID expression may be shut off.

Nevertheless, AID expression and a poor prognosis are correlated in several human B-cell lymphomas/leukemias (Table 1). As mentioned above, AID expression is associated with the UM B-CLL subset, which has a poorer prognosis than the M B-CLL subset (Heintel et al., 2004; McCarthy et al., 2003). A report that AID expression in B-CLL is associated with aberrant SHM in the c-myc, Pax5, and RhoH genes and with transformation into a more aggressive lymphoma (Reiniger et al., 2006) further supports the potential role of AID as a new prognostic marker for B-CLL.

In addition, significantly higher expression of AID was observed in a subgroup of DLBCL cases with a significantly poorer prognosis (Lossos et al., 2004; Pasqualucci et al., 2004). DLBCLs are categorized into three subgroups based on gene expression profiles: the GC B-cell-like (GCB), the activated B-cell-like (ABC), and the type III DLBCL subgroups. The ABC subgroup has poorer overall survival than the other two (Alizadeh et al., 2000; Rosenwald et al., 2002), and the level of AID expression is significantly higher in this subgroup than in the other two, although AID is highly expressed in all three of them (Lossos et al., 2004; Pasqualucci et al., 2001). Similarly, the association between AID expression and a poor prognosis was examined in primary cutaneous large B-cell lymphomas (PCLBCLs), which have two main groups: primary cutaneous follicle center lymphoma (PCFCL), which is indolent, and PCLBCL, leg type (PCLBCL-leg), which has an intermediate prognosis (Willemze et al., 2005). While aberrant SHM in the Bcl-6, Pax5, RhoH, and/ or c-myc genes was observed in cases of both PCFCL and PCLBCL-leg, the expression level of AID was significantly higher in PCLBCL-leg than in PCFCL (Dijkman et al., 2006). This observation is consistent with the fact that PCFCL and PCLBCL-leg have gene expression profiles similar to those of GCB and ABC-DLBCL, respectively (Hoefnagel et al., 2005).

Finally, two out of seven FL cases with clinical and histological progression showed elevated AID expression and selective outgrowth of AID-expressing clones during the transformation into DLBCL, suggesting that AID is involved in the transformation from indolent FL to aggressive DLBCL (Smit et al., 2003). These observations suggest that AID may play a role in tumor evolution, and AID expression may be useful as a new prognostic marker in certain human B-cell malignancies. A large-scale study investigating the correlation between AID expression and poor prognosis, and studies to determine the mechanism behind this correlation will pave the way for diagnostic and therapeutic applications targeting AID in these diseases.

5. Mechanism of AID Expression in Normal and Malignant B Cells

5.1. Regulation of AID Expression in Normal B Cells

Under physiological conditions, AID expression is tightly regulated, and only transiently and specifically induced in activated B cells in GCs to trigger SHM and CSR. This tight regulation is important, not only for the proper control of CSR and SHM but also for the prevention of potential oncogenesis by aberrant AID expression. Although the precise mechanism of this regulation has not been completely elucidated, AID expression in normal B cells is known to be facilitated by the concerted action of factors that induce CSR, including cytokines (like IL-4 and TGF-β) and the CD40 ligand (CD40L) (Muramatsu et al., 1999). BLyS and APRIL, which are expressed by dendritic cells, also synergize with IL-4, IL-10, or TGF-β to induce AID expression in B cells (Litinskiy et al., 2002). In addition, a bacterial component, LPS, is a potent inducer of AID in murine B cells (Muramatsu et al., 1999).

Several studies have suggested that the specific expression of AID in activated B cells results from a complex combination of both positive and negative transcriptional regulators. For instance, the AID expression induced by IL-4 and CD40 signals requires the binding of STAT6 and NF-κB to the 5' upstream region of the AID gene (Dedeoglu et al., 2004; Zhou et al., 2003). A basic helix-loop-helix (bHLH) transcription factor, E47, is reported to directly activate AID expression, possibly by binding the highly conserved intronic E-box sites in the AID gene (Sayegh et al., 2003). In contrast, the antagonist HLH proteins Id2 and Id3 repress AID expression (Gonda et al., 2003; Sayegh et al., 2003). In addition, a B lineage-specific transcription factor, Pax5, which is also antagonized by Id proteins (Roberts et al., 2001), seems to be involved in the lineage-specific expression of AID (Gonda et al., 2003). These observations indicate that the Id proteins probably play an important role in the negative regulation of AID expression. Interestingly, Blimp-1, a transcriptional repressor that drives the terminal differentiation of GC B cells into plasma cells by extinguishing the mature B-cell gene expression program (Shaffer et al., 2002), represses Pax5 expression (Lin et al., 2002), and induces Id2 expression (Shaffer et al., 2002). Thus, Blimp-1 potentially works as a molecular switch to repress AID expression after B cells have completed CSR and/or SHM. On the other hand, the minimal promoter of the mouse AID gene was found to be ubiquitously active, and a functionally important GA box within the minimal promoter binds the Sp-family of ubiquitous transcription factors, Sp1 and Sp3 (Yadav et al., 2006). These results suggest that both tissue-specific and ubiquitous mechanisms are involved in the precise regulation of AID gene expression.

5.2. Mechanism of AID Expression in B-Cell Malignancy

The mechanism by which AID is constitutively expressed in B-cell lymphomas/leukemias is being gradually revealed. In normal B cells, the expression of GC-related genes, including AID, is shut off by transcriptional regulation as B cells differentiate into plasma cells. As mentioned above, Blimp-1 extinguishes the expression of genes required for GC-cell functions, including Bcl-6 and AID, and it induces plasma-cell genes such as XBP-1 (Shaffer et al., 2002). Thus, the continuous expression of AID in lymphoma cells could be partly due to the downregulation of Blimp-1 function. Indeed, the expression of AID inversely correlates with the expression of Blimp-1 in cases of MALT lymphoma and immunocytoma (Greeve et al., 2003). Furthermore, a report showed that the Blimp-1 gene is inactivated by structural alterations in ~25% of ABC-DLBCL cases, and the Blimp-1 protein is abnormally absent in a large number of additional cases, despite the presence of the Blimp-1 mRNA (Pasqualucci et al., 2006). The inactivation of Blimp-1 may account for the high expression level of AID in ABC-DLBCL, which is mostly characterized by the down-regulation of GC-specific expression markers and the upregulation of markers for post-GC plasmacytic differentiation (Alizadeh et al., 2000; Lossos et al., 2004; Pasqualucci et al., 2004; Rosenwald et al., 2002).

The mechanism of AID induction in human B-cell malignancies, particularly in those arising from cells that never inhabited the GC, has not been sufficiently studied yet. However, several studies indicate that AID can be induced directly in B cells outside GCs by various pathogens in a T-cell-independent manner. Bacterial LPS directly induces AID expression in murine B cells, probably through binding to Toll-like receptor (TLR) 4 (Muramatsu et al., 1999; Poltorak et al., 1998). Human papillomavirus-like particles also directly induce AID expression and CSR in murine B cells through the TLR4-MyD88 pathway (Yang et al., 2005). Moreover, infection by viruses such as Epstein–Barr virus (EBV) and *Hepatitis C virus* (HCV), which cause or are associated with human B-lineage malignancy, induces AID expression in B-lineage cells at various differentiation stages.

EBV infection has been shown to induce AID expression (Epeldegui et al., 2007; He et al., 2003) as well as CSR (He et al., 2003) and mutations in cellular proto-oncogenes (Bcl-6 and p53) (Epeldegui et al., 2007) in human peripheral blood B cells *in vitro*. EBV is one of the most common human viruses, mainly infecting B cells and, to a lesser extent, T cells and epithelial cells (Kuppers, 2003). Although EBV usually persists as an asymptomatic latent infection, it is associated with several B-cell lymphomas such as endemic BL and Hodgkin's lymphoma, as well as some T-cell lymphomas and epithelial tumors (Kuppers,

2003). It is also well known that EBV can transform and immortalize human B cells *in vitro*, generating lymphoblastoid cell lines.

In latently infected B cells, nine EBV-encoded latent proteins—six EBV nuclear antigens (EBNAs) and three latent membrane proteins (LMPs)—are expressed in various combinations, and B cells infected with EBV *in vitro* express all of the latent EBV genes (Kuppers, 2003). Among them, LMP1 and EBNA2 have been shown to regulate AID expression in B cells (Epeldegui *et al.*, 2007; He *et al.*, 2003; Tobollik *et al.*, 2006). LMP1 functionally resembles a constitutively active CD40 (Devergne *et al.*, 1996; Kilger *et al.*, 1998; Mosialos *et al.*, 1995; Sylla *et al.*, 1998), and induces both AID expression and CSR in B cells in cooperation with BAFF and APRIL, which are also induced in B cells by LMP1 (He *et al.*, 2003). Meanwhile, EBNA2, together with EBNA-LP, is expressed before other latent viral genes in B cells *in vitro* (Alfieri *et al.*, 1991; Rooney *et al.*, 1989), and acts as a constitutively active Notch through interactions with RBP-J (Grossman *et al.*, 1994; Henkel *et al.*, 1994; Zimber-Strobl and Strobl, 2001; Zimber-Strobl *et al.*, 1994), thereby upregulating several viral genes, including LMP1, as well as cellular genes involved in the transformation of infected cells (Abbot *et al.*, 1990; Calender *et al.*, 1987; Fahraeus *et al.*, 1990; Wang *et al.*, 1987). In contrast to LMP1, EBNA2 inhibits AID expression in several different B cell lines, and this negative effect of EBNA2 on AID expression seems to be dominant over the positive effect of LMP1 in some situations (Tobollik *et al.*, 2006).

BL cells are usually characterized by AID expression and ongoing SHM (Section 4). Interestingly, there seems to be a counter-selection for EBNA2 expression during EBV-associated Burkitt's lymphomagenesis, because EBV-positive BL cells normally do not express any EBV-encoded latent proteins except for EBNA1, and several cases have had a deletion of the EBNA2 gene that abrogated EBNA2 expression (Kelly *et al.*, 2002). While the antagonistic effect of EBNA2 on c-myc function must also be considered (Pajic *et al.*, 2001), the strong inhibitory effect of EBNA2 on AID expression may partly account for the counter-selection for EBNA2 expression during lymphomagenesis. In contrast, as described above, HRS cells of CHL lack both AID expression and ongoing SHM in most cases, although in ~40% of cases of CHL in the Western world, the HRS cells are EBV-positive, usually $LMP1^+EBNA2^-$ (Kuppers, 2003). Therefore, the relative contribution of EBV to AID expression seems to differ among different types of EBV-associated lymphoma, probably depending on the developmental stage of the lymphoma cells and the combination of EBV latent genes expressed.

Furthermore, HCV infection induces AID expression in human peripheral B cells, at least partly through the interaction between its envelope glycoprotein,

E2, and CD81, a cellular receptor for HCV comprising the multimeric B-cell antigen receptor complex together with CD19 and CD21 molecules (Machida et al., 2004, 2005). HCV infection of B cells also induces both DSBs and SHM in several cellular genes, such as IgV and p53, as well as the expression of error-prone DNA polymerases ι and ζ (Machida et al., 2004). Both AID and these error-prone DNA polymerases contribute to HCV-induced SHM in cellular genes, but their relative contribution seems to vary for different target genes (Machida et al., 2004, 2005). Persisting HCV infection mainly causes chronic hepatitis, liver cirrhosis, and HCC, and it is associated with B-cell proliferative diseases such as mixed cryoglobulinemia and non-Hodgkin's B-cell lymphomas (Ferri et al., 1994; Silvestri et al., 1996). The IgH/Bcl-2 translocation has been frequently observed in HCV-infected patients with mixed cryoglobulinemia (Kitay-Cohen et al., 2000), and ongoing SHM in the IgV gene is frequently found in HCV-associated immunocytoma (Ivanovski et al., 1998). Therefore, it is reasonable to speculate that HCV-induced AID contributes to the development of HCV-associated B-cell lymphomas by causing chromosomal translocations and mutations.

More strikingly, AID can be induced in bone marrow-derived pre-B cells by Abelson murine leukemia virus (A-MuLV) infection (Gourzi et al., 2006). Such ectopically expressed AID seems to be functional because the JH4 and λ5 genes are frequently mutated in A-MuLV-infected wild-type bone-marrow cells but not in AID-deficient cells (Gourzi et al., 2006). A-MuLV is a transforming retrovirus that transforms early B cells *in vitro* and causes pro-B or pre-B cell leukemia *in vivo* (Rosenberg, 1982). In contrast to the predicted roles of AID in the virus-associated B-lymphomagenesis described above, AID deficiency increases the susceptibility to viral transformation by A-MuLV both *in vitro* and *in vivo*, suggesting that AID helps protect B cells from A-MuLV-induced leukemiagenesis (Gourzi et al., 2006). This protection has been attributed to delayed cell-cycle progression and increased susceptibility to NK cell killing, which are probably caused by the phosphorylation of checkpoint kinase-1 and the upregulation of NKG2D ligand, respectively (Gourzi et al., 2006). Although more detailed analyses are needed to confirm the involvement of NK cells in the protection against A-MuLV, the possibility that AID plays a role in innate defense through its genotoxic activity is intriguing.

In summary, some viral infections induce functional AID expression in B lineage cells at various developmental stages outside of the GCs. Further investigations will reveal the importance of AID expression in the pathogenesis of virus-associated lymphomas/leukemias (Fig. 1).

6. AID Expression in Normal and Malignant Nonlymphoid Cells

As described earlier, AID expression is typically restricted to GC B cells undergoing CSR and SHM. However, several reports show that AID is expressed even in nonlymphoid cells. Pluripotent tissues also express AID (Morgan *et al.*, 2004; Schreck *et al.*, 2006). A high level of AID transcripts, comparable to that in lymph nodes, was detected in mouse oocytes, and weaker expression of AID transcripts was found in embryonic germ cells, primordial germ cells, and embryonic stem cells (Morgan *et al.*, 2004). Immunohistochemical analyses further showed that AID is strongly expressed in normal spermatocytes in the human testis (Schreck *et al.*, 2006). These results suggest that AID may play physiological roles in developmental processes in pluripotent tissues. Although it remains speculative, it is an exciting possibility that AID may be involved in epigenetic reprogramming and meiosis in these cells (Morgan *et al.*, 2004; Schreck *et al.*, 2006).

Interestingly, most adult human testicular germ cell tumors (GCTs) have an increased copy number of chromosome 12p, to which the human AID gene maps, and this chromosomal marker has been suggested as one of the earliest genetic changes associated with the pathogenesis of testicular GCTs (Chaganti and Houldsworth, 2000). Although premalignant intratubular germ cell neoplasia, the precursor lesion of testicular cancers, and seminomas consistently lack AID expression, AID is expressed in ∼10% of mixed nonseminomatous GCTs (Schreck *et al.*, 2006). This result suggests that the continued expression of AID is not involved in the neoplastic process of GCTs. Nevertheless, it is still of interest to know whether the expressed AID is functional and if it plays a role in GCT cells.

Accumulating evidence indicates that AID is expressed in nonlymphoid tumor cells. Constitutively expressed AID transcripts were detected in six of six well-defined epithelial breast cancer cell lines, and the expression level was comparable to that found in B-cell lymphoma Ramos cells (Babbage *et al.*, 2006). Four of five human hepatoma cell lines also constitutively expressed variable amounts of AID transcripts (Kou *et al.*, 2006). In addition, AID transcripts were expressed in both human HCCs and the surrounding noncancerous liver tissues with underlying liver cirrhosis or chronic hepatitis, but were almost absent from normal liver tissue (Kou *et al.*, 2006). Furthermore, these authors showed that hepatocytes isolated from nontumorous liver tissues with active hepatitis expressed AID at a level comparable to infiltrating lymphocytes. They further confirmed AID expression by immunohistochemistry in hepatocytes in cirrhotic liver tissue, and in neoplastic cells in HCC liver tissues.

Thus, AID seems to be upregulated in hepatocytes in chronically inflamed, damaged liver.

Currently, it is unclear how AID expression is triggered in these nonlymphoid cells. B cells are induced to express AID in response to various stimuli, including LPS, cytokines, and viral infection (Section 5); AID expression in nonlymphoid cells may be induced by the same or similar signaling pathways. Indeed, AID expression was enhanced or induced in human hepatoma cell lines (HepG2 and PLC/PRF/5) and in cultured primary human hepatocytes by TGF-β treatment, which is known to upregulate AID expression in B cells (Kou et al., 2006; Muramatsu et al., 1999). Interestingly, both the cancerous and surrounding noncancerous liver tissues from patients with HCV-associated HCC tended to express higher amounts of AID than tissues from HCC patients with *Hepatitis B virus* (HBV) infection or whose HCC was of unknown etiology (Kou et al., 2006). It remains to be examined whether HCV infection triggers AID expression directly in hepatocytes as it does in B cells (Machida et al., 2004) and/or via factors secreted by inflammatory cells. Even if the former is the case, it cannot be ruled out that HCV infection induces AID expression through different pathways in B cells and hepatocytes because the binding of the HCV envelope glycoprotein E2 to CD81, a cellular receptor for HCV, induces AID expression in B cells but not in HepG2 cells (Machida et al., 2005).

The above results show that AID potentially plays roles in both physiological and pathophysiological conditions in cells other than B cells. In particular, AID expression in nonlymphoid cells may contribute to neoplastic transformation and/or malignant progression of these cells because ectopically expressed AID causes tumorigenesis in nonlymphoid tissues, including lung epithelium, liver, and skin, possibly by causing aberrant mutations in oncogenes (Okazaki et al., 2003; I.M.O., unpublished data). It has long been thought that persistent inflammation is associated with an increased risk of tumor development. Indeed, >15% of human malignancies can be attributed to chronic inflammation (Coussens and Werb, 2002; Li et al., 2005; Lu et al., 2006). The tumor-promoting inflammatory microenvironment appears to be established by a wide range of leukocytes, including neutrophils, dendritic cells, macrophages, eosinophils, mast cells, and lymphocytes, which together contribute to tumor development through complex and yet-to-be unraveled mechanisms (Coussens and Werb, 2002; Li et al., 2005; Lu et al., 2006). Because AID expression can be induced under inflammatory conditions (Kou et al., 2006), it is possible that AID participates in the complex mechanisms underlying inflammation-associated cancer development (Fig. 1). A thorough understanding of the mechanisms of AID induction and the roles of AID in normal and malignant nonlymphoid cells awaits further analyses.

7. Concluding Remarks

The identification of AID as a key enzyme required for the CSR and SHM of the Ig gene has led us to investigate the molecular mechanisms linking the deregulation of these processes with the genomic instability observed in many B-cell lymphomas, including chromosomal translocations and mutations. Both basic and clinical research studies highlight the importance of AID in the pathogenesis of B-cell lymphomas. Because AID is likely to be involved not only in tumorigenesis but also in the tumor evolution of B-cell lymphomas, the inhibition of AID expression could be a promising therapeutic target for human B-cell leukemias/lymphomas. Inhibition of AID might not cause serious complications, given that patients with the autosomal-recessive form of hyper-IgM syndrome (HIGM2), which is caused by AID deficiency, show few lethal clinical manifestations (Revy *et al.*, 2000). The blockade of AID would suppress further DNA breakage, which presumably facilitates the clonal evolution that leads to rapid tumor evolution through additional mutations and chromosomal translocations. Human B-cell leukemias and lymphomas with poor prognoses often show rapid clonal evolution, which induces resistance to the chemotherapy (Schiffer, 2001). If such clonal evolution is ameliorated by the inhibition of AID expression, these tumors might be controllable by other therapeutic modalities such as intensive chemotherapy, immunotherapy, and other target therapies.

Acknowledgments

We thank Drs. N. A. Begum, V. Shivarov, and L. M. Kato for helpful advice and critical reading of the chapter. I.M.O. and A.K. are research fellows of the Japan Society for the Promotion of Science.

References

Abbot, S. D., Rowe, M., Cadwallader, K., Ricksten, A., Gordon, J., Wang, F., Rymo, L., and Rickinson, A. B. (1990). Epstein-Barr virus nuclear antigen 2 induces expression of the virus-encoded latent membrane protein. *J. Virol.* **64**, 2126–2134.

Adams, J. M., Harris, A. W., Pinkert, C. A., Corcoran, L. M., Alexander, W. S., Cory, S., Palmiter, R. D., and Brinster, R. L. (1985). The c-myc oncogene driven by immunoglobulin enhancers induces lymphoid malignancy in transgenic mice. *Nature* **318**, 533–538.

Albesiano, E., Messmer, B. T., Damle, R. N., Allen, S. L., Rai, K. R., and Chiorazzi, N. (2003). Activation-induced cytidine deaminase in chronic lymphocytic leukemia B cells: Expression as multiple forms in a dynamic, variably sized fraction of the clone. *Blood* **102**, 3333–3339.

Alfieri, C., Birkenbach, M., and Kieff, E. (1991). Early events in Epstein-Barr virus infection of human B lymphocytes. *Virology* **181**, 595–608.

Alizadeh, A. A., Eisen, M. B., Davis, R. E., Ma, C., Lossos, I. S., Rosenwald, A., Boldrick, J. C., Sabet, H., Tran, T., Yu, X., Powell, J. I., Yang, L., *et al.* (2000). Distinct types of diffuse large B-cell lymphoma identified by gene expression profiling. *Nature* **403**, 503–511.

Babbage, G., Garand, R., Robillard, N., Zojer, N., Stevenson, F. K., and Sahota, S. S. (2004). Mantle cell lymphoma with t(11;14) and unmutated or mutated VH genes expresses AID and undergoes isotype switch events. *Blood* **103**, 2795–2798.

Babbage, G., Ottensmeier, C. H., Blaydes, J., Stevenson, F. K., and Sahota, S. S. (2006). Immunoglobulin heavy chain locus events and expression of activation-induced cytidine deaminase in epithelial breast cancer cell lines. *Cancer Res.* **66**, 3996–4000.

Braeuninger, A., Kuppers, R., Strickler, J. G., Wacker, H. H., Rajewsky, K., and Hansmann, M. L. (1997). Hodgkin and Reed-Sternberg cells in lymphocyte predominant Hodgkin disease represent clonal populations of germinal center-derived tumor B cells. *Proc. Natl. Acad. Sci. USA* **94**, 9337–9342.

Calender, A., Billaud, M., Aubry, J. P., Banchereau, J., Vuillaume, M., and Lenoir, G. M. (1987). Epstein-Barr virus (EBV) induces expression of B-cell activation markers on *in vitro* infection of EBV-negative B-lymphoma cells. *Proc. Natl. Acad. Sci. USA* **84**, 8060–8064.

Cerutti, A., Zan, H., Kim, E. C., Shah, S., Schattner, E. J., Schaffer, A., and Casali, P. (2002). Ongoing *in vivo* immunoglobulin class switch DNA recombination in chronic lymphocytic leukemia B cells. *J. Immunol.* **169**, 6594–6603.

Chaganti, R. S., and Houldsworth, J. (2000). Genetics and biology of adult human male germ cell tumors. *Cancer Res.* **60**, 1475–1482.

Coussens, L. M., and Werb, Z. (2002). Inflammation and cancer. *Nature* **420**, 860–867.

Damle, R. N., Wasil, T., Fais, F., Ghiotto, F., Valetto, A., Allen, S. L., Buchbinder, A., Budman, D., Dittmar, K., Kolitz, J., Lichtman, S. M., Schulman, P., *et al.* (1999). Ig V gene mutation status and CD38 expression as novel prognostic indicators in chronic lymphocytic leukemia. *Blood* **94**, 1840–1847.

Dedeoglu, F., Horwitz, B., Chaudhuri, J., Alt, F. W., and Geha, R. S. (2004). Induction of activation-induced cytidine deaminase gene expression by IL-4 and CD40 ligation is dependent on STAT6 and NFkappaB. *Int. Immunol.* **16**, 395–404.

Devergne, O., Hatzivassiliou, E., Izumi, K. M., Kaye, K. M., Kleijnen, M. F., Kieff, E., and Mosialos, G. (1996). Association of TRAF1, TRAF2, and TRAF3 with an Epstein-Barr virus LMP1 domain important for B-lymphocyte transformation: Role in NF-kappaB activation. *Mol. Cell. Biol.* **16**, 7098–7108.

Difilippantonio, M. J., Petersen, S., Chen, H. T., Johnson, R., Jasin, M., Kanaar, R., Ried, T., and Nussenzweig, A. (2002). Evidence for replicative repair of DNA double-strand breaks leading to oncogenic translocation and gene amplification. *J. Exp. Med.* **196**, 469–480.

Dijkman, R., Tensen, C. P., Buettner, M., Niedobitek, G., Willemze, R., and Vermeer, M. H. (2006). Primary cutaneous follicle center lymphoma and primary cutaneous large B-cell lymphoma, leg type, are both targeted by aberrant somatic hypermutation but demonstrate differential expression of AID. *Blood* **107**, 4926–4929.

Dudley, D. D., Chaudhuri, J., Bassing, C. H., and Alt, F. W. (2005). Mechanism and control of V(D)J recombination versus class switch recombination: Similarities and differences. *Adv. Immunol.* **86**, 43–112.

Epeldegui, M., Hung, Y. P., McQuay, A., Ambinder, R. F., and Martinez-Maza, O. (2007). Infection of human B cells with Epstein-Barr virus results in the expression of somatic hypermutation-inducing molecules and in the accrual of oncogene mutations. *Mol. Immunol.* **44**, 934–942.

Fahraeus, R., Jansson, A., Ricksten, A., Sjoblom, A., and Rymo, L. (1990). Epstein-Barr virus-encoded nuclear antigen 2 activates the viral latent membrane protein promoter by modulating the activity of a negative regulatory element. *Proc. Natl. Acad. Sci. USA* **87**, 7390–7394.

Faili, A., Aoufouchi, S., Gueranger, Q., Zober, C., Leon, A., Bertocci, B., Weill, J. C., and Reynaud, C. A. (2002). AID-dependent somatic hypermutation occurs as a DNA single-strand event in the BL2 cell line. *Nat. Immunol.* **3**, 815–821.

Ferri, C., Caracciolo, F., Zignego, A. L., La Civita, L., Monti, M., Longombardo, G., Lombardini, F., Greco, F., Capochiani, E., Mazzoni, A., Mazzaro, C., and Pasero, G. (1994). Hepatitis C virus infection in patients with non-Hodgkin's lymphoma. *Br. J. Haematol.* **88**, 392–394.

Forconi, F., Sahota, S. S., Raspadori, D., Ippoliti, M., Babbage, G., Lauria, F., and Stevenson, F. K. (2004). Hairy cell leukemia: At the crossroad of somatic mutation and isotype switch. *Blood* **104**, 3312–3317.

Franco, S., Gostissa, M., Zha, S., Lombard, D. B., Murphy, M. M., Zarrin, A. A., Yan, C., Tepsuporn, S., Morales, J. C., Adams, M. M., Lou, Z., Bassing, C. H., *et al.* (2006). H2AX prevents DNA breaks from progressing to chromosome breaks and translocations. *Mol. Cell* **21**, 201–214.

Gladdy, R. A., Taylor, M. D., Williams, C. J., Grandal, I., Karaskova, J., Squire, J. A., Rutka, J. T., Guidos, C. J., and Danska, J. S. (2003). The RAG-1/2 endonuclease causes genomic instability and controls CNS complications of lymphoblastic leukemia in p53/Prkdc-deficient mice. *Cancer Cell* **3**, 37–50.

Gonda, H., Sugai, M., Nambu, Y., Katakai, T., Agata, Y., Mori, K. J., Yokota, Y., and Shimizu, A. (2003). The balance between Pax5 and Id2 activities is the key to AID gene expression. *J. Exp. Med.* **198**, 1427–1437.

Gordon, M. S., Kanegai, C. M., Doerr, J. R., and Wall, R. (2003). Somatic hypermutation of the B cell receptor genes B29 (Igbeta, CD79b) and mb1 (Igalpha, CD79a). *Proc. Natl. Acad. Sci. USA* **100**, 4126–4131.

Gourzi, P., Leonova, T., and Papavasiliou, F. N. (2006). A role for activation-induced cytidine deaminase in the host response against a transforming retrovirus. *Immunity* **24**, 779–786.

Greeve, J., Philipsen, A., Krause, K., Klapper, W., Heidorn, K., Castle, B. E., Janda, J., Marcu, K. B., and Parwaresch, R. (2003). Expression of activation-induced cytidine deaminase in human B-cell non-Hodgkin lymphomas. *Blood* **101**, 3574–3580.

Greiner, A., Tobollik, S., Buettner, M., Jungnickel, B., Herrmann, K., Kremmer, E., and Niedobitek, G. (2005). Differential expression of activation-induced cytidine deaminase (AID) in nodular lymphocyte-predominant and classical Hodgkin lymphoma. *J. Pathol.* **205**, 541–547.

Grossman, S. R., Johannsen, E., Tong, X., Yalamanchili, R., and Kieff, E. (1994). The Epstein-Barr virus nuclear antigen 2 transactivator is directed to response elements by the J kappa recombination signal binding protein. *Proc. Natl. Acad. Sci. USA* **91**, 7568–7572.

Hamblin, T. (2002). Chronic lymphocytic leukaemia: One disease or two? *Ann. Hematol.* **81**, 299–303.

Hardianti, M. S., Tatsumi, E., Syampurnawati, M., Furuta, K., Saigo, K., Kawano, S., Kumagai, S., Nakamura, F., and Matsuo, Y. (2004a). Expression of activation-induced cytidine deaminase (AID) in Burkitt lymphoma cells: Rare AID-negative cell lines with the unmutated rearranged VH gene. *Leuk. Lymphoma* **45**, 155–160.

Hardianti, M. S., Tatsumi, E., Syampurnawati, M., Furuta, K., Saigo, K., Nakamachi, Y., Kumagai, S., Ohno, H., Tanabe, S., Uchida, M., and Yasuda, N. (2004b). Activation-induced cytidine deaminase expression in follicular lymphoma: Association between AID expression and ongoing mutation in FL. *Leukemia* **18**, 826–831.

Hardianti, M. S., Tatsumi, E., Syampurnawati, M., Furuta, K., Suzuki, A., Saigo, K., Kawano, S., Takenokuchi, M., Kumagai, S., Matsuo, Y., Koizumi, T., and Takeuchi, M. (2005). Presence of somatic hypermutation and activation-induced cytidine deaminase in acute lymphoblastic leukemia L2 with t(14;18)(q32;q21). *Eur. J. Haematol.* **74**, 11–19.

Harris, A. W., Pinkert, C. A., Crawford, M., Langdon, W. Y., Brinster, R. L., and Adams, J. M. (1988). The E mu-myc transgenic mouse. A model for high-incidence spontaneous lymphoma and leukemia of early B cells. *J. Exp. Med.* **167**, 353–371.
He, B., Raab-Traub, N., Casali, P., and Cerutti, A. (2003). EBV-encoded latent membrane protein 1 cooperates with BAFF/BLyS and APRIL to induce T cell-independent Ig heavy chain class switching. *J. Immunol.* **171**, 5215–5224.
Heintel, D., Kroemer, E., Kienle, D., Schwarzinger, I., Gleiss, A., Schwarzmeier, J., Marculescu, R., Le, T., Mannhalter, C., Gaiger, A., Stilgenbauer, S., Dohner, H., *et al.* (2004). High expression of activation-induced cytidine deaminase (AID) mRNA is associated with unmutated IGVH gene status and unfavourable cytogenetic aberrations in patients with chronic lymphocytic leukaemia. *Leukemia* **18**, 756–762.
Henkel, T., Ling, P. D., Hayward, S. D., and Peterson, M. G. (1994). Mediation of Epstein-Barr virus EBNA2 transactivation by recombination signal-binding protein J kappa. *Science* **265**, 92–95.
Hoefnagel, J. J., Dijkman, R., Basso, K., Jansen, P. M., Hallermann, C., Willemze, R., Tensen, C. P., and Vermeer, M. H. (2005). Distinct types of primary cutaneous large B-cell lymphoma identified by gene expression profiling. *Blood* **105**, 3671–3678.
Honjo, T., Kinoshita, K., and Muramatsu, M. (2002). Molecular mechanism of class switch recombination: Linkage with somatic hypermutation. *Annu. Rev. Immunol.* **20**, 165–196.
Imai, K., Slupphaug, G., Lee, W. I., Revy, P., Nonoyama, S., Catalan, N., Yel, L., Forveille, M., Kavli, B., Krokan, H. E., Ochs, H. D., Fischer, A., *et al.* (2003). Human uracil-DNA glycosylase deficiency associated with profoundly impaired immunoglobulin class-switch recombination. *Nat. Immunol.* **4**, 1023–1028.
Ito, S., Nagaoka, H., Shinkura, R., Begum, N., Muramatsu, M., Nakata, M., and Honjo, T. (2004). Activation-induced cytidine deaminase shuttles between nucleus and cytoplasm like apolipoprotein B mRNA editing catalytic polypeptide 1. *Proc. Natl. Acad. Sci. USA* **101**, 1975–1980.
Ivanovski, M., Silvestri, F., Pozzato, G., Anand, S., Mazzaro, C., Burrone, O. R., and Efremov, D. G. (1998). Somatic hypermutation, clonal diversity, and preferential expression of the VH 51p1/VL kv325 immunoglobulin gene combination in hepatitis C virus-associated immunocytomas. *Blood* **91**, 2433–2442.
Janz, S. (2006). Myc translocations in B cell and plasma cell neoplasms. *DNA Repair (Amst.)* **5**, 1213–1224.
Kanzler, H., Kuppers, R., Hansmann, M. L., and Rajewsky, K. (1996). Hodgkin and Reed-Sternberg cells in Hodgkin's disease represent the outgrowth of a dominant tumor clone derived from (crippled) germinal center B cells. *J. Exp. Med.* **184**, 1495–1505.
Kelly, G., Bell, A., and Rickinson, A. (2002). Epstein-Barr virus-associated Burkitt lymphomagenesis selects for downregulation of the nuclear antigen EBNA2. *Nat. Med.* **8**, 1098–1104.
Kilger, E., Kieser, A., Baumann, M., and Hammerschmidt, W. (1998). Epstein-Barr virus-mediated B-cell proliferation is dependent upon latent membrane protein 1, which simulates an activated CD40 receptor. *EMBO J.* **17**, 1700–1709.
Kitay-Cohen, Y., Amiel, A., Hilzenrat, N., Buskila, D., Ashur, Y., Fejgin, M., Gaber, E., Safadi, R., Tur-Kaspa, R., and Lishner, M. (2000). Bcl-2 rearrangement in patients with chronic hepatitis C associated with essential mixed cryoglobulinemia type II. *Blood* **96**, 2910–2912.
Klapper, W., Szczepanowski, M., Heidorn, K., Muschen, M., Liedtke, S., Sotnikova, A., Andersen, N. S., Greeve, J., and Parwaresch, R. (2006). Immunoglobulin class-switch recombination occurs in mantle cell lymphomas. *J. Pathol.* **209**, 250–257.

Klein, U., Tu, Y., Stolovitzky, G. A., Mattioli, M., Cattoretti, G., Husson, H., Freedman, A., Inghirami, G., Cro, L., Baldini, L., Neri, A., Califano, A., et al. (2001). Gene expression profiling of B cell chronic lymphocytic leukemia reveals a homogeneous phenotype related to memory B cells. *J. Exp. Med.* **194,** 1625–1638.

Kolar, G. R., Mehta, D., Pelayo, R., and Capra, J. D. (2006). A novel human B cell subpopulation representing the initial population to express AID. *Blood.* DOI: 10-1182/blood-2006-07-037150.

Kotani, A., Okazaki, I. M., Muramatsu, M., Kinoshita, K., Begum, N. A., Nakajima, T., Saito, H., and Honjo, T. (2005). A target selection of somatic hypermutations is regulated similarly between T and B cells upon activation-induced cytidine deaminase expression. *Proc. Natl. Acad. Sci. USA* **102,** 4506–4511.

Kotani, A., Kakazu, N., Tsuruyama, T., Okazaki, I. M., Muramatsu, M., Kinoshita, K., Nagaoka, H., Yabe, D., and Honjo, T. (2007). AID promotes B-cell lymphomagenesis in Emu-cmyc transgenic mice. *Proc. Natl. Acad. Sci. USA* **104,** 1616–1620.

Kou, T., Marusawa, H., Kinoshita, K., Endo, Y., Okazaki, I. M., Ueda, Y., Kodama, Y., Haga, H., Ikai, I., and Chiba, T. (2006). Expression of activation-induced cytidine deaminase in human hepatocytes during hepatocarcinogenesis. *Int. J. Cancer* **120,** 469–476.

Kovalchuk, A. L., Kim, J. S., Park, S. S., Coleman, A. E., Ward, J. M., Morse, H. C., III, Kishimoto, T., Potter, M., and Janz, S. (2002). IL-6 transgenic mouse model for extraosseous plasmacytoma. *Proc. Natl. Acad. Sci. USA* **99,** 1509–1514.

Kuppers, R. (2003). B cells under influence: Transformation of B cells by Epstein-Barr virus. *Nat. Rev. Immunol.* **3,** 801–812.

Kuppers, R. (2005). Mechanisms of B-cell lymphoma pathogenesis. *Nat. Rev. Cancer* **5,** 251–262.

Kuppers, R., and Dalla-Favera, R. (2001). Mechanisms of chromosomal translocations in B cell lymphomas. *Oncogene* **20,** 5580–5594.

Kuppers, R., Schwering, I., Brauninger, A., Rajewsky, K., and Hansmann, M. L. (2002). Biology of Hodgkin's lymphoma. *Ann. Oncol.* **13**(Suppl. 1), 11–18.

Li, Q., Withoff, S., and Verma, I. M. (2005). Inflammation-associated cancer: NF-kappaB is the lynchpin. *Trends Immunol.* **26,** 318–325.

Lin, K. I., Angelin-Duclos, C., Kuo, T. C., and Calame, K. (2002). Blimp-1-dependent repression of Pax-5 is required for differentiation of B cells to immunoglobulin M-secreting plasma cells. *Mol. Cell. Biol.* **22,** 4771–4780.

Litinskiy, M. B., Nardelli, B., Hilbert, D. M., He, B., Schaffer, A., Casali, P., and Cerutti, A. (2002). DCs induce CD40-independent immunoglobulin class switching through BLyS and APRIL. *Nat. Immunol.* **3,** 822–829.

Lossos, I. S., Levy, R., and Alizadeh, A. A. (2004). AID is expressed in germinal center B-cell-like and activated B-cell-like diffuse large-cell lymphomas and is not correlated with intraclonal heterogeneity. *Leukemia* **18,** 1775–1779.

Lu, H., Ouyang, W., and Huang, C. (2006). Inflammation, a key event in cancer development. *Mol. Cancer Res.* **4,** 221–233.

Machida, K., Cheng, K. T., Sung, V. M., Shimodaira, S., Lindsay, K. L., Levine, A. M., Lai, M. Y., and Lai, M. M. (2004). Hepatitis C virus induces a mutator phenotype: Enhanced mutations of immunoglobulin and protooncogenes. *Proc. Natl. Acad. Sci. USA* **101,** 4262–4267.

Machida, K., Cheng, K. T., Pavio, N., Sung, V. M., and Lai, M. M. (2005). Hepatitis C virus E2-CD81 interaction induces hypermutation of the immunoglobulin gene in B cells. *J. Virol.* **79,** 8079–8089.

Marafioti, T., Hummel, M., Foss, H. D., Laumen, H., Korbjuhn, P., Anagnostopoulos, I., Lammert, H., Demel, G., Theil, J., Wirth, T., and Stein, H. (2000). Hodgkin and reed-sternberg cells represent an expansion of a single clone originating from a germinal center B-cell with functional immunoglobulin gene rearrangements but defective immunoglobulin transcription. *Blood* **95**, 1443–1450.

Martin, A., and Scharff, M. D. (2002). Somatic hypermutation of the AID transgene in B and non-B cells. *Proc. Natl. Acad. Sci. USA* **99**, 12304–12308.

Martin, A., Bardwell, P. D., Woo, C. J., Fan, M., Shulman, M. J., and Scharff, M. D. (2002). Activation-induced cytidine deaminase turns on somatic hypermutation in hybridomas. *Nature* **415**, 802–806.

McBride, K. M., Barreto, V., Ramiro, A. R., Stavropoulos, P., and Nussenzweig, M. C. (2004). Somatic hypermutation is limited by CRM1-dependent nuclear export of activation-induced deaminase. *J. Exp. Med.* **199**, 1235–1244.

McCarthy, H., Wierda, W. G., Barron, L. L., Cromwell, C. C., Wang, J., Coombes, K. R., Rangel, R., Elenitoba-Johnson, K. S., Keating, M. J., and Abruzzo, L. V. (2003). High expression of activation-induced cytidine deaminase (AID) and splice variants is a distinctive feature of poor-prognosis chronic lymphocytic leukemia. *Blood* **101**, 4903–4908.

Migliazza, A., Martinotti, S., Chen, W., Fusco, C., Ye, B. H., Knowles, D. M., Offit, K., Chaganti, R. S., and Dalla-Favera, R. (1995). Frequent somatic hypermutation of the 5′ noncoding region of the BCL6 gene in B-cell lymphoma. *Proc. Natl. Acad. Sci. USA* **92**, 12520–12524.

Mitelman, F. (2000). Recurrent chromosome aberrations in cancer. *Mutat. Res.* **462**, 247–253.

Morgan, H. D., Dean, W., Coker, H. A., Reik, W., and Petersen-Mahrt, S. K. (2004). Activation-induced cytidine deaminase deaminates 5-methylcytosine in DNA and is expressed in pluripotent tissues: Implications for epigenetic reprogramming. *J. Biol. Chem.* **279**, 52353–52360.

Mosialos, G., Birkenbach, M., Yalamanchili, R., VanArsdale, T., Ware, C., and Kieff, E. (1995). The Epstein-Barr virus transforming protein LMP1 engages signaling proteins for the tumor necrosis factor receptor family. *Cell* **80**, 389–399.

Mottok, A., Hansmann, M. L., and Brauninger, A. (2005). Activation induced cytidine deaminase expression in lymphocyte predominant Hodgkin lymphoma. *J. Clin. Pathol.* **58**, 1002–1004.

Muramatsu, M., Sankaranand, V. S., Anant, S., Sugai, M., Kinoshita, K., Davidson, N. O., and Honjo, T. (1999). Specific expression of activation-induced cytidine deaminase (AID), a novel member of the RNA-editing deaminase family in germinal center B cells. *J. Biol. Chem.* **274**, 18470–18476.

Muramatsu, M., Kinoshita, K., Fagarasan, S., Yamada, S., Shinkai, Y., and Honjo, T. (2000). Class switch recombination and hypermutation require activation-induced cytidine deaminase (AID), a potential RNA editing enzyme. *Cell* **102**, 553–563.

Muto, T., Muramatsu, M., Taniwaki, M., Kinoshita, K., and Honjo, T. (2000). Isolation, tissue distribution, and chromosomal localization of the human activation-induced cytidine deaminase (AID) gene. *Genomics* **68**, 85–88.

Muto, T., Okazaki, I. M., Yamada, S., Tanaka, Y., Kinoshita, K., Muramatsu, M., Nagaoka, H., and Honjo, T. (2006). Negative regulation of activation-induced cytidine deaminase in B cells. *Proc. Natl. Acad. Sci. USA* **103**, 2752–2757.

Neri, A., Barriga, F., Knowles, D. M., Magrath, I. T., and Dalla-Favera, R. (1988). Different regions of the immunoglobulin heavy-chain locus are involved in chromosomal translocations in distinct pathogenetic forms of Burkitt lymphoma. *Proc. Natl. Acad. Sci. USA* **85**, 2748–2752.

Neuberger, M. S., and Milstein, C. (1995). Somatic hypermutation. *Curr. Opin. Immunol.* **7**, 248–254.

Okazaki, I. M., Kinoshita, K., Muramatsu, M., Yoshikawa, K., and Honjo, T. (2002). The AID enzyme induces class switch recombination in fibroblasts. *Nature* **416**, 340–345.

Okazaki, I. M., Hiai, H., Kakazu, N., Yamada, S., Muramatsu, M., Kinoshita, K., and Honjo, T. (2003). Constitutive expression of AID leads to tumorigenesis. *J. Exp. Med.* **197**, 1173–1181.

Oppezzo, P., Vuillier, F., Vasconcelos, Y., Dumas, G., Magnac, C., Payelle-Brogard, B., Pritsch, O., and Dighiero, G. (2003). Chronic lymphocytic leukemia B cells expressing AID display dissociation between class switch recombination and somatic hypermutation. *Blood* **101**, 4029–4032.

Pajic, A., Staege, M. S., Dudziak, D., Schuhmacher, M., Spitkovsky, D., Eissner, G., Brielmeier, M., Polack, A., and Bornkamm, G. W. (2001). Antagonistic effects of c-myc and Epstein-Barr virus latent genes on the phenotype of human B cells. *Int. J. Cancer* **93**, 810–816.

Pasqualucci, L., Neumeister, P., Goossens, T., Nanjangud, G., Chaganti, R. S., Kuppers, R., and Dalla-Favera, R. (2001). Hypermutation of multiple proto-oncogenes in B-cell diffuse large-cell lymphomas. *Nature* **412**, 341–346.

Pasqualucci, L., Guglielmino, R., Houldsworth, J., Mohr, J., Aoufouchi, S., Polakiewicz, R., Chaganti, R. S., and Dalla-Favera, R. (2004). Expression of the AID protein in normal and neoplastic B cells. *Blood* **104**, 3318–3325.

Pasqualucci, L., Compagno, M., Houldsworth, J., Monti, S., Grunn, A., Nandula, S. V., Aster, J. C., Murty, V. V., Shipp, M. A., and Dalla-Favera, R. (2006). Inactivation of the PRDM1/BLIMP1 gene in diffuse large B cell lymphoma. *J. Exp. Med.* **203**, 311–317.

Petiniot, L. K., Weaver, Z., Barlow, C., Shen, R., Eckhaus, M., Steinberg, S. M., Ried, T., Wynshaw-Boris, A., and Hodes, R. J. (2000). Recombinase-activating gene (RAG) 2-mediated V(D)J recombination is not essential for tumorigenesis in Atm-deficient mice. *Proc. Natl. Acad. Sci. USA* **97**, 6664–6669.

Poltorak, A., He, X., Smirnova, I., Liu, M. Y., Van Huffel, C., Du, X., Birdwell, D., Alejos, E., Silva, M., Galanos, C., Freudenberg, M., Ricciardi-Castagnoli, P., *et al.* (1998). Defective LPS signaling in C3H/HeJ and C57BL/10ScCr mice: Mutations in Tlr4 gene. *Science* **282**, 2085–2088.

Potter, M. (2003). Neoplastic development in plasma cells. *Immunol. Rev.* **194**, 177–195.

Potter, M., and Wiener, F. (1992). Plasmacytomagenesis in mice: Model of neoplastic development dependent upon chromosomal translocations. *Carcinogenesis* **13**, 1681–1697.

Rada, C., Williams, G. T., Nilsen, H., Barnes, D. E., Lindahl, T., and Neuberger, M. S. (2002). Immunoglobulin isotype switching is inhibited and somatic hypermutation perturbed in UNG-deficient mice. *Curr. Biol.* **12**, 1748–1755.

Ramiro, A. R., Jankovic, M., Eisenreich, T., Difilippantonio, S., Chen-Kiang, S., Muramatsu, M., Honjo, T., Nussenzweig, A., and Nussenzweig, M. C. (2004). AID is required for c-myc/IgH chromosome translocations *in vivo*. *Cell* **118**, 431–438.

Ramiro, A. R., Jankovic, M., Callen, E., Difilippantonio, S., Chen, H. T., McBride, K. M., Eisenreich, T. R., Chen, J., Dickins, R. A., Lowe, S. W., Nussenzweig, A., and Nussenzweig, M. C. (2006). Role of genomic instability and p53 in AID-induced c-myc-Igh translocations. *Nature* **440**, 105–109.

Reiniger, L., Bodor, C., Bognar, A., Balogh, Z., Csomor, J., Szepesi, A., Kopper, L., and Matolcsy, A. (2006). Richter's and prolymphocytic transformation of chronic lymphocytic leukemia are associated with high mRNA expression of activation-induced cytidine deaminase and aberrant somatic hypermutation. *Leukemia* **20**, 1089–1095.

Revy, P., Muto, T., Levy, Y., Geissmann, F., Plebani, A., Sanal, O., Catalan, N., Forveille, M., Dufourcq-Labelouse, R., Gennery, A., Tezcan, I., Ersoy, F., *et al.* (2000). Activation-induced cytidine deaminase (AID) deficiency causes the autosomal recessive form of the Hyper-IgM syndrome (HIGM2). *Cell* **102**, 565–575.

Roberts, E. C., Deed, R. W., Inoue, T., Norton, J. D., and Sharrocks, A. D. (2001). Id helix-loop-helix proteins antagonize pax transcription factor activity by inhibiting DNA binding. *Mol. Cell. Biol.* **21,** 524–533.

Rooney, C., Howe, J. G., Speck, S. H., and Miller, G. (1989). Influence of Burkitt's lymphoma and primary B cells on latent gene expression by the nonimmortalizing P3J-HR-1 strain of Epstein-Barr virus. *J. Virol.* **63,** 1531–1539.

Rosenberg, N. (1982). Abelson leukemia virus. *Curr. Top. Microbiol. Immunol.* **101,** 95–126.

Rosenwald, A., Alizadeh, A. A., Widhopf, G., Simon, R., Davis, R. E., Yu, X., Yang, L., Pickeral, O. K., Rassenti, L. Z., Powell, J., Botstein, D., Byrd, J. C., *et al.* (2001). Relation of gene expression phenotype to immunoglobulin mutation genotype in B cell chronic lymphocytic leukemia. *J. Exp. Med.* **194,** 1639–1647.

Rosenwald, A., Wright, G., Chan, W. C., Connors, J. M., Campo, E., Fisher, R. I., Gascoyne, R. D., Muller-Hermelink, H. K., Smeland, E. B., Giltnane, J. M., Hurt, E. M., Zhao, H., *et al.* (2002). The use of molecular profiling to predict survival after chemotherapy for diffuse large-B-cell lymphoma. *N. Engl. J. Med.* **346,** 1937–1947.

Rucci, F., Cattaneo, L., Marrella, V., Sacco, M. G., Sobacchi, C., Lucchini, F., Nicola, S., Bella, S. D., Villa, M. L., Imberti, L., Gentili, F., Montagna, C., *et al.* (2006). Tissue-specific sensitivity to AID expression in transgenic mouse models. *Gene* **377,** 150–158.

Sayegh, C. E., Quong, M. W., Agata, Y., and Murre, C. (2003). E-proteins directly regulate expression of activation-induced deaminase in mature B cells. *Nat. Immunol.* **4,** 586–593.

Schiffer, C. A. (2001). Treatment of high-grade lymphoid malignancies in adults. *Semin. Hematol.* **38,** 22–26.

Schreck, S., Buettner, M., Kremmer, E., Bogdan, M., Herbst, H., and Niedobitek, G. (2006). Activation-induced cytidine deaminase (AID) is expressed in normal spermatogenesis but only infrequently in testicular germ cell tumours. *J. Pathol.* **210,** 26–31.

Schroeder, H. W., Jr., and Dighiero, G. (1994). The pathogenesis of chronic lymphocytic leukemia: Analysis of the antibody repertoire. *Immunol. Today* **15,** 288–294.

Shaffer, A. L., Lin, K. I., Kuo, T. C., Yu, X., Hurt, E. M., Rosenwald, A., Giltnane, J. M., Yang, L., Zhao, H., Calame, K., and Staudt, L. M. (2002). Blimp-1 orchestrates plasma cell differentiation by extinguishing the mature B cell gene expression program. *Immunity* **17,** 51–62.

Shen, H. M., Peters, A., Baron, B., Zhu, X., and Storb, U. (1998). Mutation of BCL-6 gene in normal B cells by the process of somatic hypermutation of Ig genes. *Science* **280,** 1750–1752.

Shiramizu, B., Barriga, F., Neequaye, J., Jafri, A., Dalla-Favera, R., Neri, A., Guttierez, M., Levine, P., and Magrath, I. (1991). Patterns of chromosomal breakpoint locations in Burkitt's lymphoma: Relevance to geography and Epstein-Barr virus association. *Blood* **77,** 1516–1526.

Shirogane, T., Fukada, T., Muller, J. M., Shima, D. T., Hibi, M., and Hirano, T. (1999). Synergistic roles for Pim-1 and c-Myc in STAT3-mediated cell cycle progression and anti-apoptosis. *Immunity* **11,** 709–719.

Silvestri, F., Pipan, C., Barillari, G., Zaja, F., Fanin, R., Infanti, L., Russo, D., Falasca, E., Botta, G. A., and Baccarani, M. (1996). Prevalence of hepatitis C virus infection in patients with lymphoproliferative disorders. *Blood* **87,** 4296–4301.

Smit, L. A., Bende, R. J., Aten, J., Guikema, J. E., Aarts, W. M., and van Noesel, C. J. (2003). Expression of activation-induced cytidine deaminase is confined to B-cell non-Hodgkin's lymphomas of germinal-center phenotype. *Cancer Res.* **63,** 3894–3898.

Suematsu, S., Matsusaka, T., Matsuda, T., Ohno, S., Miyazaki, J., Yamamura, K., Hirano, T., and Kishimoto, T. (1992). Generation of plasmacytomas with the chromosomal translocation t(12;15) in interleukin 6 transgenic mice. *Proc. Natl. Acad. Sci. USA* **89,** 232–235.

Sylla, B. S., Hung, S. C., Davidson, D. M., Hatzivassiliou, E., Malinin, N. L., Wallach, D., Gilmore, T. D., Kieff, E., and Mosialos, G. (1998). Epstein-Barr virus-transforming protein latent infection membrane protein 1 activates transcription factor NF-kappaB through a pathway that includes the NF-kappaB-inducing kinase and the IkappaB kinases IKKalpha and IKKbeta. *Proc. Natl. Acad. Sci. USA* **95,** 10106–10111.

Tobollik, S., Meyer, L., Buettner, M., Klemmer, S., Kempkes, B., Kremmer, E., Niedobitek, G., and Jungnickel, B. (2006). Epstein-barr-virus nuclear antigen 2 inhibits AID expression during EBV-driven B cell growth. *Blood* **108,** 3859–3864.

Unniraman, S., Zhou, S., and Schatz, D. G. (2004). Identification of an AID-independent pathway for chromosomal translocations between the Igh switch region and Myc. *Nat. Immunol.* **5,** 1117–1123.

Vanasse, G. J., Halbrook, J., Thomas, S., Burgess, A., Hoekstra, M. F., Disteche, C. M., and Willerford, D. M. (1999). Genetic pathway to recurrent chromosome translocations in murine lymphoma involves V(D)J recombinase. *J. Clin. Invest.* **103,** 1669–1675.

Wang, F., Gregory, C. D., Rowe, M., Rickinson, A. B., Wang, D., Birkenbach, M., Kikutani, H., Kishimoto, T., and Kieff, E. (1987). Epstein-Barr virus nuclear antigen 2 specifically induces expression of the B-cell activation antigen CD23. *Proc. Natl. Acad. Sci. USA* **84,** 3452–3456.

Willemze, R., Jaffe, E. S., Burg, G., Cerroni, L., Berti, E., Swerdlow, S. H., Ralfkiaer, E., Chimenti, S., Diaz-Perez, J. L., Duncan, L. M., Grange, F., Harris, N. L., *et al.* (2005). WHO-EORTC classification for cutaneous lymphomas. *Blood* **105,** 3768–3785.

Willis, T. G., and Dyer, M. J. (2000). The role of immunoglobulin translocations in the pathogenesis of B-cell malignancies. *Blood* **96,** 808–822.

Yadav, A., Olaru, A., Saltis, M., Setren, A., Cerny, J., and Livak, F. (2006). Identification of a ubiquitously active promoter of the murine activation-induced cytidine deaminase (AICDA) gene. *Mol. Immunol.* **43,** 529–541.

Yang, R., Murillo, F. M., Delannoy, M. J., Blosser, R. L., Yutzy, W. H. T., Uematsu, S., Takeda, K., Akira, S., Viscidi, R. P., and Roden, R. B. (2005). B lymphocyte activation by human papillomavirus-like particles directly induces Ig class switch recombination via TLR4-MyD88. *J. Immunol.* **174,** 7912–7919.

Yoshikawa, K., Okazaki, I. M., Eto, T., Kinoshita, K., Muramatsu, M., Nagaoka, H., and Honjo, T. (2002). AID enzyme-induced hypermutation in an actively transcribed gene in fibroblasts. *Science* **296,** 2033–2036.

Zhu, C., Mills, K. D., Ferguson, D. O., Lee, C., Manis, J., Fleming, J., Gao, Y., Morton, C. C., and Alt, F. W. (2002). Unrepaired DNA breaks in p53-deficient cells lead to oncogenic gene amplification subsequent to translocations. *Cell* **109,** 811–821.

Zhou, C., Saxon, A., and Zhang, K. (2003). Human activation-induced cytidine deaminase is induced by IL-4 and negatively regulated by CD45: Implication of CD45 as a Janus kinase phosphatase in antibody diversification. *J. Immunol.* **170,** 1887–1893.

Zimber-Strobl, U., and Strobl, L. J. (2001). EBNA2 and Notch signalling in Epstein-Barr virus mediated immortalization of B lymphocytes. *Semin. Cancer Biol.* **11,** 423–434.

Zimber-Strobl, U., Strobl, L. J., Meitinger, C., Hinrichs, R., Sakai, T., Furukawa, T., Honjo, T., and Bornkamm, G. W. (1994). Epstein-Barr virus nuclear antigen 2 exerts its transactivating function through interaction with recombination signal binding protein RBP-J kappa, the homologue of Drosophila Suppressor of Hairless. *EMBO J.* **13,** 4973–4982.

Pathophysiology of B-Cell Intrinsic Immunoglobulin Class Switch Recombination Deficiencies

Anne Durandy,[*,†,‡,§] Nadine Taubenheim,[*,†,‡] Sophie Peron,[*,†,‡] and Alain Fischer[*,†,‡,§,¶]

[*]Inserm, U768, Paris F-75015, France
[†]Univ René Descartes-Paris 5, Paris F-75006, France
[‡]Hôpital Necker-Enfants Malades, 149 rue de Sèvres 75015 Paris, France
[§]Assistance Publique Hôpitaux de Paris, Hôpital Necker-Enfants Malades, 149 rue de Sèvres 75015 Paris, France
[¶]Unité d'immunologie et Hématologie Pédiatrique, Hôpital Necker-Enfants Malades, 149 rue de Sèvres 75015 Paris, France

Abstract 275
1. Introduction 276
2. Ig-CSR Deficiency Type 1 Caused by Activation-Induced Cytidine Deaminase Deficiency 279
3. Ig-CSR Deficiency Type 2 Caused by UNG Deficiency 289
4. Molecularly Undefined Ig-CSR Deficiency with Normal SHM 292
5. Concluding Remarks 296
   References 298

Abstract

B-cell intrinsic immunoglobulin class switch recombination (Ig-CSR) deficiencies, previously termed hyper-IgM syndromes, are genetically determined conditions characterized by normal or elevated serum IgM levels and an absence or very low levels of IgG, IgA, and IgE. As a function of the molecular mechanism, the defective CSR is variably associated to a defect in the generation of somatic hypermutations (SHMs) in the Ig variable region. The study of Ig-CSR deficiencies contributed to a better delineation of the mechanisms underlying CSR and SHM, the major events of antigen-triggered antibody maturation. Four Ig-CSR deficiency phenotypes have been so far reported: the description of the activation-induced cytidine deaminase (AID) deficiency (Ig-CSR deficiency 1), caused by recessive mutations of AICDA gene, characterized by a defect in CSR and SHM, clearly established the role of AID in the induction of the Ig gene rearrangements underlying CSR and SHM. A CSR-specific function of AID has, however, been detected by the observation of a selective CSR defect caused by mutations affecting the C-terminus of AID. Ig-CSR deficiency 2 is the consequence of uracil-N-glycosylase (UNG) deficiency. Because UNG, a molecule of the base excision repair machinery, removes uracils from DNA and AID deaminates cytosines into uracils, that observation indicates that the AID-UNG pathway directly targets DNA of switch regions from the Ig heavy-chain locus to induce the CSR process. Ig-CSR deficiencies 3 and 4 are characterized by a selective CSR defect resulting from blocks at distinct steps of CSR. A further understanding of the CSR machinery is expected from their molecular definition.

1. Introduction

B-cell intrinsic immunoglobulin class switch recombination (Ig-CSR) deficiencies are rare primary immunodeficiencies, usually denominated hyper-IgM syndromes, the frequency of which is evaluated to 1 in 100,000 births. All are characterized by a defective Ig-CSR, as shown by the serum Ig level determination: IgM levels are either normal or increased, contrasting with a strong decrease or an absence of IgG, IgA, and IgE (Notarangelo et al., 1992). All mature B cells carry membrane IgM and IgD or IgM only, since no switched Ig (IgG or IgA) is produced. As a function of the molecular defect, the defective CSR is associated or not with a defective generation of somatic hypermutations (SHMs) into the Ig variable (V) region. The definition of different Ig-CSR deficiencies made it possible a better delineation of the mechanisms underlying CSR and SHM, both required for maturation of antibody responses.

Maturation of the antibody repertoire results in the production of antibodies of various isotypes with high affinity for antigen, a process that is required for providing an efficient humoral response. Antibody maturation occurs in the germinal centers of the secondary lymphoid organs following antigen and T-cell-driven activation: (1) the CSR results in the production of antibodies of different isotypes (IgG, IgA, and IgE) with the same V specificity, and therefore the same antigen affinity (Iwasato et al., 1990; Kinoshita and Honjo, 2000; Matsuoka et al., 1990). CSR is necessary for adaptative antibody response since the different Ig isotypes exhibit distinct biological activities: IgG has a longer half-life than IgM (21 and 5 days, respectively), binds to Fcγ receptors increasing phagocytosis of phagocytic cells and activates the complement system. IgA, which is mostly produced in mucosae, is a first means of defense toward pathogens. IgE plays a major role against antihelmintic infection. (2) The SHM introduces with high-frequency ($1/10^3$ bp/cell cycle) stochastic mutations mostly in the V region of the Ig, a genetic modification that is followed by the positive selection of B cells carrying a B-cell receptor (BCR) with high affinity for antigen (Jacobs et al., 2001; Storb et al., 1998). This process requires interaction with follicular dendritic cells (Frazer et al., 1997; Rajewsky, 1996). SHM-induced self-reactive B cells are either deleted or inactivated by receptor revision (Itoh et al., 2000; Meffre et al., 1998; Wilson et al., 2000). CSR and SHM occur simultaneously in germinal centers under BCR/CD40 activation but neither is a prerequisite for the other because IgM may be mutated while

IgG or IgA can remain unmutated (Jacob and Kelsoe, 1992; Kaartinen et al., 1983; Liu et al., 1996).

The description of an X-linked Ig-CSR deficiency caused by mutations in the gene encoding the CD40 ligand molecule (CD40L, CD154) (Allen et al., 1993; Aruffo et al., 1993; Disanto et al., 1993; Korthauer et al., 1993), a molecule highly expressed on follicular helper T cells (Breitfeld et al., 2000), has demonstrated the essential role of the CD40 signaling pathway in B cells for both events of antibody maturation. CD40L interacts with CD40 constitutively expressed on B cells, but also on monocytes and dendritic cells (Castle et al., 1993; Fuleihan et al., 1993; Nonoyama et al., 1993). Due to a CD40 transactivation defect, the B cells of patients with this syndrome cannot proliferate or form germinal centers in secondary lymphoid organs or produce IgG and IgA *in vivo*. However, B cells are intrinsically normal as they can be induced to proliferate and to undergo CSR to generate IgG, IgA, and IgE on *in vitro* activation by CD40 agonists and appropriate cytokines (Durandy et al., 1993). The defective CSR is often associated with decreased SHM (Agematsu et al., 1998), an observation that indicates that CD40L/CD40 interaction is necessary for induction of both events in germinal centers. CD40− deficiency has been observed in a few patients as an autosomal recessive inherited disease and diagnosed on the lack of CD40 expression on B cells and monocytes. The clinical and immunologic findings are identical to those of CD40L deficiency, with the exception that the B cells cannot undergo CSR on *in vitro* sCD40L+ cytokine activation (Ferrari et al., 2001). CD40 signaling pathway in B cells necessary for CSR and SHM involves NF-κB, as shown by the observation that hypomorphic mutations of the gene encoding the NF-κB essential modulator or NEMO (IKKγ), a regulatory unit of the IKKα, IKKβ and IKKγ complex, can also lead in some patients to a CSR deficiency. Presumably because of the heterogeneity of the mutations, the *in vitro* CD40-mediated CSR and the SHM are found variably defective (Jain et al., 2004; Durandy, unpublished data). Such variability could be also related to the fact that CD40 activation induces two NF-κB pathways: the NF-κB1 (p50 and its precursor p106) that requires IKKα, IKKβ and IKKγ complex, and the NF-κB2 (p52 and its precursor p100) that does not (Coope et al., 2002).

Surprisingly, CD40L deficiency is in some occasions associated with detectable IgA amounts, despite a complete absence of CD40L expression. This observation points to CD40L-independent pathway(s) triggering CSR. CSR can occur through the B-cell-activating factor receptor (BAFF-R) and the transmembrane activator and calcium-modulating cyclophilin-interacting protein (TACI). Following exposure to BAFF or the proliferation-inducing ligand (APRIL), and in the presence of appropriate cytokines and BCR engagement, B cells undergo an entirely CD40-independent CSR leading to the production of IgG and IgA. This CSR can occur in the splenic marginal zone or intestinal lamina propria (Litinskiy et al., 2002). The role of BAFF and APRIL in CSR has been emphasized by the observation of IgG and/or IgA defects in patients deficient in TACI (Castigli et al., 2005; Salzer et al., 2005). Other T-cell molecules also play a role, such as the inducible costimulator molecule (ICOS), also expressed on follicular T cells in germinal centers. Indeed, ICOS deficiency, first described as a rare cause of common variable immunodeficiency (Grimbacher et al., 2003), can lead to a defective CSR likely because of defective germinal center reaction (Warnatz et al., 2006). Another molecule, the complement protein C4b-binding protein (C4BP), can also play a role in B-cell survival and CSR. It has been shown to bind CD40, to colocalize with B cells in secondary follicles and to induce CSR toward IgE in presence of IL-4 in an NF-κB-dependent signaling pathway (Blom et al., 2003; Brodeur et al., 2003; Morio et al., 1995).

SHMs have been shown also to occur in IgM+CD27+ B cells in the absence of CD40L expression (Weller et al., 2001). These mutated IgM B cells very likely produce antibodies against encapsulated bacteria in the splenic marginal zone (Kruetzmann et al., 2003). This B-cell subset displays similarity to murine B-1a B cells, which secrete natural antibodies and are required for the T-cell-independent antibody response to polysaccharide antigens (Martin and Kearney, 2000; Wardemann et al., 2002). Pyk2-deficient mice, which lack marginal zone B cells, exhibit an impaired antibody response to polysaccharides (Fagarasan and Honjo, 2000; Guinamard et al., 2000). The mechanism underlying the generation of SHM in the absence of CD40L/CD40 signaling remains unknown (Weller et al., 2004). Another evidence for the possible occurrence of SHM outside the germinal centers is the observation that self-reactive-mutated B cells are usually generated in the T zone-red pulp border of the spleen rather than in the germinal centers (William et al., 2002).

Besides these Ig-CSR deficiencies secondary to defective T- and B-cell interaction or B-cell CD40 signaling pathway, half of Ig-CSR deficiencies are caused by an intrinsic B-cell defect which directly impairs the complex machinery of the CSR process (Callard et al., 1994; Durandy et al., 1997). These Ig-CSR deficiencies are characterized by a selective CSR defect resulting from blocks at distinct steps of CSR. Patients are prone to infections with bacterial pathogens but not to opportunistic infections, in contrast to patients affected by Ig-CSR deficiency caused by a defective CD40 signaling pathway. The prognosis is therefore much better for these patients, although continuous Ig substitution treatment is required. Unlike patients with defective CD40 signaling pathway or ICOS deficiency, patients with these Ig-CSR deficiencies frequently present with enlargement of lymphoid organs such as the spleen, tonsils, and lymph nodes.

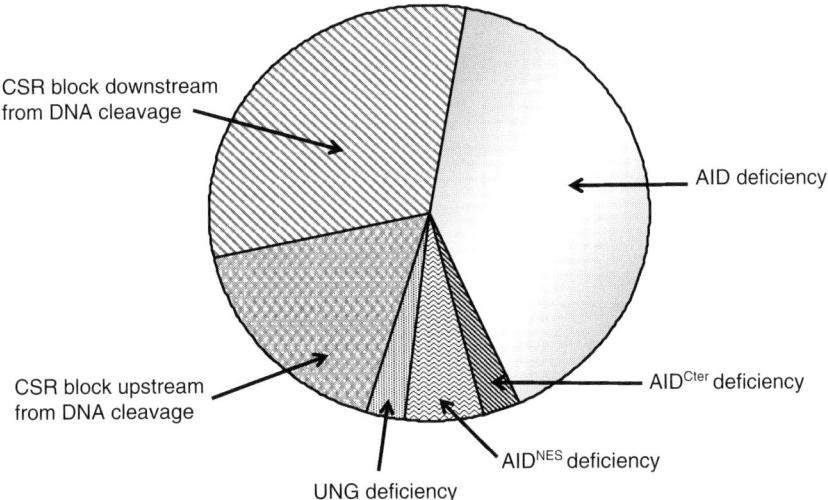

Figure 1 Relative frequency of the four different subsets of B-cell intrinsic Ig-CSR deficiencies. Frequency was evaluated according to the number of affected families.

As in the other Ig-CSR deficiencies, patients have normal or high serum IgM levels, contrasting with markedly reduced serum IgG and IgA levels. Consistent with serum Ig levels, IgG antibodies specific for pathogens or immunization antigens are absent, whereas isohemagglutinins and antipolysaccharidic antigen antibodies of the IgM isotype are detected. It is, at present, unclear whether the ability of patients' B cells to produce antipolysaccharide antibodies provides a significant protection against infections by *Streptococcus pneumoniae* and *Haemophilus influenzae*.

The dissection of B-cell abnormalities and molecular definition of these B intrinsic Ig-CSR deficiencies has made possible to delineate some of the molecular events involved in the antibody maturation processes. Four different subsets are defined (Fig. 1).

2. Ig-CSR Deficiency Type 1 Caused by Activation-Induced Cytidine Deaminase Deficiency

This Ig-CSR deficiency was found to be the consequence of a defect in the activation-induced cytidine deaminase (AID), a molecule specifically expressed in activated B cells.

2.1. Classical AID Deficiency

2.1.1. Phenotype

Sixty-two patients from 43 unrelated families and different ethnic backgrounds were referred for investigation because of susceptibility to bacterial infections, mostly of the upper respiratory and digestive tracts. Impressive enlargement of the tonsils and lymph nodes was observed in 47 patients, leading in some to multiple biopsies. Pathological examination revealed the presence of giant germinal centers (5–10 times larger than normal) filled with highly proliferating B cells (Fig. 2). Proliferating B cells coexpress at plasma membrane IgM, IgD, and CD38, all phenotypic characteristics of a small B-cell subset known as germinal center founder cells (Lebecque et al., 1997). These cells correspond to a transitional stage between follicular mantle and germinal center B cells, at the stage at which SHM of the IgV region gene and antigen-driven selection occur. The expression of CD95 on B cells and the presence of numerous macrophages filled with apoptotic bodies appeared to rule out a defect in apoptosis to account for germinal center enlargement, which is presumably the consequence of an intense B-cell proliferation (Revy et al., 2000). IgM-mediated autoimmunity was not infrequent (12 patients), mostly affecting blood cells (autoimmune hemolytic anemia or thrombocytopenia). Other autoimmune manifestations were rarely observed, including rheumatoid arthritis (one case), autoimmune hepatitis (two cases), uveitis (one case), diabetes (one case), and systemic lupus erymathous disease (one case). One patient suffered

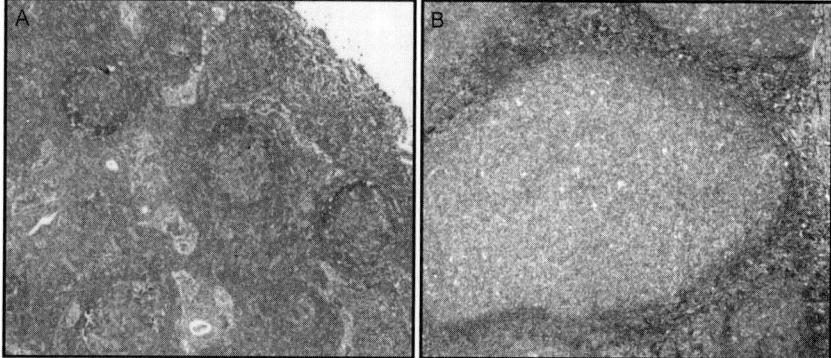

Figure 2 Giant germinal centers in AID deficiency. (A) Reactive cervical lymph node from an age-matched control. (B) Cervical lymph node from an AID-deficient patient (p.68X+p.H56-E58 del). Immunochemistry with an AID-specific monoclonal antibody.

from inflammatory bowel disease (Quartier et al., 2004). Malignancies were not reported with the exception of an Ewing sarcoma.

These patients suffered from a drastically defective CSR, as IgG, IgA, and IgE levels were barely detectable in serum, in contrast to elevated IgM levels in all cases, except in six who were diagnosed and treated early in life. Although serum IgM levels decreased in most patients after Ig substitution was initiated, they frequently remained above normal values. Isohemagglutinins and antipolysaccharide IgM antibodies were detected, contrasting to the complete absence of IgG antibody production in response to immunization antigens or microorganisms. In vitro, B cells normally proliferated, produced large amounts of IgM, and upregulated the CD23 activation marker when activated by sCD40L+ appropriate cytokines. In contrast, they could not undergo CSR to generate IgG, IgA, or IgE on the same stimulation (Durandy et al., 1997). Analysis of the successive events of the in vitro CSR enabled to place the block inside the CSR pathway. The first step of CSR resulting in the generation of Ig germ line transcripts was detectable, whereas the further steps were not: double-stranded DNA breaks (DSB) in Sμ regions, as judged by a very sensitive ligation-mediated PCR technique (Catalan et al., 2003), could not be detected, excision and functional Ig transcripts were equally undetectable, and no switched Ig isotype could be found in culture supernatants (Revy et al., 2000). Therefore, the CSR defect was shown to be located downstream from the transcription step and upstream from the DSB creation (Table 1; Fig. 3).

All peripheral blood B cells expressed membrane IgM and most (90%) coexpressed IgD. A normal percentage (20–50%) carried CD27, a marker that has been related to the memory-mutated phenotype of B cells (Klein et al., 1998). Such cells could have undergone SHM in normal conditions. SHM was investigated in the VH3–23 Ig region of purified CD19+/CD27+ B cells from 29 patients. SHM was found constantly absent or drastically decreased (0- < 1.2%) as compared to age-matched controls (2.5–6.3% mutations/bp) (Fig. 4B). Analysis of the nucleotide substitution of the few observed mutations did not reveal any obviously abnormal pattern.

2.1.2. AICDA Mutations

The observation of consanguineous families led to check for a genetic locus cosegregating with the disease. A homozygosity mapping was performed in eight families, which determined a 4.5-cM region on chromosome 12p13 with a lod score of 10.45, a locus in which *AICDA* gene encoding the B-cell-specific molecule AID (Muramatsu et al., 1999) was localized (Muto et al., 2000). We therefore sequenced *AICDA* and found biallelic mutations scattered all along the gene, affecting as well the nuclear localization signal (NLS), the active

Table 1 Phenotype of B-Cell Intrinsic Ig-CSR Deficiencies[a]

Deficiency	Inheritance	Relative frequency (%)	CSR step block	CD27+ B cells	SHM	Autoimmunity	Lymphoma
AID	AR	43	Upstream for DSB	N	0 or ↘	+	–
AID^{Cter}	AR	3	ND	N	N	–	–
AID^{NES}	AD	6	Downstream for DSB	N	N	–	–
UNG	AR	3	Upstream for DSB	N	N (bias)	+	Possible
AID cofactor?	AR?	18	Upstream for DSB	N	N	+	–
DNA repair?	AR?	33	Downstream for DSB	↓	N	+	+

[a]ND, not done; N, normal; AR, autosomal recessive; AD, autosomal dominant.

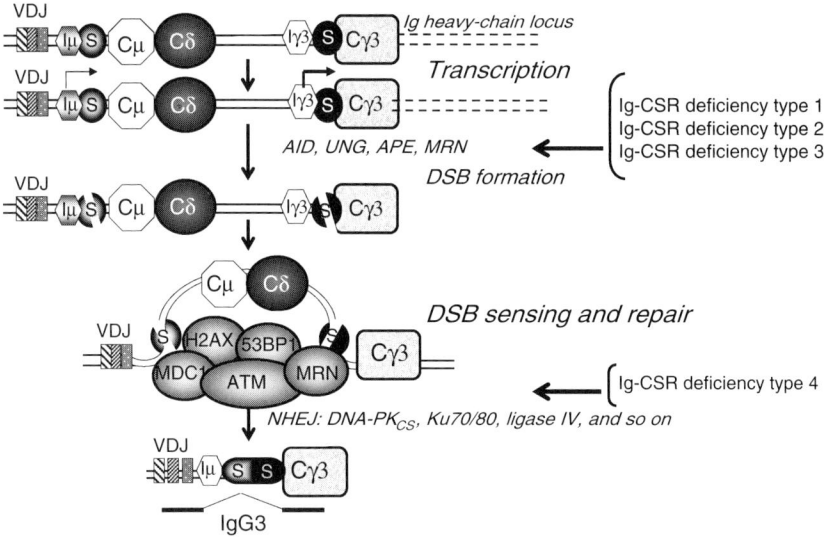

Figure 3 Schematic representation of Ig-CSR and its defects. A schematic representation of the successive steps of CSR toward IgG3 as an example is shown. The transcription step is induced by cytokines. AID induces the DNA lesion by deamination of cytidine into uracil residues. The uracil misintegrated into DNA are removed by UNG2, resulting in an abasic site that is eventually cleaved by an apyrimidinic endonuclease (APE) or the MRN complex (M, MRE11 for meiotic recombination homologue 11; R, hRAD50; N, NBS1 for Nijmegen Breakage syndrome 1). The precise mechanisms leading to DSB in switch (S) regions are not perfectly understood. Multimolecular complexes including phosphorylated γ H2AX, the p53-binding protein (53BP1), the ataxia telangiectasia mutated (ATM), the complex MRN, and MDC1 (DNA damage checkpoint 1) recognize and repair the CSR-induced DSB, in association with the NHEJ enzymes. Defects in the Ig-CSR processes are shown.

cytidine deaminase domain, and the APOBEC1-like domain (Fig. 4A). Eighteen were either missense mutations or in-frame small insertions or deletions, while five led to a premature stop codon, and one was a large deletion of all the coding sequence. Mutations were found mostly in the homozygous state (32 families) or compound heterozygous mutations (11 families) (Durandy *et al.*, 2006; Quartier *et al.*, 2004). Some of them were recurrent and found in unrelated families but no clear mutation hot spot was observed. Of note, we did not detect mutations located either at the phosphorylation sites (S38 and T27) or the dimerization domain (G47–G54) that have been respectively described (Basu *et al.*, 2005; Wang *et al.*, 2006).

In vivo data obtained with these natural human mutations were corroborated by three different *in vitro* assays: analysis of cytidine deaminase activity

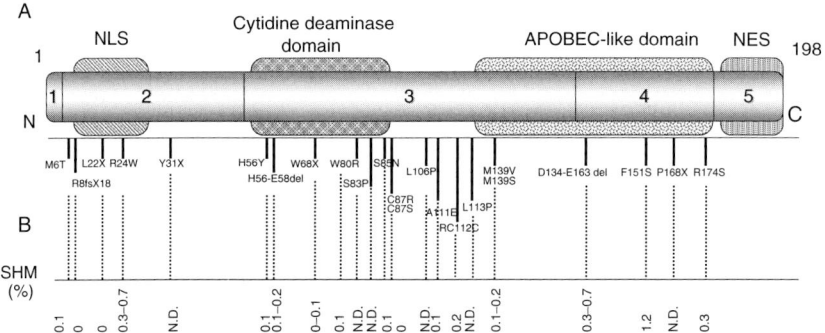

Figure 4 Autosomal recessive Ig-CSR deficiency due to mutations in *AICDA* gene. (A) Twenty-three different mutations (18 missense mutations or in-frame small deletions, 5 nonsense mutations or frameshift deletions) were observed in 62 patients from 43 unrelated families. Mutations were found homozygous in 32 families; others presented with compounded mutations. (B) SHM frequency was studied in 29 patients on VH3-23 region of IgM on CD19+CD27+ purified B-cell population. Results are expressed as the percentage of mutated nucleotides on all studied nucleotides. Age-matched controls, 2.5–6.3%; ND, not done. When several patients carrying same mutations were tested, the results show the range of SHM observed.

on DNA after transfection in *Escherichia coli*, as described by Petersen-Mahrt *et al.* (2002), induction of CSR after expression in AID$^{-/-}$ murine splenic B cells, and study of SHM on an appropriate substrate after transduction in fibroblasts (Okazaki *et al.*, 2002). Mutants located in the NLS (p.R8fsX18, p.R24W), in the cytidine deaminase domain (p.H56Y, p.H56-E58 del, p.W68X, p.W80R), in the domain located between the cytidine deaminase domain and the APOBEC1-like domain (p.L106P, p.D143-E163 del), and in the APOBEC1-like domain (p.M139V) exerted no detectable cytidine deaminase activity in *E. coli*, with the exception of p.M139V in which a residual activity was found (Ta *et al.*, 2003). All mutants exerted neither CSR in B cells nor SHM activity in fibroblasts. The expression of the *AICDA* mutants, assessed after transfection in 293T cells, was found positive except for in p.R8fsX18, p.W86X, and p.D143-E163 del (Ta *et al.*, 2003). However, endogeneous AID expression was either decreased or even undetectable by Western blot analysis in EBV B-cell lines from all these patients and in germinal centers by immunohistochemistry in available biopsies, suggesting that, in most cases, mutations lead to an unstable protein (Durandy, unpublished data).

The description of a defect of both CSR and SHM in AID deficiency, in concordance with the phenotype concomitantly described in AID-deficient mice (Muramatsu *et al.*, 2000), provided the key findings to determine the master role of AID in CSR and SHM.

2.2. AID Deficiency Associated with Preserved SHM

In three other patients with AID deficiency, a normal frequency and pattern of SHM were observed, contrasting with a drastically impaired *in vivo* and *in vitro* CSR (Table 1; Fig. 5A). The giant germinal centers usually observed in secondary lymphoid organs in the other AID-deficient patients were not detected as noted in a biopsy specimen obtained in one case. This preliminary observation suggests a direct role for SHM in the control of B-cell proliferation inside

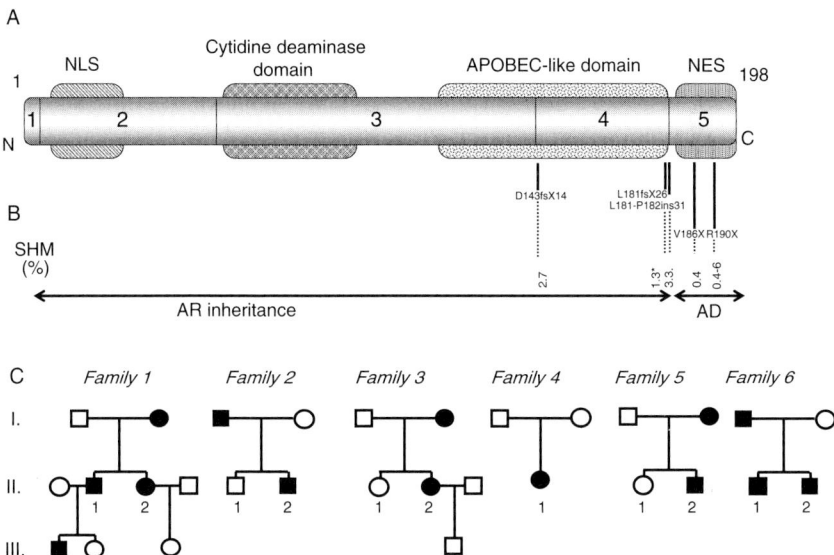

Figure 5 Ig-CSR deficiencies due to mutations in *AICDA* C-terminus. (A) *AICDA* C-terminal mutations. Three patients carried mutation on splice sites in intron 4, the consequences of which were different. In one patient, a homozygous mutation led to the in-frame insertion of 31 nucleotides between exon 4 and exon 5 (p.L181-182 ins31). In the two other patients, the splice site mutation was heterozygous and associated with a missense mutation located either in the region between the cytidine deaminase domain and the APOBEC-like domains (p.R112C) or in the cytidine deaminase domain (p.S83P). The predicted protein was, in one case, frameshift replacement of the C-terminus by 26 amino acids (p.L181fsX26) and in the other case, deletion of exon 4 and frameshift replacement by 4 amino acids (D143-L181fsX4). Both mutations abrogated the NES. Fourteen patients from 6 families carried heterozygous nonsense mutations located in the NES: R190X in 11 patients (5 unrelated families) and V186X in 3 patients (1 family). (B) SHM was performed on CD19+CD27+ B-cell population, except in * in which SHM was studied on CD19+ B-cell population (controls: 0.5–5%). AR, autosomal recessive; AD, autosomal dominant. (C) Autosomal dominant transmission of AICDA pedigrees of autosomal dominant AID deficiencies: p.R190X/+ (families 1–5), p.V186X/+ (family 6).

the germinal centers. Strikingly, these three patients carried mutations located in the C-terminal part of *AICDA* (AID^{Cter}) (Fig. 5A). In one, a homozygous mutation in the splice acceptor site of intron 4 leads to the in-frame insertion of 31 amino acids (p.L181-P182ins31), leading to expression of an abnormally large protein. Two other patients exhibited compound mutations: (1) a missense mutation in domain located between the cytidine deaminase domain and the APOBEC1-like domain (p.R112C) and a mutation in the splice donor site of intron 4, leading to a 26 amino acid frameshift replacement of the C-terminus leading to the NES sequence loss (p.L181fsX26), (2) a mutation in the cytidine deaminase domain (p.S83P) and a splice donor site mutation of intron 4 resulting in deletion of exon 4 and frameshift insertion of four amino acids also excluding the NES (p.D143fsX4). In *in vitro* assays, the p.L181-182ins.31 mutant exerted a slightly reduced cytidine deaminase activity in *E. coli* that is likely the consequence of decreased expression of the protein. Both p.L181-182ins.31 and p.L181fsX26 mutants were shown to induce SHM in fibroblasts but not CSR in AID$^{-/-}$ B cells, although, as expected, the p.R112C, an *AICDA* mutation located in the APOBEC1-like domain, was unable to sustain both CSR and SHM (Ta *et al.*, 2003). Interestingly, these three mutations located in the C-terminal part of AID (p.L181-182ins.31, p.L181fsX26, and p.D143fsX4) do not exert a dominant negative effect since heterozygous carriers exhibited normal serum Ig levels (Durandy, unpublished data).

The observation of normal SHM but defective CSR induced by these natural mutants was confirmed by the analysis of an artificial mutant deleted of the last 10 amino acids. This mutant was found to catalyze SHM, gene conversion but not CSR (Barreto *et al.*, 2003). No data concerning the occurrence of CSR-induced mutations and DSB in S regions are up to now available in patients causing mutations in AID^{Cter}. However, results found with the artificial mutant strongly suggest that AID has a CSR-specific activity possibly by binding through its C-terminus to one or several CSR-specific cofactor(s). Such an interaction could account for the AID selectivity in targeting DNA in S regions of Ig genes of germinal center B cells. Alternatively, because the artificial mutant, although unable to induce CSR when transduced into AID$^{-/-}$ mice splenic B cells, led to a normal frequency and pattern of mutations in the Sμ region, the CSR cofactor could also be involved in the CSR-specific DNA repair (Barreto *et al.*, 2003). Two proteins, DNA-dependent protein kinase (DNA-PK$_{CS}$) and murine double minute 2 (MDM2), have been reported as binding the C-terminus of AID (MacDuff *et al.*, 2006; Wu *et al.*, 2005). They could represent CSR-specific AID cofactors since (1) the nonhomologous end joining (NHEJ) repair pathway to which DNA-PK$_{CS}$ belongs has been shown to be required for CSR but dispensable for SHM (Rolink *et al.*, 1996) and (2) MDM2 binds the Nijmegen breakage syndrome 1 (NBS1) molecule

(Alt et al., 2005), a molecule necessary for the CSR-induced DNA repair (Reina-San-Martin et al., 2005). MDM2 has been shown to be required for gene conversion in the chicken DT-40 cell line, but no data on CSR are available. Such an interaction between AID and MDM2 could suggest that the AID-induced DNA breaks are sensed to induce appropriate DNA repair, following NBS1 recruitment.

Conversely, several artificial murine *AICDA* mutants with mutations located in the NLS in AID N-terminus have been shown to exert, as expected, a normal cytidine deaminase activity after transfection in *E. coli*, but strikingly a normal CSR activity when transduced in murine splenic AID$^{-/-}$ B cells, contrasting with a defective SHM induction in fibroblasts (Shinkura et al., 2003). This feature, which is not only related to impaired NLS, raises the hypothesis that an interaction of AID N-terminus with SHM cofactor(s) could exist. However, we could not confirm this observation in six Ig-CSR-deficient patients harboring homozygous missense mutations in the N-terminus of AID immediately upstream from the NLS (p.M6T) or within the NLS (p.R24W) (Fig. 4A). All present with both a typical CSR defect as shown by their Ig levels and *in vitro* B-cell activation and a complete lack of SHM. This observation suggests several possibilities: (1) the recruitment of cofactors could be not identical in humans and mice or (2) these natural mutants lead either to an unstable protein or to a protein unable to properly shuttle into the nucleus. However, AID was detectable by Western blot in a p.R24W-mutated EBV-B-cell line. Finally, one cannot exclude that an immunodeficiency consisting in defective antibody affinity maturation but normal CSR could be caused by AID mutations located at the N-terminus remains to be described. It implies that AID-mutated protein is expressed and traffics normally between cytoplasm and nucleus on activation.

2.3. Autosomal Dominant Transmission of AID Deficiency

In 14 patients from 6 unrelated families, we observed an Ig-CSR deficiency, the inheritance of which was suggestive of an autosomal dominant transmission (Fig. 5C). It was characterized by variable susceptibility to infections and serum Ig level abnormalities: serum IgM was increased, IgG was absent or only decreased, and IgA was undetectable. Interestingly, these patients carry heterozygous nonsense mutations located in the nuclear export signal (NES): p.R190X in five families (Imai et al., 2005) and p.V186X in one (Fig. 5A). Both normal and mutated allele transcripts were equally expressed in activated B cells as judged by semiquantitative RT-PCR amplification. Although the *in vitro* CSR was drastically defective, the DSB were normally found in Sμ regions, localizing the CSR defect downstream from the DNA cleavage, a finding compatible with the hypothesis that CSR-specific AID-cofactor(s) is (are) involved in CSR-DNA repair of S regions (Table 1).

SHM frequency was normal, except in two patients (2 II-2 and 6 II-2) in whom SHM was undetectable (Fig. 5C). The reason of this defect remains unknown. Because the available AID-specific monoclonal antibody recognizes its 10 last amino acids, it was not possible to check for the presence of the truncated protein. However, full-length AID protein was observed in the available p.R190X EBV B-cell lines.

The variable immunodeficiency found in p.R190X or p.V186X heterozygous patients is not caused by haploinsufficiency, considering the normal Ig levels observed in subjects carrying heterozygous mutations located elsewhere in *AICDA* gene (Imai *et al.*, 2005). Two nonmutually exclusive hypotheses can, thus, be proposed to account for this dominant negative effect: (1) The truncation affects the NES domain of the protein, leading to nuclear accumulation of the mutant allele, which could interfere with normal AID trafficking and function. While wild-type AID is only detected in the cytoplasm of activated B cells and is able to shuttle into the nucleus for a short period on activation, the p.R190X-mutated allele was found mostly in the nucleus after overexpression in AID-deficient B cells (Ito *et al.*, 2004). However, the observation that two different splice site mutations leading also to NES truncation are responsible for an autosomal recessive CSR defect, with conserved SHM (see above), suggests that the loss of NES may not be sufficient to create a dominant negative mutant. (2) The mutated allele, incorporated in an AID homomultimeric complex, disrupts AID activity. It has been reported that AID forms homomultimeric complexes *in vitro* (Ta *et al.*, 2003), even in the absence of its C-terminal part, as shown by detectable *in vitro* multimerization of artificial mutants truncated for the last 10 amino acids (Barreto *et al.*, 2003). An AID motif involved in homodimerization has been delineated between p.G47 and p.G54 and thus is present in these C-terminal mutants (Wang *et al.*, 2006). One possibility to consider is that intact AID multimers could be necessary to recruit CSR-specific AID cofactor(s).

Molecular target of AID has been a matter of debate. As the sequence of AID shares similarity with that of the RNA-editing enzyme APOBEC1, it has been suggested that AID edits an mRNA encoding a substrate common to CSR and SHM, probably an endonuclease (Chen *et al.*, 2001; Honjo *et al.*, 2002; Kinoshita and Honjo, 2001). The requirement for *de novo* protein synthesis downstream from AID expression in CSR could suggest the synthesis of a recombinase, and is consistent with the RNA-editing model (Doi *et al.*, 2003). The findings of a CSR-specific deficiency associated with given AICDA mutations would, in this context, suggest that AID can edit two different endonucleases, making it more complex and less likely. Alternatively, several lines of evidence indicate that AID is a DNA-editing enzyme. Transfection of AID into *E. coli* results in deamination of DNA deoxycytidine residues into deoxyuridine (Petersen-Mahrt *et al.*, 2002). Furthermore, it has been demonstrated that AID can induce deoxycytidine deamination on single-stranded DNA in cell-free experimental conditions (Bransteitter *et al.*, 2003; Chaudhuri *et al.*, 2003; Dickerson *et al.*, 2003; Ramiro *et al.*, 2003). However, these data were obtained in nonphysiological conditions, involving overexpression in *E. coli* or in *in vitro* assays, in which the well-known RNA-editing protein APOBEC1 has a similar effect (Harris *et al.*, 2002; Petersen-Mahrt and Neuberger, 2003). The description of the *in vivo* consequences on antibody maturation of the defect in uracil-N-glycosylase (UNG), an enzyme that recognizes uracil residues on DNA, as described below, is, however, only compatible with a DNA-editing activity of AID.

3. Ig-CSR Deficiency Type 2 Caused by UNG Deficiency

We reported three patients from three families, two being consanguineous, affected by a severe Ig-CSR deficiency with high levels of IgM and very low levels or absence of IgG and IgA, leading to recurrent bacterial infections (Imai *et al.*, 2003b). Two of the three patients presented with lymphadenopathies, one with autoimmunity (hemolytic anemia). The CSR defect was also observed *in vitro* as shown by the complete lack of production of IgG, IgA, or IgE by patients' B cells on activation by sCD40L+ appropriate cytokines, although their B cells proliferate in the same culture conditions. As observed in most cases of AID deficiency, the CSR defect occurs downstream from the germ line transcript induction and upstream from the DSB occurrence (Imai *et al.*, 2003b) (Table 1). In contrast with what is observed in most patients affected by AID deficiency, the frequency of SHM was found normal in the CD19+CD27+ B-cell population. However, the pattern of SHM was strikingly abnormal in the three patients since a slight increase in mutations targeting G/C residues (75%) as compared to controls (63%) was observed. It was associated with a drastic skewed nucleotide substitution pattern on G/C since nearly all found mutations were transitions (G > A, C > T 95%) whereas, in controls, transitions represent only 60% of mutations. Conversely, transition frequency was normal on A/T nucleotides (50%) (Imai *et al.*, 2003b).

Because the Ig-CSR deficiency phenotype observed in these patients resembled the phenotype described as a consequence of homozygous *UNG* gene inactivation in mice (Rada *et al.*, 2002), although in the latter a much milder CSR defect was found, we explored the possibility of UNG deficiency in the patients. In humans, as in mice, UNG has two different promotors and two alternative splice products, resulting in two isoforms: UNG1, the mitochondrial

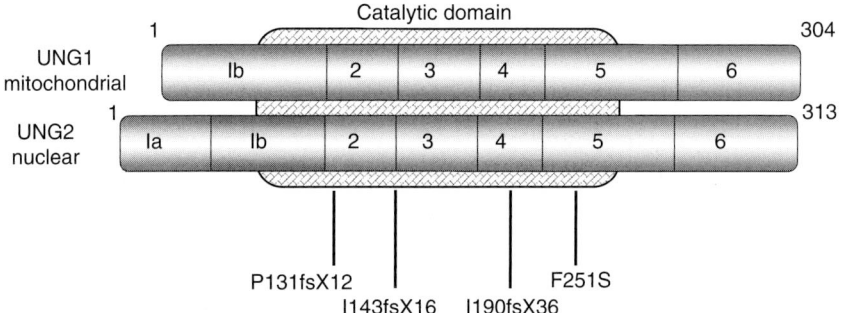

Figure 6 Autosomal recessive Ig-CSR deficiency due to mutations in *UNG* gene. Three patients presented with mutations located in the catalytic domain of both UNG1 and UNG2. Number of amino acids are those of UNG2. One patient carried two heterozygous small frameshift deletions (p.P131fsX12 + p.I190fsX36), the two other were homozygous for a small frameshift deletion (p.I143fsX16) or a missense mutation (p.F251S), respectively. In three patients, UNG1 and UNG2 were undetectable in EBV B-cell lines by immunoprecipitation.

isoform, is ubiquitously expressed while UNG2, the nuclear isoform, is only expressed in proliferating cells (Nilsen *et al.*, 2000; Otterlei *et al.*, 1998), including B cells activated for CSR (Imai *et al.*, 2003b). The above-mentioned *de novo* protein synthesis-dependent step downstream from AID activity in CSR described in murine splenic B cells (Doi *et al.*, 2003) could, thus, possibly correspond to UNG2 induction. We found mutations in all three patients: two heterozygous small deletions leading to premature stop codons (p.P131fsX12 + p.I190fsX36 in nuclear UNG2) in one patient, a homozygous missense mutation (p.F251S) in another patient, and a homozygous small deletion leading to a stop codon in the third one (p.I143fsX16) (Fig. 6). All four mutations were located in the active site of UNG1 and UNG2.

UNG mutations, as studied in EBV B-cell lines, led to an absence of any detectable protein by immunoprecipitation using a polyclonal antibody to UNG1 and UNG2, and no UNG activity neither in cytoplasmic nor in nuclear extracts (Imai *et al.*, 2003b; Kavli *et al.*, 2005). In accordance with this observation, accumulation of genomic uracil residues was present in the three EBV B-cell lines, while undetectable in controls. These results indicate that no other UNG, such as SMUG1 (Di Noia *et al.*, 2006), can compensate for the absence of UNG2, at least in EBV B cells. In contrast, although lacking the UNG1 isoform, patients do not present with metabolic abnormalities, suggesting a compensatory activity exerted by other uracil-DNA glycosylases in mitochondria.

The description of a drastic CSR defect and a skewed pattern of SHM in the absence of UNG is only compatible with a DNA-editing activity of AID. Hence, in the proposed model, AID deaminates dC on DNA to generate dU residues (Di Noia and Neuberger, 2002; Rada et al., 2002). Following the deglycosylation and removal of the misintegrated dU residues by UNG, an abasic site is created, which can be attacked by an apyrimidinic endonuclease, resulting in DNA breaks (Fig. 3). It has been shown *in vitro* that the MRE11/hRad50/NBS1 complex could exert this endonucleasic activity (Larson et al., 2005). In the absence of UNG2 and of abasic site, the DNA cleavage cannot occur, leading to a defect in CSR and a skewed pattern of SHM because SHMs occur by replication of U:G residues leading to transitions (G > A, C > T) only or by their repair by the mismatch repair (MMR) enzymes (MSH2, MSH6) leading to transitions and transversions on bystander nucleotidic residues (Di Noia and Neuberger, 2002; Rada et al., 2004; Xue et al., 2006). The discrepancy between the drastic CSR defect observed in UNG-deficient humans and the more subtle defect observed in UNG$^{-/-}$ mice could be related to a variable involvement of MMR in CSR in both species (Ehrenstein and Neuberger, 1999; Schrader et al., 1999).

An identical phenotype was observed in the three patients, although two patients carried *UNG* mutations encoding truncated proteins, and the third one a missense mutation (p.F251S in UNG2). To assess the consequences of this last mutation on protein expression and activity, it was shown that, although the mutant protein was weakly expressed after transfection into *E. coli*, the purified protein exerted a normal enzymatic activity. However, when coexpressed in HeLa cells, the p.F251S mutant interacted with wtUNG1, an interaction that led to its abnormal translocation from nucleus to mitochondria and its rapid degradation (Kavli et al., 2005). Such a mechanism can very likely underlie the accumulation of genomic uracil residues as well as the drastic Ig-CSR deficiency observed in the patient. This result is of importance since it has been reported that the mouse counterpart of this mutant (denoted F242S) can remove uracil and restore CSR when transduced in UNG$^{-/-}$ B cells (Begum et al., 2004). One explanation for this discrepancy could be that the UNG2 F251S mutant effect depends on the balance between its expression level and that of UNG1. Overexpression of *UNG2* mutant, in the absence of UNG1 in UNG$^{-/-}$ B cells, does not lead to abnormal redirection to mitochondria and degradation, thus enabling CSR since the protein is active.

It has also been proposed that enzymatically dead UNG is required for CSR, suggesting that UNG is either involved in the recruitment of DNA repair molecules or play a role by folding the CSR-induced DSB (Honjo et al., 2004). However, this hypothesis does not fit with (1) the defective occurrence of DSB in Sμ regions in UNG-deficient B cells on activation to CSR (Imai et al., 2003b) and (2) the accumulation of genomic uracils found in UNG-deficient EBV B-cell lines (Kavli *et al.*, 2005).

UNG deficiency, as detected so far in three patients, is not associated with other clinical features than Ig-CSR deficiency. However, UNG is part of the DNA base excision repair involved in the repair of spontaneously occurring base lesions and therefore constitutes an antimutagenic defense strategy. UNG-deficient mice do develop B-cell lymphomas when aging (Nilsen *et al.*, 2003). It is, thus, possible that UNG deficiency predisposes to such tumors in adulthood. Another consequence of UNG deficiency has been reported in UNG-deficient mice since postischemic brain injury is much more severe than in control mice, a likely consequence of the mitochondrial DNA repair defect (Endres *et al.*, 2004).

Therefore, the complete absence of UNG leads in humans to a unique Ig-CSR deficiency characterized by defective CSR and a skewed pattern of SHM, an observation providing a clue to demonstrate the DNA-editing activity of AID.

4. Molecularly Undefined Ig-CSR Deficiency with Normal SHM

Half cases of the Ig-CSR deficiency caused by an intrinsic B-cell defect are neither related to AID nor UNG deficiency and remain molecularly unelucidated (Fig. 1). We had the opportunity to study the clinical and immunologic phenotype of 52 patients affected by an Ig-CSR deficiency, previously published as HIGM4, although its molecular defect is still undefined (Imai *et al.*, 2003a). Although most cases were sporadic, the observation of patients in a few multiplex or consanguineous families is compatible with an autosomal recessive inheritance. The clinical phenotype is very similar to that of AID deficiency, including susceptibility to bacterial infections of the respiratory tract and the gut and autoimmunity. Autoimmune hemolytic anemia and thrombocytopenia were not infrequent (eight cases) while other autoimmune manifestations (uveitis and systemic lupus erythematous) were noted in a few cases (1 and 2, respectively). Lymphoid hyperplasia was less frequent and milder than in AID deficiency, characterized by moderate follicular hyperplasia, whereas the giant germinal centers typical of AID deficiency were not observed.

The CSR defect appears to be milder than in AID deficiency since residual levels of IgG could be detected in the serum from 18 patients of 52. *In vitro*, B cells from these patients (expressing IgM and IgD or IgM only), although able to proliferate, to produce IgM, and to up-regulate CD23, did not undergo CSR on activation by sCD40L and appropriate cytokines. *AICDA, UNG2,* and Ig germ line transcripts were normally induced on CSR induction, whereas Ig excision circles and functional transcripts were undetectable. Even B cells from patients with residual serum IgG levels lacked functional γ transcripts, indicating that either the *in vitro* test is less sensitive than the *in vivo* Ig level determination or a residual CSR had occurred *in vivo* as a result of repeated stimulations, or via another signaling pathway. The overexpression of BAFF or APRIL on activated dendritic cells stimulates marginal zone B cells to undergo CSR in a CD40-independent pathway—a compensatory mechanism absent in AID-deficient cells which cannot undergo CSR whatever the stimulation.

Isohemagglutinins and IgM antipolysaccharide antibodies were present in normal amounts but no IgG antibodies against immunization agents or infectious antigens were detected (Imai *et al.*, 2003a). SHM was found normal in frequency and pattern, an observation not in favor of AID or UNG deficiencies, a diagnosis definitively excluded by both gene sequencing and protein expression studies.

Further analysis of the precise location of the CSR block led to the delineation of two different groups.

4.1. Ig-CSR Deficiency Type 3 Characterized by a CSR Block Located Upstream from the Sµ Region DNA Cleavage

This subset, up to now observed in 17 patients, is always associated with a normal fraction of CD19+CD27+ "memory" B-cell population. This phenotype is similar to the one of patients carrying mutations in the C-terminus of AID.

The Ig-CSR deficiency, herein described, could be the consequence of a defective targeting of AID on S regions since the CSR-induced DSB are shown not to occur in Sµ regions from patients' B cells, localizing the CSR defect, as in AID deficiency, downstream from the transcription step and upstream from the DNA cleavage (Table 1; Fig. 3). An interaction between the 32-kD subunit of the DNA-binding replication protein A (RPA) complex and AID has been reported as essential for AID binding to both DNA in S and V regions (Chaudhuri *et al.*, 2004). However, this interaction is likely unaffected in this Ig-CSR deficiency since SHMs are normally found.

Another possibility could be a defect in AID phosphorylation. Indeed, AID phosphorylation by protein kinase A (PKA) on S38 and T27 amino acids has been shown to be required for AID interaction with RPA, binding to double-stranded DNA and activity in CSR. Artificial mutants carrying alanine substitutions on S38 and T27 amino acids are unable to induce CSR when transduced in AID$^{-/-}$ murine splenic B cells (Basu *et al.*, 2005). However, the same requirement of AID phosphorylation for interaction with RPA and SHM has been also described (McBride *et al.*, 2006). Other additional post-transcriptional modification of AID, required for CSR and dispensable for SHM, could thus be responsible for this Ig-CSR deficiency if defective.

An alternative mechanism could also consist in AID inaccessibility to S regions because of a defect in an activation-dependent change in chromatin unrelated to transcription.

4.2. Ig-CSR Deficiency Type 4 Characterized by a CSR Block Downstream from the Sµ Region DNA Cleavage

The clinical phenotype of this subset differs by the occurrence of B-cell lymphomas (5 of 35 patients). In one available biopsy of an affected cervical lymph node, numerous monoclonal immunoblastic B cells, strongly expressing AID, were observed in interfollicular areas surrounding follicles of various sizes (Durandy, unpublished data). Lymphoma was not associated with EBV.

In contrast to most cases of AID deficiency, the DSB were normally detected in Sµ regions in CSR-activated B cells, although the *in vitro* CSR was defective. However, the next step, DNA repair, was impaired since excision circles and functional transcripts of switched isotypes were not found (Table 1; Fig. 3). The occurrence of DSB in Sµ regions ruled out a defect in AID targeting to S regions. SHMs were found normal in frequency and pattern within the CD27+CD19+ B-cell-purified population. Of note, however, this B-cell subset was strikingly decreased as compared to controls (<10% of B cells). Several hypotheses can be discussed to account for this unique phenotype.

4.2.1. A Defect in the Repair of the AID-Induced DNA Lesion in S Regions

The occurrence of B-cell lymphomas, the decreased number of CD27+ B cells, and the CSR defect located downstream from the DNA breaks suggest that a DNA repair defect during the CSR process could be responsible for this Ig-CSR deficiency. The discrepancy between the findings of defective *in vivo* and *in vitro* CSR and normal generation of SHM also fits with this hypothesis because CSR and SHM are known to use different pathways for DNA repair. The NHEJ pathway, which repairs DSB, is involved in CSR-DNA repair (Casellas *et al.*, 1998; Manis *et al.*, 1998; Rolink *et al.*, 1996). Nevertheless, a defect in one of the NHEJ components is unlikely to account for this condition because NHEJ proteins are also required for V(D)J recombination of both T- and B-cell receptors. Patients exhibited normal numbers of T and B cells, with functional antigen receptors, unlike other NHEJ-defective patients such as Artemis-deficient patients (Moshous *et al.*, 2001) or Cernunnos-deficient patients (Buck *et al.*, 2006). One may postulate that another DNA repair pathway is involved, as suggested by the observation of normal CSR in SCID mice, despite the lack of DNA-PK activity (Bosma *et al.*, 2002). A defect in one such repair enzyme could be responsible for this Ig-CSR deficiency.

It has been described that CSR-induced DSB in S regions induce DNA repair foci involving phosphorylated histone γH2AX and the MRE11/hRad50/NBS1 (MRE11, meiotic recombination homologue 11) complex at Ig loci (Petersen et al., 2001). A defective CSR with normal SHM has been reported in H2AX-knockout mice (Petersen et al., 2001) but a deficiency in H2AX has been ruled out in patients by gene sequencing and normal DNA repair foci formation (Durandy, unpublished data). Mutations in the NBS1 and MRE11 genes could be excluded because they are responsible for the Nijmegen breakage syndrome (Varon et al., 1998) and ataxia-telangiectasia-like disorder (Stewart et al., 1999), respectively, features of which being not found in the studied condition. Ataxia-telangiectasia mutated (ATM) plays also a role in CSR-DNA repair as shown by the typical Ig-CSR deficiency condition observed in some patients (Weemaes et al., 1984), characterized by abnormal S region junctions, and normal SHM (Pan-Hammarstrom et al., 2003).

The p53-binding protein (53BP1), which participates to the early step of DSB repair by facilitating end joinings, has also been described as being required for CSR and dispensable for SHM (Manis et al., 2004; Ward et al., 2004). However, 53bp1-deleted mice also present with a partial T-cell deficiency (Ward et al., 2003), not found in patients. Nevertheless, the gene encoding 53BP1 was sequenced and found normal in the patients affected with this Ig-CSR deficiency. The DNA damage checkpoint protein 1 (MDC1), which plays a role in genomic stability and DSB repair, has been reported to be involved in CSR, but at a lower magnitude as shown by the only slight CSR defect observed in mdc1$^{-/-}$ mice (Lou et al., 2006). MDC1 involvement was also excluded by gene sequencing (Durandy, unpublished data).

Although the MMR enzymes play a role in CSR, at least in mice (Ehrenstein and Neuberger, 1999; Schrader et al., 1999; Stavnezer and Schrader, 2005), it is unlikely that a defect in one of these molecules could account for the phenotype, herein, described because (1) UNG-dependent CSR should be preserved and (2) no other cancers were detected in these patients.

Therefore, we could not up to now find a defect in any molecule known to be directly involved in DNA repair of S regions in this Ig-CSR deficiency, raising the hypothesis that survival signals to switching B cells or responses to the consequences of DNA damage within the germinal centers could be deficient in this condition.

4.2.2. A Defect in Switched B-Cell Differentiation or Survival

A defect in B-cell differentiation could also be responsible for this Ig-CSR deficiency. For example, Bach2, which is a repressor of the expression of the plasma cell differentiation factors Blimp1 and XBP-1, plays a critical role in

CSR and SHM in mice (Muto et al., 2004). Bach2-deficient mice exhibit a CSR defect but a more profound SHM defect than found in patients. Lymph nodes are depleted of germinal centers and CSR-activated B cells do not express *AID* transcripts, both observations not found in the studied condition. Finally, the involvement of Bach2 in this Ig-CSR deficiency has been ruled out by gene sequencing (Durandy, unpublished data).

A defect in survival signals delivered to switched B cells could also explain this phenotype. Molecular interactions are known to be required for B-cell survival, including BAFF interaction with its BCR, BAFF-R. The natural mutant mouse strain A/WySnJ, BAFF-R-knockout mice, and mice treated with the BAFF-neutralizing BAFF-R-Fc protein disclose B-cell depletion and an impaired T-cell-dependent antibody response (Kayagaki et al., 2002; Schiemann et al., 2001; Thompson et al., 2001). The decreased number of CD27+ B cells and the defective IgG and IgA production in patients fit with this model. However, the observed *in vitro* defective CD40-dependent CSR cannot be accounted for by a BAFF-R or BAFF abnormality, though a defect in another unknown factor can, however, be postulated.

Another hypothesis could be an inappropriate response to DNA damage. In other cells than germinal center B cells, DSB activate p53 and p21, resulting in cell cycle arrest and apoptosis. In germinal centers, in contrast, the p53 response to DNA damage is negatively regulated directly by its highly expressed transcriptional regulator Bcl-6, while p21-induced cell cycle arrest is suppressed through interaction of its transcriptional activator Miz1 with Bcl-6. Both of these events enable intense proliferation of B cells undergoing CSR (Phan et al., 2005). In accordance with this observation, Bcl-6-deficient mice are depleted of germinal centers because of a strong B-cell apoptosis (Ye et al., 1997). Such a defect in transcriptional repression of proteins involved in cell cycle arrest induced by DNA damage could also underline this Ig-CSR deficiency. Investigation of this pathway is ongoing. However, this hypothesis does not fit with the normal generation of SHM which also results from a DNA damage, but possibly does not involve similar breaks.

In any case, the molecular definition of these Ig-CSR deficiencies would be essential for a better understanding of the complex mechanisms of CSR, up to now not completely elucidated, and for the delineation of the human diseases, although rare, characterized by a CSR deficiency.

5. Concluding Remarks

The precise description of the different Ig-CSR deficiency conditions is essential for a medical point of view since prognosis, thus follow-up of patients, may differ according to the defect. All Ig-CSR deficiencies are characterized by a profound CSR defect, but they differ for SHM generation, raising the question of the role of mutated IgM in defense against infections and in inducing or not autoimmunity. Indeed, AID deficiency is most often characterized by a drastic defect in SHM, while SHMs are present with a skewed pattern in UNG deficiency and normal in AID C-terminal deficiency and the other Ig-CSR deficiencies. At first glance, susceptibility to infections appears identical in the four groups, suggesting that mutated IgM may not play a significant role in efficient immunity to bacteria. However, this requires to be looked in details during the intervals patients are not treated by parenteral injections of immunoglobulins. Careful assessment of susceptibility to infections in animal models may provide useful information on the role of (un)mutated IgM antibodies in anti-infectious immunity. AID-deficient mice do survive after a secondary infection by influenza virus, although they present a severe morbidity, indicating that even unmutated IgM antibodies can contribute to control that particular viral infection (Harada et al., 2003). The protective role of IgM, even unmutated, is emphasized by the overall milder clinical phenotype observed in Ig-CSR deficiencies, as compared to agammaglobulinemia, resulting in the fact that Ig-CSR deficiencies are diagnosed much later up to adulthood (Imai et al., 2005; Quartier et al., 2004).

The role of SHM-modulating autoimmunity can be also discussed. Patients affected with an Ig-CSR deficiency due to an intrinsic B-cell defect present with autoimmune manifestations, some of them being clearly related to IgM autoantibodies. Autoimmunity is likely not simply related to IgM serum levels since autoimmune manifestations are significantly less frequent in CD40L deficiency in which IgM levels are equally elevated. Autoimmunity apparently occurs with the same frequency in AID deficiency characterized by a lack of SHM and in other Ig-CSR deficiencies with normal SHM generation. Although IgM autoimmune antibodies themselves have not been checked for SHM, our observation suggests that autoimmunity can be supported by germ line Ig sequences in accordance with occurrence of autoimmunity in AID deficiency.

Occurrence of B-cell lymphomas is another special concern associated with some of the Ig-CSR deficiencies. Such cancers are not intrinsically linked to Ig-CSR deficiency itself since they were not reported in 62 cases of AID deficiency. They are detected in Ig-CSR deficiency associated with a defective DNA repair of either the AID-induced lesion (as observed in UNG-deficient mice, also in humans?) or the UNG/AP-endonuclease-induced DNA breaks (as observed in Ig-CSR deficiency type 4).

The ongoing delineation of inherited Ig-CSR deficiency syndromes is shedding new light on the process of physiological antibody maturation in humans. Natural mutants observed in human immunodeficiencies have, in some cases, been described before generation of the appropriate mouse model.

The genetic definition of the X-linked CD40L deficiency was determined before the generation of CD40L-deficient mice. Both observations provided clear evidence for the essential role played in antibody maturation by the CD40 signaling pathway.

The study of B intrinsic Ig-CSR deficiencies has contributed to a better understanding of the complex mechanisms underlying the CSR and the SHM. The phenotype of AID-deficient patients and mice, which have been concomitantly described, has demonstrated the master role of this newly described B-cell-specific molecule in both events of antibody maturation, the CSR and SHM. Data obtained in humans have contributed to establish that AID acts upstream from the occurrence of the DSB in S regions. The description of an Ig-CSR deficiency caused by UNG deficiency provided strong evidence for a DNA-editing activity for AID, first suggested by *in vitro* data. Additional data have shown that AID could act in antibody maturation not only by its cytidine deaminase activity but as a potential docking protein recruiting cofactors. Study of natural as well as artificially engineered mutants in humans strongly suggests that the C-terminus of AID could bind specific CSR cofactors, involved in DNA repair rather than in AID targeting. In addition, the description that peculiar AID mutants can exert a dominant negative effect fit with the *in vitro* observation of AID homomultimerization. Finally, the study of the up to now unelucidated Ig-CSR deficiencies could also help to resolve some of the issues that remain obscure in the Ig-CSR process. One also should not exclude the description of new phenotypes possibly related to CSR deficiencies, for instance selective Ig isotype deficiencies, up to now not elucidated (Hanson et al., 1988).

Acknowledgments

This work was supported by grants from the Institut National de la Santé et de la Recherche Médicale (INSERM), l'Assistance Publique des Hôpitaux de Paris (AP-HP), l'Association de la Recherche contre le Cancer (ARC), la Ligue Contre le Cancer, CEE contract EURO-POLICY-PID (coordinator: C.I.E. Smith), The Institut des Maladies Rares (GIS) and l'Agence Nationale de la Recherche (ANR), and l'Institut National du Cancer (INCa) N°PL021. We thank Mrs. M. Sifouane for secretarial assistance and Ms. M. Forveille for skillful technical help.

References

Agematsu, K., Nagumo, H., Shinozaki, K., Hokibara, S., Yasui, K., Terada, K., Kawamura, N., Toba, T., Nonoyama, S., Ochs, H. D., and Komiyama, A. (1998). Absence of IgD-CD27(+) memory B cell population in X-linked hyper-IgM syndrome. *J. Clin. Invest.* **102**(4), 853–860.

Allen, R. C., Armitage, R. J., Conley, M. E., Rosenblatt, H., Jenkins, N. A., Copeland, N. G., Bedell, M. A., Edelhoff, S., Disteche, C. M., Simoneaux, D. K., Fanslow, W. C., Belmont, J., et al. (1993). CD40 ligand gene defects responsible for X-linked hyper-IgM syndrome. *Science* **259**(5097), 990–993.

Alt, J. R., Bouska, A., Fernandez, M. R., Cerny, R. L., Xiao, H., and Eischen, C. M. (2005). Mdm2 binds to Nbs1 at sites of DNA damage and regulates double strand break repair. *J. Biol. Chem.* **280**(19), 1877–1881.

Aruffo, A., Farrington, M., Hollenbaugh, D., Li, X., Milatovich, A., Nonoyama, S., Bajorath, J., Grosmaire, L. S., Stenkamp, R., Neubauer, M., Roberts, R. L., Noelle, R. J., et al. (1993). The CD40 ligand, gp39, is defective in activated T cells from patients with X-linked hyper-IgM syndrome. *Cell* **72**(2), 291–300.

Barreto, V., Reina-San-Martin, B., Ramiro, A. R., McBride, K. M., and Nussenzweig, M. C. (2003). C-terminal deletion of AID uncouples class switch recombination from somatic hypermutation and gene conversion. *Mol. Cell* **12**(2), 501–508.

Basu, U., Chaudhuri, J., Alpert, C., Dutt, S., Ranganath, S., Li, G., Schrum, J. P., Manis, J. P., and Alt, F. W. (2005). The AID antibody diversification enzyme is regulated by protein kinase A phosphorylation. *Nature* **438**(7067), 508–511.

Begum, N. A., Kinoshita, K., Kakazu, N., Muramatsu, M., Nagaoka, H., Shinkura, R., Biniszkiewicz, D., Boyer, L. A., Jaenisch, R., and Honjo, T. (2004). Uracil DNA glycosylase activity is dispensable for immunoglobulin class switch. *Science* **305**(5687), 1160–1163.

Blom, A. M., Kask, L., and Dahlback, B. (2003). CCP1-4 of the C4b-binding protein alpha-chain are required for factor I mediated cleavage of complement factor C3b. *Mol. Immunol.* **39**(10), 547–556.

Bosma, G. C., Kim, J., Urich, T., Fath, D. M., Cotticelli, M. G., Ruetsch, N. R., Radic, M. Z., and Bosma, M. J. (2002). DNA-dependent protein kinase activity is not required for immunoglobulin class switching. *J. Exp. Med.* **196**(11), 1483–1495.

Bransteitter, R., Pham, P., Scharff, M. D., and Goodman, M. F. (2003). Activation-induced cytidine deaminase deaminates deoxycytidine on single-stranded DNA but requires the action of RNase. *Proc. Natl. Acad. Sci. USA* **100**(7), 4102–4107.

Breitfeld, D., Ohl, L., Kremmer, E., Ellwart, J., Sallusto, F., Lipp, M., and Forster, R. (2000). Follicular B helper T cells express CXC chemokine receptor 5, localize to B cell follicles, and support immunoglobulin production. *J. Exp. Med.* **192**(11), 1545–1552.

Brodeur, S. R., Angelini, F., Bacharier, L. B., Blom, A. M., Mizoguchi, E., Fujiwara, H., Plebani, A., Notarangelo, L. D., Dahlback, B., Tsitsikov, E., and Geha, R. S. (2003). C4b-binding protein (C4BP) activates B cells through the CD40 receptor. *Immunity* **18**(6), 837–848.

Buck, D., Malivert, L., De Chasseval, R., Barraud, A., Fondaneche, M. C., Sanal, O., Plebani, A., Stephan, J. L., Hufnagel, M., Le Deist, F., Fischer, A., Durandy, A., et al. (2006). Cernunnos, a novel nonhomologous end-joining factor, is mutated in human immunodeficiency with microcephaly. *Cell* **124**(2), 287–299.

Callard, R. E., Smith, S. H., Herbert, J., Morgan, G., Padayachee, M., Lederman, S., Chess, L., Kroczek, R. A., Fanslow, W. C., and Armitage, R. J. (1994). CD40 ligand (CD40L) expression and B cell function in agammaglobulinemia with normal or elevated levels of IgM (HIM). Comparison of X-linked, autosomal recessive, and non-X-linked forms of the disease, and obligate carriers. *J. Immunol.* **153**(7), 3295–3306.

Casellas, R., Nussenzweig, A., Wuerffel, R., Pelanda, R., Reichlin, A., Suh, H., Qin, X. F., Besmer, E., Kenter, A., Rajewsky, K., and Nussenzweig, M. C. (1998). Ku80 is required for immunoglobulin isotype switching. *EMBO J.* **17**(8), 2404–2411.

Castigli, E., Wilson, S. A., Garibyan, L., Rachid, R., Bonilla, F., Schneider, L., and Geha, R. S. (2005). TACI is mutant in common variable immunodeficiency and IgA deficiency. *Nat. Genet.* **37**(8), 829–834.

Castle, B. E., Kishimoto, K., Stearns, C., Brown, M. L., and Kehry, M. R. (1993). Regulation of expression of the ligand for CD40 on T helper lymphocytes. *J. Immunol.* **151**(4), 1777–1788.

Catalan, N., Selz, F., Imai, K., Revy, P., Fischer, A., and Durandy, A. (2003). The block in immunoglobulin class switch recombination caused by activation-induced cytidine deaminase deficiency occurs prior to the generation of DNA double strand breaks in switch mu region. *J. Immunol.* **171**(5), 2504–2509.

Chaudhuri, J., Tian, M., Khuong, C., Pinaud, E., and Alt, F. W. (2003). Transcription-targeted DNA deamination by the AID antibody diversification enzyme. *Nature* **422**(6933), 726–730.

Chaudhuri, J., Khuong, C., and Alt, F. W. (2004). Replication protein A interacts with AID to promote deamination of somatic hypermutation targets. *Nature* **430**(7003), 992–998.

Chen, X., Kinoshita, K., and Honjo, T. (2001). Variable deletion and duplication at recombination junction ends: Implication for staggered double-strand cleavage in class-switch recombination. *Proc. Natl. Acad. Sci. USA* **98**(24), 13860–13865.

Coope, H. J., Atkinson, P. G., Huhse, B., Belich, M., Janzen, J., Holman, M. J., Klaus, G. G., Johnston, L. H., and Ley, S. C. (2002). CD40 regulates the processing of NF-kappaB2 p100 to p52. *EMBO J.* **21**(20), 5375–5385.

Di Noia, J., and Neuberger, M. S. (2002). Altering the pathway of immunoglobulin hypermutation by inhibiting uracil-DNA glycosylase. *Nature* **419**(6902), 43–48.

Di Noia, J. M., Rada, C., and Neuberger, M. S. (2006). SMUG1 is able to excise uracil from immunoglobulin genes: Insight into mutation versus repair. *EMBO J.* **25**(3), 585–595.

Dickerson, S. K., Market, E., Besmer, E., and Papavasiliou, F. N. (2003). AID mediates hypermutation by deaminating single stranded DNA. *J. Exp. Med.* **197**(10), 1291–1296.

Disanto, J. P., Bonnefoy, J. Y., Gauchat, J. F., Fischer, A., and De Saint Basile, G. (1993). CD40 ligand mutations in x-linked immunodeficiency with hyper-IgM. *Nature* **361**(6412), 541–543.

Doi, T., Kinoshita, K., Ikegawa, M., Muramatsu, M., and Honjo, T. (2003). *De novo* protein synthesis is required for the activation-induced cytidine deaminase function in class-switch recombination. *Proc. Natl. Acad. Sci. USA* **100**(5), 2634–2638.

Durandy, A., Schiff, C., Bonnefoy, J. Y., Forveille, M., Rousset, F., Mazzei, G., Milili, M., and Fischer, A. (1993). Induction by anti-CD40 antibody or soluble CD40 ligand and cytokines of IgG, IgA and IgE production by B cells from patients with X-linked hyper IgM syndrome. *Eur. J. Immunol.* **23**(9), 2294–2299.

Durandy, A., Hivroz, C., Mazerolles, F., Schiff, C., Bernard, F., Jouanguy, E., Revy, P., Disanto, J. P., Gauchat, J. F., Bonnefoy, J. Y., Casanova, J. L., and Fischer, A. (1997). Abnormal CD40-mediated activation pathway in B lymphocytes from patients with hyper-IgM syndrome and normal CD40 ligand expression. *J. Immunol.* **158**(6), 2576–2584.

Durandy, A., Péron, S., Taubenheim, N., and Fischer, A. (2006). Activation-induced cytidine deaminase: Structure-function relationship as based on the study of mutants. *Hum. Mutat.* **27**(12), 1185–1191.

Ehrenstein, M. R., and Neuberger, M. S. (1999). Deficiency in Msh2 affects the efficiency and local sequence specificity of immunoglobulin class-switch recombination: Parallels with somatic hypermutation. *EMBO J.* **18**(12), 3484–3490.

Endres, M., Biniszkiewicz, D., Sobol, R. W., Harms, C., Ahmadi, M., Lipski, A., Katchanov, J., Mergenthaler, P., Dirnagl, U., Wilson, S. H., Meisel, A., and Jaenisch, R. (2004). Increased postischemic brain injury in mice deficient in uracil-DNA glycosylase. *J. Clin. Invest.* **113**(12), 1711–1721.

Fagarasan, S., and Honjo, T. (2000). T-independent immune response: New aspects of B cell biology. *Science* **290**(5489), 89–92.

Ferrari, S., Giliani, S., Insalaco, A., Al-Ghonaium, A., Soresina, A. R., Loubser, M., Avanzini, M. A., Marconi, M., Badolato, R., Ugazio, A. G., Levy, Y., Catalan, N., *et al.* (2001). Mutations of CD40 gene cause an autosomal recessive form of immunodeficiency with hyper IgM. *Proc. Natl. Acad. Sci. USA* **98**(22), 12614–12619.

Frazer, J. K., Legros, J., De Bouteiller, O., Liu, Y. J., Banchereau, J., Pascual, V., and Capra, J. D. (1997). Identification and cloning of genes expressed by human tonsillar B lymphocyte subsets. *Ann. NY Acad. Sci.* **815**, 316–318.

Fuleihan, R., Ramesh, N., Loh, R., Jabara, H., Rosen, R. S., Chatila, T., Fu, S. M., Stamenkovic, I., and Geha, R. S. (1993). Defective expression of the CD40 ligand in X chromosome-linked immunoglobulin deficiency with normal or elevated IgM. *Proc. Natl. Acad. Sci. USA* **90**(6), 2170–2173.

Grimbacher, B., Hutloff, A., Schlesier, M., Glocker, E., Warnatz, K., Drager, R., Eibel, H., Fischer, B., Schaffer, A. A., Mages, H. W., Kroczek, R. A., and Peter, H. H. (2003). Homozygous loss of ICOS is associated with adult-onset common variable immunodeficiency. *Nat. Immunol.* **4**(3), 261–268.

Guinamard, R., Okigaki, M., Schlessinger, J., and Ravetch, J. V. (2000). Absence of marginal zone B cells in Pyk-2-deficient mice defines their role in the humoral response. *Nat. Immunol.* **1**(1), 31–36.

Hanson, L. A., Soderstrom, R., Avanzini, A., Bengtsson, U., Bjorkander, J., and Soderstrom, T. (1988). Immunoglobulin subclass deficiency. *Pediatr. Infect. Dis. J.* **7**(Suppl. 5), S17–S21.

Harada, Y., Muramatsu, M., Shibata, T., Honjo, T., and Kuroda, K. (2003). Unmutated immunoglobulin M can protect mice from death by influenza virus infection. *J. Exp. Med.* **197**(12), 1779–1785. (Epub 2003 Jun 9.)

Harris, R. S., Petersen-Mahrt, S. K., and Neuberger, M. S. (2002). RNA editing enzyme APOBEC1 and some of its homologs can act as DNA mutators. *Mol. Cell* **10**(5), 1247–1253.

Honjo, T., Kinoshita, K., and Muramatsu, M. (2002). Molecular mechanism of class switch recombination: Linkage with somatic hypermutation. *Annu. Rev. Immunol.* **20**, 165–196.

Honjo, T., Muramatsu, M., and Fagarasan, S. (2004). AID: How does it aid antibody diversity? *Immunity* **20**(6), 659–668.

Imai, K., Catalan, N., Plebani, A., Marodi, L., Sanal, O., Kumaki, S., Nagendran, V., Wood, P., Glastre, C., Sarrot-Reynauld, F., Forveille, M., Revy, P., *et al.* (2003a). Hyper-IgM syndrome type 4 with a B-lymphocyte intrinsic selective deficiency in immunoglobulin class switch recombination. *J. Clin. Invest.* **112**, 136–142.

Imai, K., Slupphaug, G., Lee, W. I., Revy, P., Nonoyama, S., Catalan, N., Yel, L., Forveille, M., Kavli, B., Krokan, H. E., Ochs, H. D., Fischer, A., *et al.* (2003b). Human uracil-DNA glycosylase deficiency associated with profoundly impaired immunoglobulin class-switch recombination. *Nat. Immunol.* **4**(10), 1023–1028.

Imai, K., Zhu, Y., Revy, P., Morio, T., Mizutani, S., Fischer, A., Nonoyama, S., and Durandy, A. (2005). Analysis of class switch recombination and somatic hypermutation in patients affected with autosomal dominant hyper-IgM syndrome type 2. *Clin. Immunol.* **115**(3), 277–285.

Ito, S., Nagaoka, H., Shinkura, R., Begum, N., Muramatsu, M., Nakata, M., and Honjo, T. (2004). Activation-induced cytidine deaminase shuttles between nucleus and cytoplasm like apolipoprotein B mRNA editing catalytic polypeptide 1. *Proc. Natl. Acad. Sci. USA* **101**(7), 1975–1980.

Itoh, K., Meffre, E., Albesiano, E., Farber, A., Dines, D., Stein, P., Asnis, S. E., Furie, R. A., Jain, R. I., and Chiorazzi, N. (2000). Immunoglobulin heavy chain variable region gene replacement As a mechanism for receptor revision in rheumatoid arthritis synovial tissue B lymphocytes. *J. Exp. Med.* **192**(8), 1151–1164.

Iwasato, T., Shimizu, A., Honjo, T., and Yamagishi, H. (1990). Circular DNA is excised by immunoglobulin class switch recombination. *Cell* **62**(1), 143–149.

Jacob, J., and Kelsoe, G. (1992). In situ studies of the primary immune response to (4-hydroxy-3-nitrophenyl)acetyl. II. A common clonal origin for periarteriolar lymphoid sheath-associated foci and germinal centers. *J. Exp. Med.* **176**(3), 679–687.

Jacobs, H., Rajewsky, K., Fukita, Y., and Bross, L. (2001). Indirect and direct evidence for DNA double-strand breaks in hypermutating immunoglobulin genes. *Philos. Trans. R. Soc. Lond. B Biol. Sci.* **356**(1405), 119–125.

Jain, A., Ma, C. A., Lopez-Granados, E., Means, G., Brady, W., Orange, J. S., Liu, S., Holland, S., and Derry, J. M. (2004). Specific NEMO mutations impair CD40-mediated c-Rel activation and B cell terminal differentiation. *J. Clin. Invest.* **114**(11), 1593–1602.

Kaartinen, M., Griffiths, G. M., Markham, A. F., and Milstein, C. (1983). mRNA sequences define an unusually restricted IgG response to 2-phenyloxazolone and its early diversification. *Nature* **304**(5924), 320–324.

Kavli, B., Andersen, S., Otterlei, M., Liabakk, N. B., Imai, K., Fischer, A., Durandy, A., Krokan, H. E., and Slupphaug, G. (2005). B cells from hyper-IgM patients carrying UNG mutations lack ability to remove uracil from ssDNA and have elevated genomic uracil. *J. Exp. Med.* **201**(12), 2011–2021.

Kayagaki, N., Yan, M., Seshasayee, D., Wang, H., Lee, W., French, D. M., Grewal, I. S., Cochran, A. G., Gordon, N. C., Yin, J., Starovasnik, M. A., and Dixit, V. M. (2002). BAFF/BLyS receptor 3 binds the B cell survival factor BAFF ligand through a discrete surface loop and promotes processing of NF-kappaB2. *Immunity* **17**(4), 515–524.

Kinoshita, K., and Honjo, T. (2000). Unique and unprecedented recombination mechanisms in class switching. *Curr. Opin. Immunol.* **12**(2), 195–198.

Kinoshita, K., and Honjo, T. (2001). Linking class-switch recombination with somatic hypermutation. *Nat. Rev. Mol. Cell Biol.* **2**(7), 493–503.

Klein, U., Rajewsky, K., and Kuppers, R. (1998). Human immunoglobulin (Ig)M+IgD+ peripheral blood B cells expressing the CD27 cell surface antigen carry somatically mutated variable region genes: CD27 as a general marker for somatically mutated (memory) B cells. *J. Exp. Med.* **188**(9), 1679–1689.

Korthauer, U., Graf, D., Mages, H. W., Briere, F., Padayachee, M., Malcolm, S., Ugazio, A. G., Notarangelo, L. D., Levinsky, R. J., and Kroczek, R. A. (1993). Defective expression of T-cell CD40 ligand causes X-linked immunodeficiency with hyper-IgM. *Nature* **361**(6412), 539–541.

Kruetzmann, S., Rosado, M. M., Weber, H., Germing, U., Tournilhac, O., Peter, H. H., Berner, R., Peters, A., Boehm, T., Plebani, A., Quinti, I., and Carsetti, R. (2003). Human immunoglobulin M memory B cells controlling *Streptococcus pneumoniae* infections are generated in the spleen. *J. Exp. Med.* **197**(7), 939–945.

Larson, E. D., Cummings, W. J., Bednarski, D. W., and Maizels, N. (2005). MRE11/RAD50 cleaves DNA in the AID/UNG-dependent pathway of immunoglobulin gene diversification. *Mol. Cell* **20**(3), 367–375.

Lebecque, S., De Bouteiller, O., Arpin, C., Banchereau, J., and Liu, Y. J. (1997). Germinal center founder cells display propensity for apoptosis before onset of somatic mutation. *J. Exp. Med.* **185**(3), 563–571.

Litinskiy, M. B., Nardelli, B., Hilbert, D. M., He, B., Schaffer, A., Casali, P., and Cerutti, A. (2002). DCs induce CD40-independent immunoglobulin class switching through BLyS and APRIL. *Nat. Immunol.* **3**(9), 822–829.

Liu, Y. J., Malisan, F., De Bouteiller, O., Guret, C., Lebecque, S., Banchereau, J., Mills, F. C., Max, E. E., and Martinez-Valdez, H. (1996). Within germinal centers, isotype switching of immunoglobulin genes occurs after the onset of somatic mutation. *Immunity* **4**(3), 241–250.

Lou, Z., Minter-Dykhouse, K., Franco, S., Gostissa, M., Rivera, M. A., Celeste, A., Manis, J. P., Van Deursen, J., Nussenzweig, A., Paull, T. T., Alt, F. W., and Chen, J. (2006). MDC1 maintains genomic stability by participating in the amplification of ATM-dependent DNA damage signals. *Mol. Cell* **21**(2), 187–200.

MacDuff, D. A., Neuberger, M. S., and Harris, R. S. (2006). MDM2 can interact with the C-terminus of AID but it is inessential for antibody diversification in DT40 B cells. *Mol. Immunol.* **43**(8), 1099–1108.

Manis, J. P., Gu, Y., Lansford, R., Sonoda, E., Ferrini, R., Davidson, L., Rajewsky, K., and Alt, F. W. (1998). Ku70 is required for late B cell development and immunoglobulin heavy chain class switching. *J. Exp. Med.* **187**(12), 2081–2089.

Manis, J. P., Morales, J. C., Xia, Z., Kutok, J. L., Alt, F. W., and Carpenter, P. B. (2004). 53BP1 links DNA damage-response pathways to immunoglobulin heavy chain class-switch recombination. *Nat. Immunol.* **5**(5), 481–487.

Martin, F., and Kearney, J. F. (2000). B-cell subsets and the mature preimmune repertoire. Marginal zone and B1 B cells as part of a "natural immune memory." *Immunol. Rev.* **175**, 70–79.

Matsuoka, M., Yoshida, K., Maeda, T., Usuda, S., and Sakano, H. (1990). Switch circular DNA formed in cytokine-treated mouse splenocytes: Evidence for intramolecular DNA deletion in immunoglobulin class switching. *Cell* **62**(1), 135–142.

McBride, K. M., Gazumyan, A., Woo, E. M., Barreto, V. M., Robbiani, D. F., Chait, B. T., and Nussenzweig, M. C. (2006). Regulation of hypermutation by activation-induced cytidine deaminase phosphorylation. *Proc. Natl. Acad. Sci. USA* **103**(23), 8798–8803.

Meffre, E., Papavasiliou, F., Cohen, P., De Bouteiller, O., Bell, D., Karasuyama, H., Schiff, C., Banchereau, J., Liu, Y. J., and Nussenzweig, M. C. (1998). Antigen receptor engagement turns off the V(D)J recombination machinery in human tonsil B cells. *J. Exp. Med.* **188**(4), 765–772.

Morio, T., Hanissian, S., and Geha, R. S. (1995). Characterization of a 23-kDa protein associated with CD40. *Proc. Natl. Acad. Sci. USA* **92**(25), 1163–1166.

Moshous, D., Callebaut, R., De Chasseval, R., Corneo, B., Cavazzana-Calvo, M., Le Deist, F., Tezcan, I., Sanal, O., Bertrand, Y., Philippe, N., Fischer, A., and De Villartay, J. P. (2001). ARTEMIS, a novel DNA double-strand break repair/V(D)J recombination protein is mutated in human severe combined immune deficiency with increased radiosensitivity (RS-SCID). *Cell* **105**, 177–186.

Muramatsu, M., Sankaranand, V. S., Anant, S., Sugai, M., Kinoshita, K., Davidson, N. O., and Honjo, T. (1999). Specific expression of activation-induced cytidine deaminase (AID), a novel member of the RNA-editing deaminase family in germinal center B cells. *J. Biol. Chem.* **274**(26), 18470–18476.

Muramatsu, M., Kinoshita, K., Fagarasan, S., Yamada, S., Shinkai, Y., and Honjo, T. (2000). Class switch recombination and hypermutation require activation-induced cytidine deaminase (AID), a potential RNA editing enzyme. *Cell* **102**(5), 553–563.

Muto, A., Tashiro, S., Nakajima, O., Hoshino, H., Takahashi, S., Sakoda, E., Ikebe, D., Yamamoto, M., and Igarashi, K. (2004). The transcriptional programme of antibody class switching involves the repressor Bach2. *Nature* **429**(6991), 566–571. (Epub 2004 May 19.)

Muto, T., Muramatsu, M., Taniwaki, M., Kinoshita, K., and Honjo, T. (2000). Isolation, tissue distribution, and chromosomal localization of the human activation-induced cytidine deaminase (AID) gene. *Genomics* **68**(1), 85–88.

Nilsen, H., Steinsbekk, K. S., Otterlei, M., Slupphaug, G., Aas, P. A., and Krokan, H. E. (2000). Analysis of uracil-DNA glycosylases from the murine Ung gene reveals differential expression in tissues and in embryonic development and a subcellular sorting pattern that differs from the human homologues. *Nucleic Acids Res.* **28**(12), 2277–2285.

Nilsen, H., Stamp, G., Andersen, S., Hrivnak, G., Krokan, H. E., Lindahl, T., and Barnes, D. E. (2003). Gene-targeted mice lacking the Ung uracil-DNA glycosylase develop B-cell lymphomas. *Oncogene* **22**(35), 5381–5386.

Nonoyama, S., Hollenbaugh, D., Aruffo, A., Ledbetter, J. A., and Ochs, H. D. (1993). B cell activation via CD40 is required for specific antibody production by antigen-stimulated human B cells. *J. Exp. Med.* **178**(3), 1097–1102.

Notarangelo, L. D., Duse, M., and Ugazio, A. G. (1992). Immunodeficiency with hyper-IgM (HIM). *Immunodefic. Rev.* **3**(2), 101–121.

Okazaki, I. M., Kinoshita, K., Muramatsu, M., Yoshikawa, K., and Honjo, T. (2002). The AID enzyme induces class switch recombination in fibroblasts. *Nature* **416**(6878), 340–345.

Otterlei, M., Haug, T., Nagelhus, T. A., Slupphaug, G., Lindmo, T., and Krokan, H. E. (1998). Nuclear and mitochondrial splice forms of human uracil-DNA glycosylase contain a complex nuclear localisation signal and a strong classical mitochondrial localisation signal, respectively. *Nucleic Acids Res.* **26**(20), 4611–4617.

Pan-Hammarstrom, Q., Dai, S., Zhao, Y., Van Dijk-Hard, I. F., Gatti, R. A., Borresen-Dale, A. L., and Hammarstrom, L. (2003). ATM is not required in somatic hypermutation of VH, but is involved in the introduction of mutations in the switch mu region. *J. Immunol.* **170**(7), 3707–3716.

Petersen, S., Casellas, R., Reina-San-Martin, B., Chen, H. T., Difilippantonio, M. J., Wilson, P. C., Hanitsch, L., Celeste, A., Muramatsu, M., Pilch, D. R., Redon, C., Ried, T., et al. (2001). AID is required to initiate Nbs1/gamma-H2AX focus formation and mutations at sites of class switching. *Nature* **414**(6864), 660–665.

Petersen-Mahrt, S. K., and Neuberger, M. S. (2003). In vitro deamination of cytosine to uracil in single-stranded DNA by APOBEC1. *J. Biol. Chem.* **278**(22), 19583–19586.

Petersen-Mahrt, S. K., Harris, R. S., and Neuberger, M. S. (2002). AID mutates E. coli suggesting a DNA deamination mechanism for antibody diversification. *Nature* **418**(6893), 99–104.

Phan, R. T., Saito, M., Basso, K., Niu, H., and Dalla-Favera, R. (2005). BCL6 interacts with the transcription factor Miz-1 to suppress the cyclin-dependent kinase inhibitor p21 and cell cycle arrest in germinal center B cells. *Nat. Immunol.* **6**(10), 1054–1060.

Quartier, P., Bustamante, J., Sanal, O., Plebani, A., Debre, M., Deville, A., Litzman, J., Levy, J., Fermand, J. P., Lane, P., Horneff, G., Aksu, G., et al. (2004). Clinical, immunologic and genetic analysis of 29 patients with autosomal recessive hyper-IgM syndrome due to activation-induced cytidine deaminase deficiency. *Clin. Immunol.* **110**(1), 22–29.

Rada, C., Williams, G. T., Nilsen, H., Barnes, D. E., Lindahl, T., and Neuberger, M. S. (2002). Immunoglobulin isotype switching is inhibited and somatic hypermutation perturbed in UNG-deficient mice. *Curr. Biol.* **12**(20), 1748–1755.

Rada, C., Di Noia, J. M., and Neuberger, M. S. (2004). Mismatch recognition and uracil excision provide complementary paths to both Ig switching and the A/T-focused phase of somatic mutation. *Mol. Cell* **16**(2), 163–171.

Rajewsky, K. (1996). Clonal selection and learning in the antibody system. *Nature* **381**(6585), 751–758.

Ramiro, A. R., Stavropoulos, P., Jankovic, M., and Nussenzweig, M. C. (2003). Transcription enhances AID-mediated cytidine deamination by exposing single-stranded DNA on the non-template strand. *Nat. Immunol.* **4**(5), 452–456.

Reina-San-Martin, B., Nussenzweig, M. C., Nussenzweig, A., and Difilippantonio, S. (2005). Genomic instability, endoreduplication, and diminished Ig class-switch recombination in B cells lacking Nbs1. *Proc. Natl. Acad. Sci. USA* **102**(5), 1590–1595.

Revy, P., Muto, T., Levy, Y., Geissmann, F., Plebani, A., Sanal, O., Catalan, N., Forveille, M., Dufourcq-Labelouse, R., Gennery, A., Tezcan, I., Ersoy, F., *et al.* (2000). Activation-induced cytidine deaminase (AID) deficiency causes the autosomal recessive form of the hyper-IgM syndrome (HIGM2). *Cell* **102**(5), 565–575.

Rolink, A., Melchers, F., and Andersson, J. (1996). The SCID but not the RAG-2 gene product is required for S mu-S epsilon heavy chain class switching. *Immunity* **5**(4), 319–330.

Salzer, U., Chapel, H. M., Webster, A. D., Pan-Hammarstrom, Q., Schmitt-Graeff, A., Schlesier, M., Peter, H. H., Rockstroh, J. K., Schneider, P., Schaffer, A. A., Hammarstrom, L., and Grimbacher, B. (2005). Mutations in TNFRSF13B encoding TACI are associated with common variable immunodeficiency in humans. *Nat. Genet.* **37**(8), 820–828.

Schiemann, B., Gommerman, J. L., Vora, K., Cachero, T. G., Shulga-Morskaya, S., Dobles, M., Frew, E., and Scott, M. L. (2001). An essential role for BAFF in the normal development of B cells through a BCMA-independent pathway. *Science* **293**(5537), 2111–2114.

Schrader, C. E., Edelmann, W., Kucherlapati, R., and Stavnezer, J. (1999). Reduced isotype switching in splenic B cells from mice deficient in mismatch repair enzymes. *J. Exp. Med.* **190**(3), 323–330.

Shinkura, R., Tian, M., Smith, M., Chua, K., Fujiwara, Y., and Alt, F. W. (2003). The influence of transcriptional orientation on endogenous switch region function. *Nat. Immunol.* **4**(5), 435–441.

Stavnezer, J., and Schrader, C. E. (2005). Mismatch repair converts AID-instigated nicks to double-strand breaks for antibody class-switch recombination. *Trends Genet.* **22**(1), 23–28.

Stewart, G. S., Maser, R. S., Stankovic, T., Bressan, D. A., Kaplan, M. I., Jaspers, N. G., Raams, A., Byrd, P. J., Petrini, J. H., and Taylor, A. M. (1999). The DNA double-strand break repair gene hMRE11 is mutated in individuals with an ataxia-telangiectasia-like disorder. *Cell* **99**(6), 577–587.

Storb, U., Peters, A., Klotz, E., Kim, N., Shen, H. M., Hackett, J., Rogerson, B., and Martin, T. E. (1998). Cis-acting sequences that affect somatic hypermutation of Ig genes. *Immunol. Rev.* **162**, 153–160.

Ta, V. T., Nagaoka, H., Catalan, N., Durandy, A., Fischer, A., Imai, K., Nonoyama, S., Tashiro, J., Ikegawa, M., Ito, S., Kinoshita, K., Muramatsu, M., *et al.* (2003). AID mutant analyses indicate requirement for class-switch-specific cofactors. *Nat. Immunol.* **4**(9), 843–848.

Thompson, J. S., Bixler, S. A., Qian, F., Vora, K., Scott, M. L., Cachero, T. G., Hession, C., Schneider, P., Sizing, I. D., Mullen, C., Strauch, K., Zafari, M., *et al.* (2001). BAFF-R, a newly identified TNF receptor that specifically interacts with BAFF. *Science* **293**(5537), 2108–2111.

Varon, R., Vissinga, C., Platzer, M., Cerosaletti, K. M., Chrzanowska, K. H., Saar, K., Beckmann, G., Seemanova, E., Cooper, P. R., Nowak, N. J., Stumm, M., Weemaes, C. M., *et al.* (1998). Nibrin, a novel DNA double-strand break repair protein, is mutated in Nijmegen breakage syndrome. *Cell* **93**(3), 467–476.

Wang, J., Shinkura, R., Muramatsu, M., Nagaoka, H., Kinoshita, K., and Honjo, T. (2006). Identification of a specific domain required for dimerization of activation-induced cytidine deaminase. *J. Biol. Chem.* **281**(28), 19115–19123.

Ward, I. M., Minn, K., Van Deursen, J., and Chen, J. (2003). p53 Binding protein 53BP1 is required for DNA damage responses and tumor suppression in mice. *Mol. Cell Biol.* **23**(7), 2556–2563.

Ward, I. M., Reina-San-Martin, B., Olaru, A., Minn, K., Tamada, K., Lau, J. S., Cascalho, M., Chen, L., Nussenzweig, A., Livak, F., Nussenzweig, M. C., and Chen, J. (2004). 53BP1 is required for class switch recombination. *J. Cell Biol.* **165**(4), 459–464.

Wardemann, H., Boehm, T., Dear, N., and Carsetti, R. (2002). B-1a B cells that link the innate and adaptive immune responses are lacking in the absence of the spleen. *J. Exp. Med.* **195**(6), 771–780.

Warnatz, K., Bossaller, L., Salzer, U., Skrabl-Baumgartner, A., Schwinger, W., Van Der Burg, M., Van Dongen, J. J., Orlowska-Volk, M., Knoth, R., Durandy, A., Draeger, R., Schlesier, M., *et al.* (2006). Human ICOS deficiency abrogates the germinal center reaction and provides a monogenic model for common variable immunodeficiency. *Blood* **107**(8), 3045–3052.

Weemaes, C. M., The, T. H., Van Munster, P. J., and Bakkeren, J. A. (1984). Antibody responses *in vivo* in chromosome instability syndromes with immunodeficiency. *Clin. Exp. Immunol.* **57**(3), 529–534.

Weller, S., Faili, A., Garcia, C., Braun, M. C., Le Deist, F. F., De Saint Basile, G. G., Hermine, O., Fischer, A., Reynaud, C. A., and Weill, J. C. (2001). CD40-CD40L independent Ig gene hypermutation suggests a second B cell diversification pathway in humans. *Proc. Natl. Acad. Sci. USA* **98**(3), 1166–1170.

Weller, S., Braun, M. C., Tan, B. K., Rosenwald, A., Cordier, C., Conley, M. E., Plebani, A., Kumararatne, D. S., Bonnet, D., Tournilhac, O., Tchernia, G., Steiniger, B., *et al.* (2004). Human blood IgM memory B cells are circulating splenic marginal zone B cells harboring a prediversified immunoglobulin repertoire. *Blood* **104**(12), 3647–3654.

William, J., Euler, C., Christensen, S., and Shlomchik, M. J. (2002). Evolution of autoantibody responses via somatic hypermutation outside of germinal centers. *Science* **297**(5589), 2066–2070.

Wilson, P. C., Wilson, K., Liu, Y. J., Banchereau, J., Pascual, V., and Capra, J. D. (2000). Receptor revision of immunoglobulin heavy chain variable region genes in normal human B lymphocytes. *J. Exp. Med.* **191**(11), 1881–1894.

Wu, X., Geraldes, P., Platt, J. L., and Cascalho, M. (2005). The double-edged sword of activation-induced cytidine deaminase. *J. Immunol.* **174**(2), 934–941.

Xue, K., Rada, C., and Neuberger, M. S. (2006). The *in vivo* pattern of AID targeting to immunoglobulin switch regions deduced from mutation spectra in msh2−/− ung−/− mice. *J. Exp. Med.* **203**(9), 2085–2094.

Ye, B. H., Cattoretti, G., Shen, Q., Zhang, J., Hawe, N., De Waard, R., Leung, C., Nouri-Shirazi, M., Orazi, A., Chaganti, R. S., Rothman, P., Stall, A. M., *et al.* (1997). The BCL-6 proto-oncogene controls germinal-centre formation and Th2-type inflammation. *Nat. Genet.* **16**(2), 161–170.

INDEX

A

Abelson murine leukemia virus (Ab-MLV) infection, 215, 262
  AID host response factor against, 229–232, 235
Ab maturation, AID-initiated mutations selection during, 143–149
Acquired immune deficiency syndrome (AIDS), 52, 141, 180, 232
β-Actin promoter, 113, 115
Activation-induced cytidine deaminase (AID), 109, 215. *See also* AID-mediated sequence diversification
  Ab maturation and, 143–149
  access to DNA during SHM and CSR, 177
  access to transcribed dsDNA
    activity of, 179–180
    RPA as cofactor, 176–178
    template *vs.* nontemplate strand activities, 178
  antibody memory, 2–28
  by antigen stimulation, 2
  APOBEC1 homology with, 12–13
  bacterial DNA, 166
  BLAST search for, 4
  binding to S regions, 167
  cis-acting determinants, 116–120
  cloning in, 4–5
  C-terminal domain of, 11
  deamination *in vitro* and transcription, 116
  dimerization for CSR, 13–14
  as DNA deaminase for antibody diversification, 38–39
  DNA deamination model, 19, 164–165
    AID mutates DNA in bacteria, 166
    function of UNG in CSR, 168–169
    putative RNA editing activities and, 163
  ssDNA-specific cytidine deaminase *in vitro*, 166–167
  UNG for DSBs, 22–24
  UNG/MMR mutations, 167–168
  in vitro deamination, 19–22
  ectopic expression in CSR, 9–10
  expression at transcriptional level, 5
  expression in
    B-cell lymphomas, 252–258
    normal and malignant nonlymphoid cells, 263–264
  expression mechanism in
    B-cell malignancy, 260–262
    normal B cells, 259
  family, 39, 41–42
  features of, 5
  functional
    domains, 11–14, 18
    homology, 12–13
    involvement in CSR, 5
  for generation of DNA lesions, 163
  in host response to viral infection
    against Ab-MLV, 229–232, 235
    epstein-barr virus, 231–235
    hepatitis C virus, 231, 234–235
  hypotheses for action of, 16
    DNA deamination model, 17, 19–24
    RNA editing model, 17–19
  initiated mutations
    in Ig genes, 127–149
    selection during Ab maturation, 143–149
  interacting molecules, 12
  involvement in DNA cleavage, 14–17, 28
  loss of CSR and SHM due to disruption in, 5–7
  mechanism of action, 39
  molecule in CSR and SHM, 4–8

INDEX

Activation-induced cytidine deaminase (AID) (*continued*)
   mutations in immunoglobulin genes, 127–149
   N-terminal domain, 11–12
   nuclear-cytoplasmic shuttling, 12–13, 18
   nuclear *vs.* cytoplasmic localization, 180–181
   phosphorylation of, 181–184
   post-transcriptional regulation of, 181–184
   putative RNA editing activities of, 163
   RNA editing hypothesis, 1, 17–19, 164
   role in
      chromosomal translocations, 249–252
      lymphomagenesis, 249–252
      tumorigenesis, 245–264
   specificity
      for CSR and SHM, 162–163
      mechanism, 179–180
   structural and functional properties of, 11–12, 43–46
   synapses DSBs
      CSR *vs.* internal S region deletions mechanisms, 184–186
      internal Sm deletions *vs.* long-range CSR, 185
      I-SceI model system, 187–189
      repair mechanism, 186–189
   targeting
      C motifs on ssDNA, 132–139
      during CSR and SHM mechanism, 179–180
      DNA elements in Ig loci, 116–117
   transgenic mouse models, 247–249
   triggered antibody hypermutation, 40
Activation-induced deaminase (AID). *See also* Activation-induced cytidine deaminase
   chromosome translocations and, 94–96
   in DNA lesion, 78–79
   function in DNA lesions, 78–79
   IL-4-induced expression in B cells, 80
   lymphomagenic lesions, 93–96
   non-Ig mutations and lymphomas and, 93–94
   nuclear transport and posttranslational modification, 82–83
   protein, 81–82
   targeting, 82–83
   transcriptional regulation, 80–81
ADAT2/ADAT3, 41–42
Adeno-associated virus (AAV) production, inhibition by APOBEC3A, 224–226
Adenocarcinomas, 248
Adenosine deaminases, 42
AICDA gene, mutations of, 275, 281, 283–285, 288
AID. *See* Activation-induced cytidine deaminase
AID/APOBEC cytidine deaminase, 216–217. *See also* Apolipoprotein B RNA-editing catalytic component
AID$^{-/-}$ B cells, 15, 23
AID controls CSR, 15
AID-cre-YFP reporter mouse, 235–236
AID deficiency, 275, 279–284, 297–298
   associated with preserved SHM, 285–287
   autosomal dominant transmission of, 287–289
   B cells, 7, 14, 182, 251
   classical deficiency
      AICDA mutations, 281, 283–285, 288
      phenotype, 280–282
AID deficient mice, 6–7, 163, 248, 250, 252
AID-dependent diversification processes, 110
AID-induced DNA lesion, 294–295
AID-mediated sequence diversification, 117
   by *cis*-acting determinants, 109–120
   DNA incorporated genome transient phase of mutability, 117–120
   histone and DNA structure responsible for, 118–119
   subnuclear compartmentalization, 119–120
   non-Ig transcription cassettes target for, 114–115
   targeting DNA elements in Ig loci, 116–117
   transcription
      AID deamination *in vitro*, 116
      for GCV/SHM in DT40 cells, 111, 113–114
      levels and frequencies correlation, 115–116
      in mammalian cells, 111–113
AID$^{-/-}$ mice, 229
AID$^{-/-}$ murine splenic B cells, 284, 286–287, 293
AID-specific mutations process, 141–143
AID-sufficient B cells, 251
AID transgenic mouse models, 247–252
Antibody diversification, activation-induced deaminase role in, 75–96
Antibody hypermutation, 40

INDEX

Antibody memory, AID as engraver of, 1–29
Anti-gH2AX antibody, 15
Antiviral cytidine deaminases. *See*
Apolipoprotein B RNA-editing catalytic component cytidine deaminases family
ApoB48, 4, 17
APOBEC. *See* Apolipoprotein B RNA-editing catalytic component family
APOBEC1, 37, 46, 49–50, 53, 55, 63, 78–79, 82, 132, 164, 166, 169, 216–217, 223, 229, 236, 283–284, 286, 288–289
 homology, 12–13, 17
 RNA editing enzyme, 1, 4, 17–18, 21, 49–50
APOBEC2, 37, 48–51, 53–54, 216, 223, 236
APOBEC3, 37, 48–63, 164, 166
 action on virus, 56–57, 220–221
 effects on mobile elements, 58
 LTR-containing endogenous retroelements and, 57–59
 non-LTR-containing endogenous retroelements and, 59–61
 retroviral hypermutation, 40
 restriction mechanism, 61–63
APOBEC3A, 56–58, 60–61, 216, 223–227
 inhibit adeno-associated virus production, 224–226
APOBEC3B, 55–58, 60–61, 216–217, 222–223, 227
APOBEC3C, 55–60, 216–217, 222–223, 227
APOBEC3D, 56, 58, 60, 216–217, 223, 227
APOBEC3E, 56, 58, 60, 216–217, 223, 227
APOBEC3F, 46, 55–60, 216, 222–224, 227, 237
 endogenous retroviruses, 226–228
 infection by foamy viruses, 224
 mutational analysis of, 48
APOBEC3G, 48, 52–63, 215–220, 223–225, 227, 235–237
 action on viruses, 220–221
 anti-ERV activity, 226–227
 antiviral activities of, 223–226
 deamination of retroviral replication and restriction of infection, 53–54
 restricts HIV infection, 52, 54–55, 217–220
APOBEC3H, 55–56, 58, 60–61
APOBEC4, 49, 51–52
APOBEC enzymes
 biochemical basis of C deamination by, 132–141
 mechanisms along ssDNA, 139–141

APOBEC proteins, 215–216
 timeline of evolution, 48–49
 Zn-dependent deaminases implications for structures of, 44–48
APOBEC gene family. *See* Apolipoprotein B RNA editing catalytic component cytidine deaminases family
Apolipoprotein B RNA-editing catalytic component cytidine deaminases family, 215–217
 adeno-associated virus production, 224–226
 antiviral activities of, 220–226
Apolipoprotein B RNA-editing catalytic component family, 37–39, 46, 48, 50–52, 63, 81, 132, 236
APRIL, 277–278, 293
Artemis-deficient B cells, 87
Artemis endonuclease, 85
Artificial switch construct in fibroblasts
 ectopic expression of AID induces
  CSR of, 9–10
  SHM of, 10–11
AsnH56Asp mutation, 144
AspH95Trp mutation, 145
Ataxia-telangiectasia mutated (ATM) kinase, 88–89, 92–93, 95–96, 186, 190–191
Ataxia-telangiectasia (A-T) syndrome, 89
ATM and Rad3-related (ATR), 91, 190–191
ATM B cells, 91–92, 192–193
ATR kinase, 88

B

BAFF. *See* B-cell-activating factor receptor
BAFF-R-knockout mice, 296
BALB/c-IL-6 transgenic mice, 250
Base excision repair (BER) enzymes, 19
B-cell-activating factor receptor, 277–278, 293, 296
B-cell chronic lymphocytic leukemia (B-CLL), 256
B-cell intrinsic immunoglobulin class switch recombination (Ig-CSR) deficiencies pathophysiology of, 275–298
B-cell malignancy, mechanism of AID expression in, 260–262
B cells, 38, 110–111, 120
 abnormalities, 234
 activation by CSR stimulants, 14, 18
 AID and, 5, 182, 251–256
 antigen receptor diversification in, 109

B cells (*continued*)
  artemis-deficient, 87
  ATM-deficient, 91, 192–193
  53BP1-deficient, 192–194
  etiology of neoplasms, 79
  germinal center, 127–131
  H2AX-deficient, 192–193
  IL-4-induced AID expression in, 80
  Ku70/80-deficient, 86
  lymphomas, 93–94, 96, 171, 180, 192, 232, 245–250, 252–256, 260, 265, 297
  MDC1-deficient, 192
  Nbs1-deficient, 192–193
  non-Hodgkin's lymphoma (NHL), 234–235
  somatic mutation in, 93
  UNG/Msh2-double-deficient, 168
Bcl-6-deficient mice, 296
BER pathway, 137, 165, 180
B Lymphocytes, genetic alterations in, 158–162
53BP1, 89, 92–93, 95–96, 186, 191, 295
53BP1-deficient B cells, 192–194
Burkitt's lymphoma (BL), 113, 246

C

C4b-binding protein (C4BP), 278
CD19, 235, 262
CD21, 235, 262
CD40, 14, 80, 86, 231–233, 261
CD81, 235, 262, 264
CD225, 235
CD8a-GFP$^+$ cells, 9
CD27+ B cells, 296
CD19+/CD27+ B cells, 281
CD4+ cells, 53, 219, 221, 233
C deamination by APOBEC enzymes, biochemical basis of, 132–141
CD4 ND5 genes, 21
CD40 ligand (CD40L), 259, 277–278, 297–298
CD40 ligand-deficient mice, 6
Cernunnos/XLF, 87–88
CH12F3-2 cells, 4, 9, 28
Chromatin immunoprecipitation (ChIP) assays, 15, 21–22, 167
Chromosome region maintenance-1 (CRM1), 82
Chromosome translocations
  activation-induced deaminase role in, 75–96
  AID role in, 94–96, 110, 249–252
Chyromicron, 17
Classical Hodgkin's lymphoma (CHL), 256

Class switch recombination (CSR), 1–2, 76–85, 109, 215–216, 245–246
  AID-induced
    B-cell-specific factor, 8–11
    C-terminal domain for, 11
    dimerization for, 13–14
    disruption in loss of, 5–7
    ectopic expression, 9–10
    as key molecule in, 4–8
  AID identification, 4–8
  APOBEC1 dimerization for, 13–14
  ATM deficiency impacts on, 91
  B cell culture, 4–8
  C and N terminal domain of AID, 11–12
  DNA damage detection and resolution, 85–93
  DNA repair systems
    damage response, 189–192
    DSB response proteins in, 192–194
    end joining, 194–197
  DSB resolution, 85–88
  ectopic expression of AID, 9–10
  evolution of, 197–198
  in fibroblasts, 9–10
  function of UNG in, 168–169
  germ line transcription and switch regions role in, 169–180
    germ line CH gene transcription role in targeting, 171–174
    IgH CH locus organization, 170
    mechanisms of transcription through, 175–178
    R-loops, 175–176
    S region function in, 170–171
  H2AX deficiency impacts on, 90
  heterologous promoters for, 111–114
  Ig promoters, 111–113
  initiation mechanism, 161
  in mammalian cells, 111–113, 118
  model for, 173
  NHEJ pathway in, 15
  NHEJ and DSB resolution during
    artemis, 87
    cernunnos/XLF, XRCC4 and DNA ligase IV, 87–88
    DNA-PK$_{CS}$, 86–87
    Ku70 and Ku80 DNA-binding subunits, 85–86
  S region
    function in, 170–171

INDEX 311

synapsis and roles of DSB response
proteins, 191
transcription for, 111, 113–114
UNG complex model during, 20
UNG function in, 24–28
catalytic site mutants effect, 24–25
replication-coupling UNG motifs
for, 25–27
WXXF motif need, 27–28
UNG/MMR mutations alter spectrum
of, 167–168
CMV promoter, 114
C-myc/IgH translocations, 94–96, 245–246,
250–251
CRE/LoxP recombination system, 92
Cryoglobulinemia, 234
CSR. See Class switch recombination
CSR block from Sm region DNA cleavage
Ig-CSR deficiency by, 293–296
CSR-deficient hyper-IgM syndromes, 88
CSR-stimulated CH12F3-2 cells, 4
C-U deamination jumping and sliding
model, 134–136
Cycloheximide, 18–19
Cytidine deaminases, 4, 37, 39, 41–47, 77, 81
Cytosine deaminases, 37, 41, 45–47, 61

D

DCMP deaminase, 41–42, 46
Diffuse large B-cell lymphomas
(DLBCLs), 180, 246, 252, 258
DNA
binding subunits Ku70 and Ku80, 85–86
damage detection and resolution during
CSR
53BP1, 92–93
g-H2AX, 89–90
NHEJ and DSB resolution, 85–88
MRN complex, 89, 91–92
response, 88–93
DNA cleavage, AID involvement in, 14–16,
19, 28
DNA deamination
for antibody diversification, 38–39
in immunity, 37–63
DNA deamination model, 1, 3, 17, 19–24, 79
of AID, 164–169
bacterial DNA mutation, 166
binding to S regions, 167
function of UNG in CSR, 168–169

ssDNA-specific cytidine deaminase
in vitro, 166–167
UNG/MMR mutations, 167–168
UNG for DSBs, 22–24
in vitro deamination, 19–22
DNA-dependent protein kinase (DNA-PK),
12, 85–86, 88, 91, 93
DNA lesions, and AID
biochemical function, 78–79
epigenetic modifications and
transcription, 77
nuclear transport and posttranslational
modification, 82–83
protein, 81–82
transcriptional regulation, 80–81
ssDNA liberation, 80
transcriptional activation, 77–78
DNA ligase IV, 87–88
DNA-PK. See DNA-dependent protein kinase
DNA-PKCS gene, 86
DNA-PK$_{CS}$ B cells, 12, 86, 88, 93
DNA-PK$_{CS}$ /– mice, 86
D145N human UNG mutant, 25
Double-stranded breaks (DSBs), 131, 157, 159
resolution during CSR, 85–88
artemis, 87
cernunnos/XLF, XRCC4 and DNA
ligase IV, 87–88
DNA-PK$_{CS}$, 86–87
Ku70 and Ku80 DNA-binding
subunits, 85–86
synapsis of AID initiated DSBs in
S region, 184–189
Double-stranded DNA (dsDNA), 80, 84, 129,
134, 136–137, 140, 162, 166, 175
DT40 cells, 111, 113–117

E

EBV-encoded nuclear antigen-2
(EBNA-2), 233–234, 261
EBV nuclear antigens (EBNAs), 261
EF1-a promoter, 113–116
Endemic Burkitt's lymphoma (eBL), 232
Endogenous retroelements
suppression by APOBEC3 family cytidine
deaminases, 226–228
non-LTR retroelements, 227–228
physiological role for, 228
Endogenous retroviruses (ERV), suppression
by APOBEC3, 226–227

Enhanced green fluorescence protein (EGFP) gene, 114
Epstein-barr virus (EBV), 260–261
  AID and, 231–235
Equine infectiousanemia virus (EIAV), APOBEC3G action on, 220
Exonuclease 1 (EXO1), 165

F

Fluorescence-activated cell sorting (FACS), 9
Fluorescence *in situ* hybridization (FISH), 23, 192–193
Follicular B-cell lymphoma (FL), 249
Frauenfelder's model of hierarchical energy landscape in proteins, 145

G

GC-derived B-cell lymphomas, 252–256
Gene conversion (GCV), 109, 110
  in DT40 cells, 113–116
  heterologous promoters for, 113–114
  transcription for, 111, 113–114
Germ cell tumors (GCTs), 263
Germ line transcript, 14
GFP reversion assay
  in B and firoblast cell line, 115–116
GFP+ cells, 114
GlyH55Val mutation, 145
Guanine deaminase, 41

H

Haemophilus influenzae, 279
H2AX cells, 15–16, 23, 89–93, 95, 163–164, 186, 190–193, 251, 295
H2AX-mice, 91, 295
HCCs. *See* Hepatocellular carcinomas
HCV cell culture (HCVcc) system, 234
HCV E2 glycoprotein, 235
Heavy chain variable (V), diversity (D) and joining (J) (V(D)J) germ line genes, 128
Hepatitis B virus (HBV), 56, 264
  APOBEC3G action on, 221–222
Hepatitis C virus (HCV), 260, 262
  AID and, 231, 234–235
Hepatocellular carcinomas, 248, 264
HIGM2. *See* Hyper-IgM syndrome type 2
Histone H3 and H4, 77, 89, 118–119, 190
HIV-1, restriction by APOBEC3G, 52, 54–55, 217–220, 223, 237
HIV Vpr-like protein, 1

H268L human UNG mutant, 25
Hodgkin and Reed-Sternberg cells, 256
Hodgkin's lymphomas, 232, 260
HTLV-1-AID transgenic mice, 248
Human B-cell malignancies, AID expression in, 252–258
  GC-derived B-cell lymphomas, 252–256
  non-GC-derived B-cell lymphomas, 256–257
  potential importance of, 257–258
Human T-cell leukemia virus-1, 57
Human T-lymphotropic virus 1, APOBEC3G action on, 221
Human UNG mutants, 25
Hyper-IgM syndrome type 2 (HIGM2), 7–8, 265, 275

I

IFNgR gene, 4
IgA+ cells, 87–88
IgG^+ B cells, 23
Ig gene diversification, 119
IKK complexes, 277
IL-4, 5, 10, 14–15, 18, 80, 86–87, 172, 231, 259
  induced AID expression in B cells, 80
IL-6, 94–95
IL-10, 259
Immunoglobulin class switch recombination (Ig-CSR) deficiency
  AICDA mutations and, 281, 283–285
  associated with SHM, 285–287
  autosomal dominant transmission of, 287–289
  caused by
    AID deficiency, 279–289, 297–298
    DNA lesion in S regions, 294–295
    CSR block, 293–296
    switched B-cell differentiation defect, 295–296
    UNG deficiency, 275, 289–292, 297–298
  with normal SHM, 292–296
  phenotype, 280–282
Immunoglobulin (Ig) genes, 2, 23, 38–39, 85, 87, 158, 164, 193, 262
  AID-initiated mutations in, 127–149
  diversification processes, 109–110
  light and heavy chain genes(IgL/IgH), 158
Immunoglobulin heavy chain class switch recombination (IgH CSR)
  deficiencies, 275
  evolution mechanism, 157–198
  initiation of, 160

INDEX

Infectious mononucleosis (IM), 232–233
Interferon-a cytokine, 222
Interleukin-4. See IL-4
Isolated lymphoid follicle (ILF), 8

J

JAK/STAT pathway, 80

K

Ku70 and Ku80
  deficient B cells, 86, 196
  deficient mice, 15, 86
  DNA-binding subunits, 85

L

Latent membrane protein-1 (LMP-1), 232–233, 261
Lck-AID transgenic mice, 248
LCLs. See Lymphoblastoid cell lines
Leukemias, 249, 265
Ligation-mediated PCR (LM-PCR), 15–16
LPS, 5, 10, 14–15, 18, 86–87, 172
Lung microadenomas, 248
Lymphoblastoid cell lines (LCLs), 232–233
Lymphocyte-predominant Hodgkin's lymphoma (LPHL), 256
Lymphocytic and histiocytic (L&H) cells, 256
Lymphoid organ hypertrophy in AID-deficient mice, mechanism of, 8
Lymphomagenesis, AID role in, 249–252
Lymphomagenic lesions and AID, 93–96
  chromosome translocations, 94–96
  non-Ig genes mutations and lymphomas, 93–94

M

MALT lymphoma, 257, 260
Mammalian cells, SHM and CSR in, 111–113
Mantle cell lymphoma (MCL), 249
M B-CLL cells, 256–258
MDC1-deficient B cells, 192
MDC gene, 4
Mdc1$^{-/-}$ mice, 295
Melanomas, 248
Mismatch repair (MMR) pathway, 79, 130–131, 137, 165, 180
MMR proteins, 165
MMTV-AID transgenic mice, 248
Mouse AID188X, 11

Mre11, Rad50, and Nbs1complex. See MRN complex
Mre11 proteins, 190
MRN complex, 89, 91–92
Msh2 and 6 proteins, 19, 22, 79, 165
Multiple myeloma (MM), 249
Murine leukemia virus (MLV), AOBEC3G action on, 220
Mutability index, 134
MYC-IgH translocations, AID role in, 180

N

Nbs1-deficient B cells, 192–193
NF-kB pathways, 80, 277–278
NIH3T3 cells, 9–10
Nijmegen breakage syndrome 1 (NBS1), 286
Nijmegen syndrome protein 1 (Nbs1), 89–90, 92, 190–192
NK cell, 233, 262
Non-GC-derived B-cell lymphomas, AID expression in, 256–257
Non-Hodgkin's lymphoma (NHL), 234–235
Nonhomologous end-Joining (NHEJ)
  during Ku70 and Ku80 DNA-binding subunits, 85–86
  during pathways, 9, 15, 95, 158, 189, 193–196, 286, 294
Non-Ig genes mutations, lymphomas and, 93–94
Nonprimate retroviruses, POBEC3G action on, 220
Normal and malignant nonlymphoid cells, AID expression in, 263–264
Normal B cells, AID expression mechanism in, 259
N204V human UNG mutant, 25

P

Pax5gene, 94
P53-binding protein 1 (53BP1), See 53BP1
Peanut agglutinin (PNA) staining, 5
Phosphatidylinositol-3-kinase, 88
3-Photon echo peak shift spectroscopy (3PEPS) technique, 145–146
PIM1gene, 94
Pms2/Mlh1 protein, 165
PNA staining. See Peanut agglutinin (PNA) staining
Polynucleotides, cytidine deaminase activity on, 37

Primary cutaneous follicle center lymphoma (PCFCL), 258
Primary cutaneous large B-cell lymphomas (PCLBCLs), 258
Protein dynamics, 145–146
Protein kinase A (PKA), 12
  phosphorylation, 83
Proto-oncogenes, mutations in, 179–180
Pyk2-deficient mice, 278

R

RAD50 proteins, 190
Replication-coupling UNG motifs for CSR, 25–27
Replication protein A (RPA), 12
Retroviral 5′ LTR, 114
RhoH gene, 94
Riboflavin deaminase, 41
RNA-editing enzymes, 42
RNA editing model, 1, 3, 17–19, 288–289
  of AID, 163–164
R-loop mechanism, 176–178
RNA polymerases (RNA pol), 12, 112–113

S

Sarcomas, 248
SCID B cells, 87
SCID mice, 86–87
Severe combined immunodeficiency (SCID), 85–86
Sheep red blood cells (SRBC) immunization, 5
SHM. See Somatic hypermutation
Simian immunodeficiency virus (SIV), 219–220
Single stranded DNA (ssDNA), 77, 82, 129, 162
  AID targets C motifs on, 132–139
  APOBEC-targeting mechanisms along, 139–141
  Apo3G and AID processive C®U deaminations on, 135, 138
  deamination of, 112
  liberation during transcription, 80
Sm region DNA cleavage, Ig-CSR deficiency by CSR block from, 293–296
Sm–Sg switch junctions, 88
Somatic hypermutation, 1–2, 76–82, 109, 215–216, 245–246, 275–276
  AID as key molecule in, 4–8
  AID identification, 4–8
  AID-induced, 127–131

AID phosphorylation role in, 183
  of artificial construct in fibroblasts, 10–11
  ATM deficiency and, 91
  B-cell and, 8–11
  C and N terminal domains of AID, 11–12
  in DT40 cells, 113–116
  ectopic expression, 9–11
  H2AX deficiency and, 90
  Ig promoters, 111–113
  initiation mechanism, 161
  loss of, 5–7
  in mammalian cells, 111–113, 118
  N-terminal domain for, 11–12
  phenomenon of, 4
  transcription for, 111, 113–114
  UNG/MMR mutations and, 167–168
SRBC-immunized mice, 5
Sterile transcript, 14
Streptococcus pneumoniae, 279
Switched B-cell differentiation defect, Ig-CSR deficiency due to, 295–296

T

TadA enzyme, 41–42
Tad1p/Tad2p/Tad3p, 41–42, 48
T cells, 5, 38, 52–53, 87, 277–278
  lymphomas, 94, 247, 260
Testicular germ cell tumors
  pathogenesis, 263
TGF-b cytokines, 80, 87, 259
Thymidine kinase promoter, 114
TLR4-MyD88 pathway, 260
Transcribed dsDNA sequences, 176–180
T7 transcription assays, 137
Transcription bubbles model, on AID activity, 136
Transcription
  for GCV/SHM in DT40 cells, 113–114
  levels and frequencies in AID-mediated sequence diversification, 115–116
  for SHM, GCV and CSR in mammalian cells, 111–113
Transmembrane activator and calcium-modulating cyclophilin-interacting protein (TACI), 277–278
TRNA deaminase, 37, 41–42, 46, 48
Tryptophan 231, mutations in, 27
Tumor biology, 253
Tumorigenesis, 110
  AID role in, 245–264

INDEX

U

UM B-CLL cells, 256–258
UNG. See Uracil DNA glycosylase
UNG/Msh2-double-deficient B cells, 168
Uracil deglicosylases (UDGs), 78
Uracil DNA glycosylase, 1, 3–4, 19
  cells, 21, 23, 25–27
  complex model during CSR, 20
  for DSBs in DNA deamination model, 22–24
  function in CSR
    catalytic site mutants effect on, 24–25
    replication-coupling motifs for, 25–27
    WXXF motifs for, 27–28
  mice, 168–169, 291

V

V(D)J recombination, 75–76, 87, 90, 92, 96, 109, 128, 158, 163, 171, 174, 188–189, 191, 193, 195–196, 216, 249–250
Vh186.2 gene, 7
Virion infectivity factor (Vif), 217–220, 225, 236–237
Viruses, APOBEC3G action on
  equine infectiousanemia virus (EIAV), 220
  hepatitis B virus (HBV), 221–222
  human T-lymphotropic virus 1 (HTLV-1), 221
  murine leukemia virus (MLV), 220
  nonprimate retroviruses, 220

W

WXXF motiffor CSR function, 27–28

X

X-linked CD40L deficiency, 298
X-linked Ig-CSR deficiency, 277
XRCC4, 85, 87–88, 197

Y

Y147A mutants, 25

Z

Zinc (Zn)-dependent deaminases, 37, 39–48
  deamination by, 44
  sequence alignment of, 47
  structure and function
    for AID/APOBECs structures, 44–48
    coordination motif, 43–44
    deaminase quaternary structures, 44
    three-dimensional structures of, 45

Contents of Recent Volumes

Volume 84

Interactions Between NK Cells and
B Lymphocytes
Dorothy Yuan

Multitasking of Helix-Loop-Helix Proteins
in Lymphopoiesis
Xiao-Hong Sun

Customized Antigens for Desensitizing
Allergic Patients
Fátima Ferreira,
Michael Wallner, and
Josef Thalhamer

Immune Response Against Dying
Tumor Cells
Laurence Zitvogel, Noelia Casares,
Marie O. Pëquignot,
Nathalie Chaput,
Mathew L. Albert,
and Guido Kroemer

HMGB1 in the Immunology
of Sepsis (Not Septic Shock)
and Arthritis
Christopher J. Czura,
Huan Yang,
Carol Ann Amella, and
Kevin J. Tracey

Selection of the T-Cell Repertoire:
Receptor-Controlled Checkpoints in
T-Cell Development
Harald Von Boehmer

The Pathogenesis of Diabetes in the
NOD Mouse
Michelle Solomon and
Nora Sarvetnick

Index

Volume 85

Cumulative Subject Index
Volumes 66–82

Volume 86

Adenosine Deaminase Deficiency:
Metabolic Basis of Immune
Deficiency and Pulmonary
Inflammation
Michael R. Blackburn and
Rodney E. Kellems

Mechanism and Control of V(D)J
Recombination Versus Class Switch
Recombination: Similarities and
Differences
Darryll D. Dudley, Jayanta Chaudhuri,
Craig H. Bassing, and Frederick W. Alt

Isoforms of Terminal
Deoxynucleotidyltransferase:
Developmental Aspects and Function
To-Ha Thai and John F. Kearney

Innate Autoimmunity
Michael C. Carroll and V. Michael Holers

Formation of Bradykinin: A Major Contributor to the Innate Inflammatory Response
Kusumam Joseph and Allen P. Kaplan

Interleukin-2, Interleukin-15, and Their Roles in Human Natural Killer Cells
Brian Becknell and Michael A. Caligiuri

Regulation of Antigen Presentation and Cross-Presentation in the Dendritic Cell Network: Facts, Hypothesis, and Immunological Implications
Nicholas S. Wilson and Jose A. Villadangos

Index

The Repair of DNA Damages/Modifications During the Maturation of the Immune System: Lessons from Human Primary Immunodeficiency Disorders and Animal Models
Patrick Revy, Dietke Buck, Françoise le Deist, and Jean-Pierre de Villartay

Antibody Class Switch Recombination: Roles for Switch Sequences and Mismatch Repair Proteins
Irene M. Min and Erik Selsing

Index

Volume 87

Role of the LAT Adaptor in T-Cell Development and T_h2 Differentiation
Bernard Malissen, Enrique Aguado, and Marie Malissen

The Integration of Conventional and Unconventional T Cells that Characterizes Cell-Mediated Responses
Daniel J. Pennington, David Vermijlen, Emma L. Wise, Sarah L. Clarke, Robert E. Tigelaar, and Adrian C. Hayday

Negative Regulation of Cytokine and TLR Signalings by SOCS and Others
Tetsuji Naka, Minoru Fujimoto, Hiroko Tsutsui, and Akihiko Yoshimura

Pathogenic T-Cell Clones in Autoimmune Diabetes: More Lessons from the NOD Mouse
Kathryn Haskins

The Biology of Human Lymphoid Malignancies Revealed by Gene Expression Profiling
Louis M. Staudt and Sandeep Dave

New Insights into Alternative Mechanisms of Immune Receptor Diversification
Gary W. Litman, John P. Cannon, and Jonathan P. Rast

Volume 88

CD22: A Multifunctional Receptor That Regulates B Lymphocyte Survival and Signal Transduction
Thomas F. Tedder, Jonathan C. Poe, and Karen M. Haas

Tetramer Analysis of Human Autoreactive CD4-Positive T Cells
Gerald T. Nepom

Regulation of Phospholipase C-γ2 Networks in B Lymphocytes
Masaki Hikida and Tomohiro Kurosaki

Role of Human Mast Cells and Basophils in Bronchial Asthma
Gianni Marone, Massimo Triggiani, Arturo Genovese, and Amato De Paulis

A Novel Recognition System for MHC Class I Molecules Constituted by PIR
Toshiyuki Takai

Dendritic Cell Biology
Francesca Granucci, Maria Foti, and Paola Ricciardi-Castagnoli

The Murine Diabetogenic Class II
  Histocompatibility Molecule I-A^{g7}:
  Structural and Functional
  Properties and Specificity of
  Peptide Selection
    Anish Suri and Emil R. Unanue

RNAi and RNA-Based Regulation of Immune
  System Function
    Dipanjan Chowdhury and Carl D. Novina

Index

Volume 89

Posttranscriptional Mechanisms Regulating
  the Inflammatory Response
    Georg Stoecklin Paul Anderson

Negative Signaling in Fc Receptor Complexes
    Marc Daëron and Renaud Lesourne

The Surprising Diversity of Lipid Antigens for
  CD1-Restricted T Cells
    D. Branch Moody

Lysophospholipids as Mediators of Immunity
    Debby A. Lin and Joshua A. Boyce

Systemic Mastocytosis
    Jamie Robyn and Dean D. Metcalfe

Regulation of Fibrosis by the Immune System
    Mark L. Lupher, Jr. and W. Michael Gallatin

Immunity and Acquired Alterations in
  Cognition and Emotion: Lessons from SLE
    Betty Diamond, Czeslawa Kowal,
    Patricio T. Huerta, Cynthia Aranow,
    Meggan Mackay, Lorraine A. DeGiorgio,
    Ji Lee, Antigone Triantafyllopoulou,
    Joel Cohen-Solal Bruce, and T. Volpe

Immunodeficiencies with Autoimmune
  Consequences
    Luigi D. Notarangelo, Eleonora Gambineri,
    and Raffaele Badolato

Index

Volume 90

Cancer Immunosurveillance and
  Immunoediting: The Roles of Immunity in
  Suppressing Tumor Development and
  Shaping Tumor Immunogenicity
    Mark J. Smyth, Gavin P. Dunn, and
    Robert D. Schreiber

Mechanisms of Immune Evasion by Tumors
    Charles G. Drake, Elizabeth Jaffee, and
    Drew M. Pardoll

Development of Antibodies
  and Chimeric Molecules for
  Cancer Immunotherapy
    Thomas A. Waldmann and John C. Morris

Induction of Tumor Immunity Following
  Allogeneic Stem Cell Transplantation
    Catherine J. Wu and Jerome Ritz

Vaccination for Treatment and
  Prevention of Cancer in Animal Models
    Federica Cavallo, Rienk Offringa,
    Sjoerd H. van der Burg,
    Guido Forni, and Cornelis J. M. Melief

Unraveling the Complex Relationship
  Between Cancer Immunity and
  Autoimmunity: Lessons from
  Melanoma and Vitiligo
    Hiroshi Uchi, Rodica Stan, Mary Jo Turk,
    Manuel E. Engelhorn, Gabrielle A. Rizzuto,
    Stacie M. Goldberg, Jedd D. Wolchok,
    and Alan N. Houghton

Immunity to Melanoma Antigens: From
  Self-Tolerance to Immunotherapy
    Craig L. Slingluff, Jr.,
    Kimberly A. Chianese-Bullock,
    Timothy N. J. Bullock, William W. Grosh,
    David W. Mullins, Lisa Nichols, Walter
    Olson, Gina Petroni, Mark Smolkin,
    and Victor H. Engelhard

Checkpoint Blockade in Cancer
  Immunotherapy
    Alan J. Korman, Karl S. Peggs, and
    James P. Allison

Combinatorial Cancer Immunotherapy
F. Stephen Hodi and Glenn Dranoff

Index

Volume 91

A Reappraisal of Humoral Immunity Based on Mechanisms of Antibody-Mediated Protection Against Intracellular Pathogens
Arturo Casadevall and Liise-anne Pirofski

Accessibility Control of V(D)J Recombination
Robin Milley Cobb, Kenneth J. Oestreich, Oleg A. Osipovich, and Eugene M. Oltz

Targeting Integrin Structure and Function in Disease
Donald E. Staunton, Mark L. Lupher, Robert Liddington, and W. Michael Gallatin

Endogenous TLR Ligands and Autoimmunity
Hermann Wagner

Genetic Analysis of Innate Immunity
Kasper Hoebe, Zhengfan Jiang, Koichi Tabeta, Xin Du, Philippe Georgel, Karine Crozat, and Bruce Beutler

TIM Family of Genes in Immunity and Tolerance
Vijay K. Kuchroo, Jennifer Hartt Meyers, Dale T. Umetsu, and Rosemarie H. DeKruyff

Inhibition of Inflammatory Responses by Leukocyte Ig-Like Receptors
Howard R. Katz

Index

Volume 92

Systemic Lupus Erythematosus: Multiple Immunological Phenotypes in a Complex Genetic Disease
Anna-Marie Fairhurst, Amy E. Wandstrat, and Edward K. Wakeland

Avian Models with Spontaneous Autoimmune Diseases
Georg Wick, Leif Andersson, Karel Hala, M. Eric Gershwin, Carlo Selmi, Gisela F. Erf, Susan J. Lamont, and Roswitha Sgonc

Functional Dynamics of Naturally Occurring Regulatory T Cells in Health and Autoimmunity
Megan K. Levings, Sarah Allan, Eva d'Hennezel, and Ciriaco A. Piccirillo

BTLA and HVEM Cross Talk Regulates Inhibition and Costimulation
Maya Gavrieli, John Sedy, Christopher A. Nelson, and Kenneth M. Murphy

The Human T Cell Response to Melanoma Antigens
Pedro Romero, Jean-Charles Cerottini, and Daniel E. Speiser

Antigen Presentation and the Ubiquitin-Proteasome System in Host–Pathogen Interactions
Joana Loureiro and Hidde L. Ploegh

Index

Volume 93

Class Switch Recombination: A Comparison Between Mouse and Human
Qiang Pan-Hammarström, Yaofeng Zhao, and Lennart Hammarström

Anti-IgE Antibodies for the Treatment of IgE-Mediated Allergic Diseases
Tse Wen Chang, Pheidias C. Wu, C. Long Hsu, and Alfur F. Hung

Immune Semaphorins: Increasing Members and Their Diverse Roles
Hitoshi Kikutani, Kazuhiro Suzuki, and Atsushi Kumanogoh

Tec Kinases in T Cell and Mast
  Cell Signaling
  Martin Felices, Markus Falk, Yoko Kosaka,
  and Leslie J. Berg

Integrin Regulation of Lymphocyte Trafficking:
  Lessons from Structural
  and Signaling Studies
  Tatsuo Kinashi

Regulation of Immune Responses and
  Hematopoiesis by the Rap1 Signal
  Nagahiro Minato, Kohei Kometani, and
  Masakazu Hattori

Lung Dendritic Cell Migration
  Hamida Hammad and Bart N. Lambrecht

Index

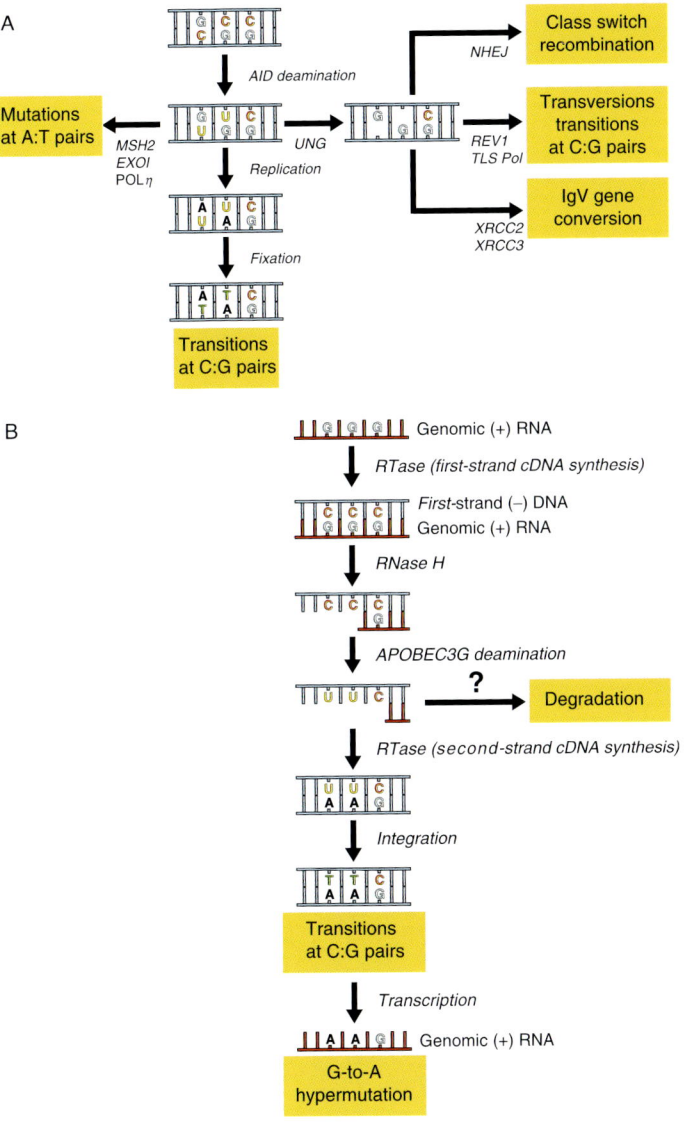

Plate 1

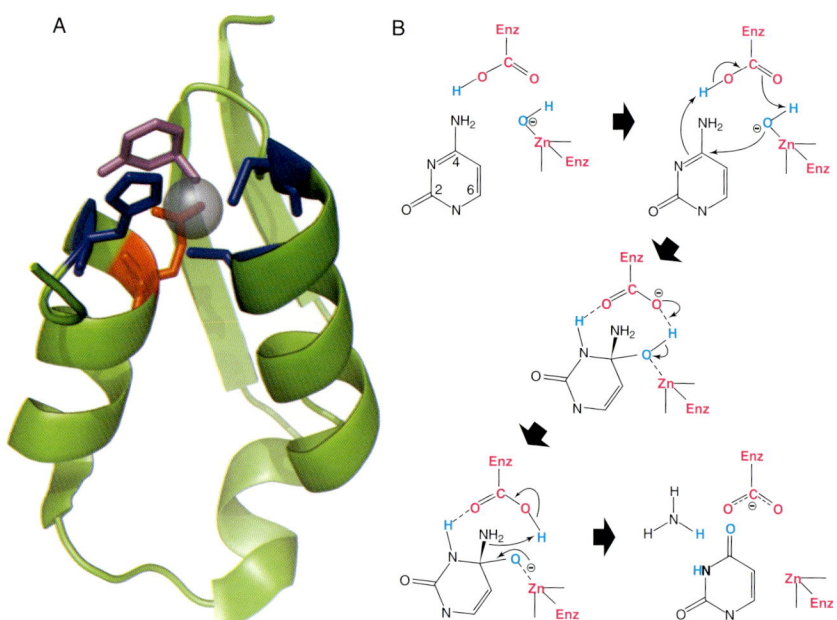

Plate 2

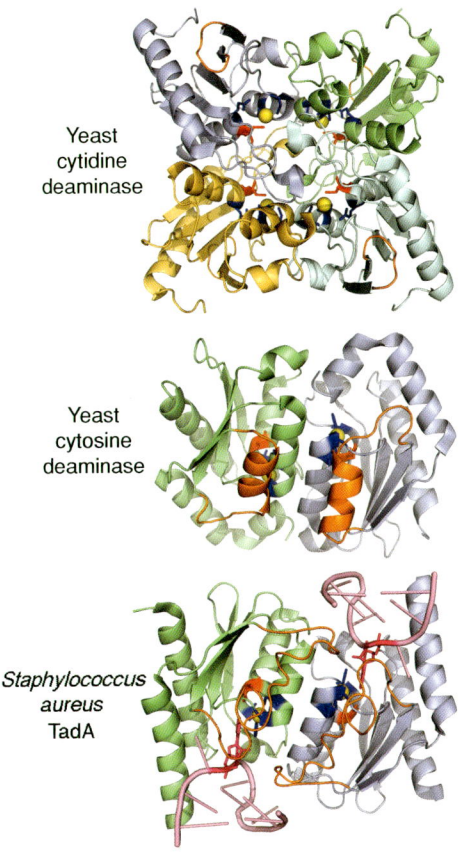

Plate 3

A

```
Yeast CDA                 ----MKVGGIEDQLEALKRAALKACELSYSPYSHFRVGCSIITNNDV----IFTGANVENASYSNCI-
Yeast CoDA                MVTGGMASKWDQKGMDIAYEEAALGYKEGVPI-----GGCIINNKDGS----VLGRGHNMRFQKGSATL
Staphylococcus aureus TadA ------MTNDIYFMTLAIEEAKKAAQLGEVPI-----GAIITKDD----EVIARAHNLRETLQQPPTA
Human AID                 ------MDSLLMNRRKFLYQFKNVRWAKGRR-ETYLCYVVRRDSATSFSLDFGYLRNKNGC-
                                                              Alpha 1              Beta 1         Beta 2
                                                           Zn-coordinating motif
Yeast CDA                 CAERSAMIQVLMAGHRSGWKCMVIGDSEDQCVSPGVCRQFINEFVVKDF----PIVMLNSTGS-
Yeast CoDA                HGEISTLENCGRLEGKVYKDTTLYTL-----SPCDMCTGAIIMYGIP----RCVVGENVNFKS
Staphylococcus aureus TadA HAEHIAIERAAKVLGSWRLEGCTLYVTL-----EPCVMCAGTIIMSRIP----RVVVGADDPKGG
Human AID                 HVELLFLRYISDWDLDPGRCYRVTWFT-----SWSPCYDCARHVADFLRGNPNLSLRIFTARLYFCEDR
                                 Alpha 2                    Beta 3                   Alpha 3    Beta 4
                                                                                              RNA-interacting
                                                                                                  loop
Yeast CDA                 ----RSKVMT----MGELLPMAFGPSHIN
Yeast CoDA                KGEKYLQTRG----HEVVVD-DERCKKIMKQFIDERPQDWFEDIGE
Staphylococcus aureus TadA CSGSLMNLLQQSNFNHRAIVDKGV--LKEACSTLLTTFFKNLRANKKSTN
Human AID                 KAEPEGLRRLHRA---GVQIAIMTFKDYFYCWNTFVENHERTFKAWEGLHENSVRLSRQLRRILLPLYEVDDLRDAFRTLGL
                                Alpha 4                        Alpha 5
```

B

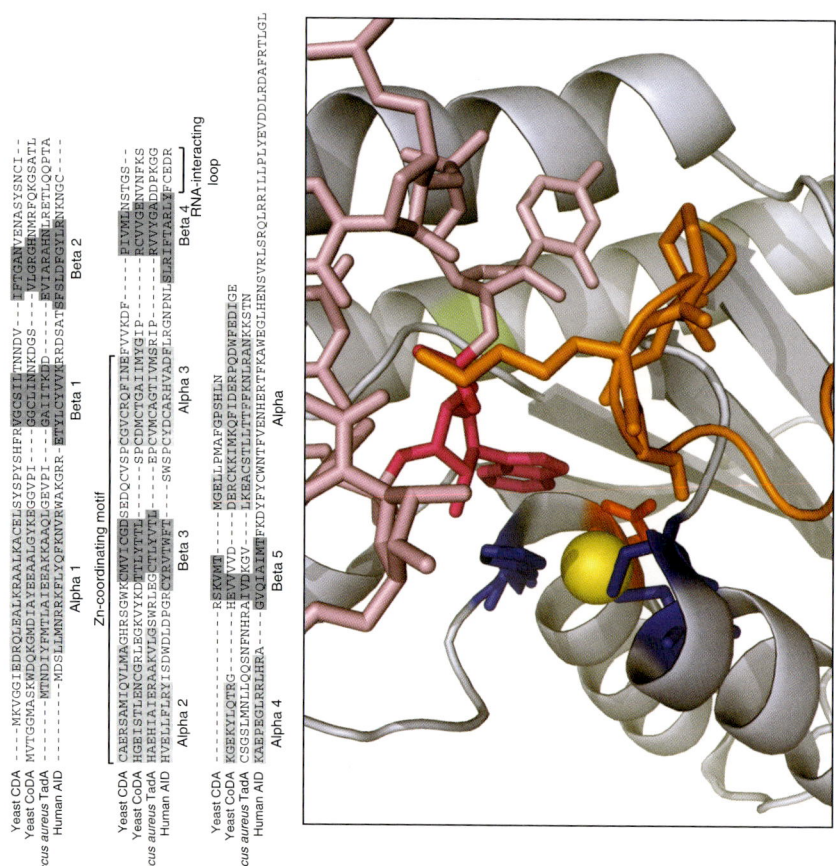

Plate 4

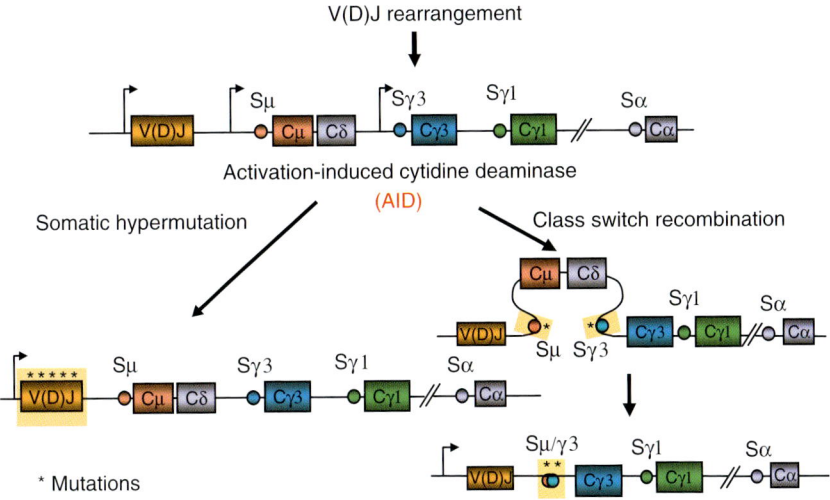

Plate 5

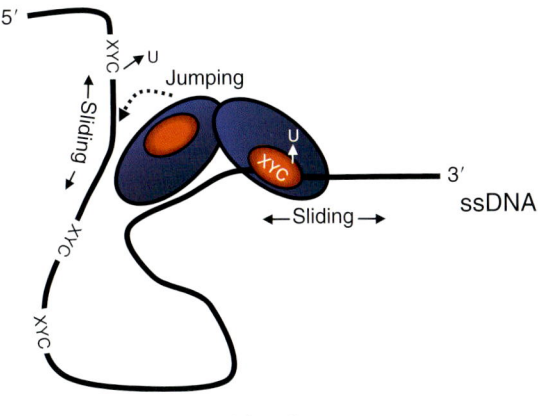

Plate 6

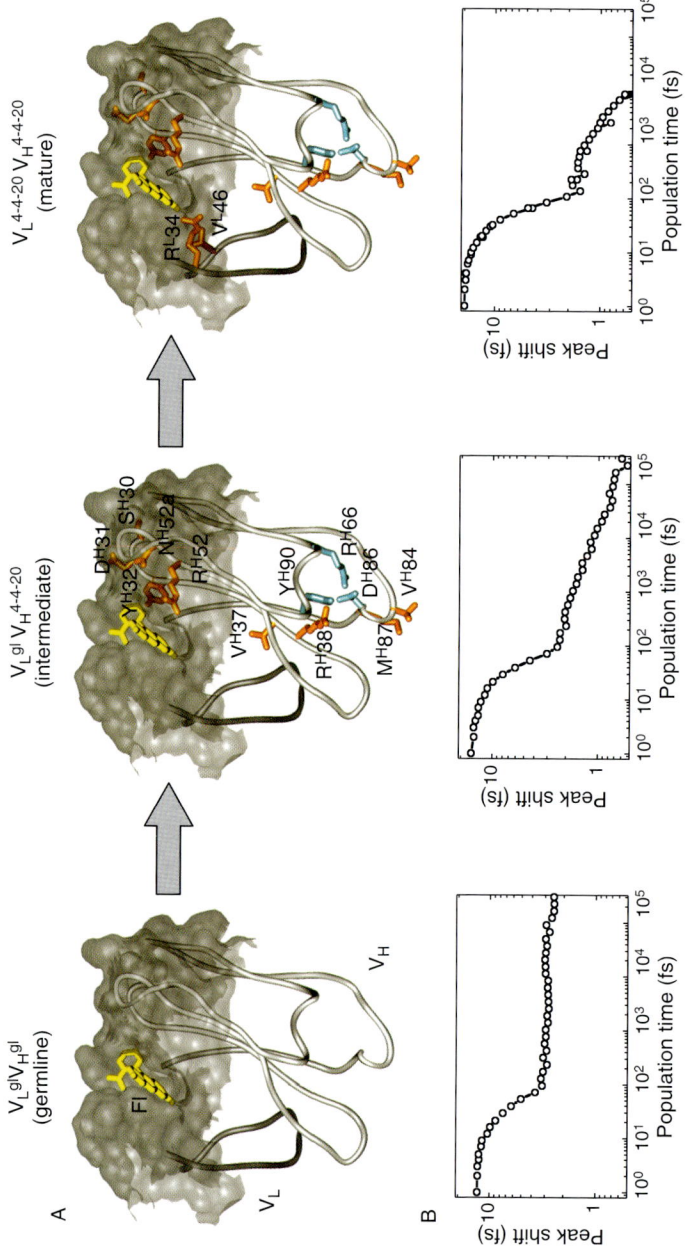

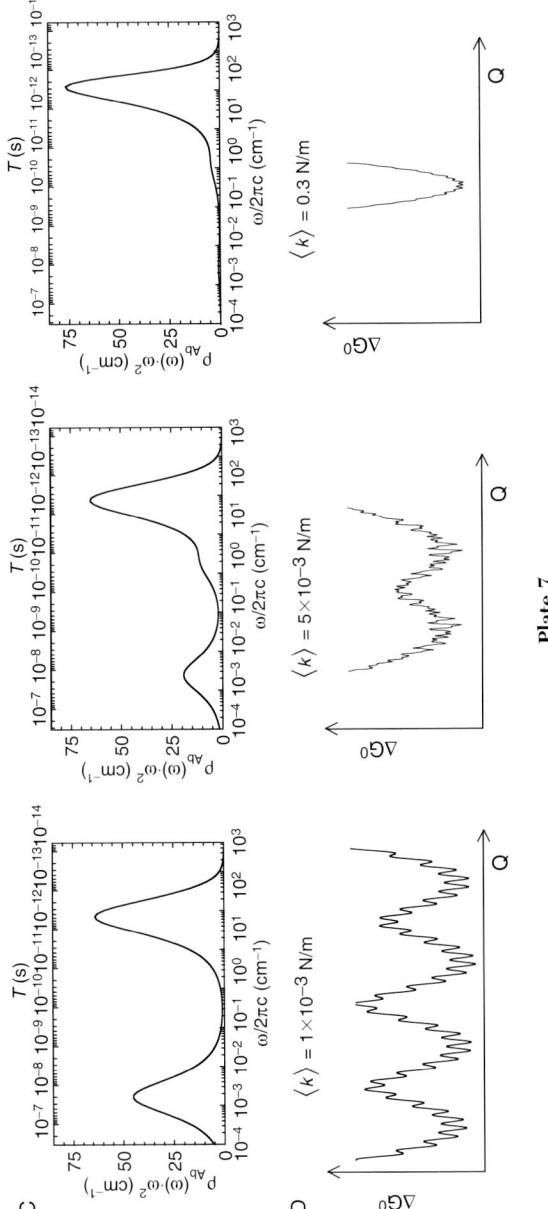

Plate 7

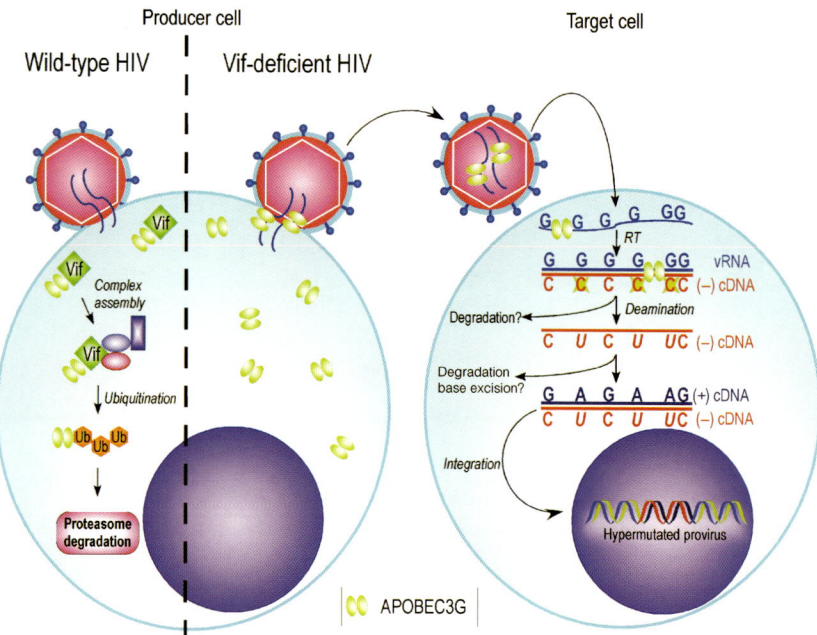

Plate 8

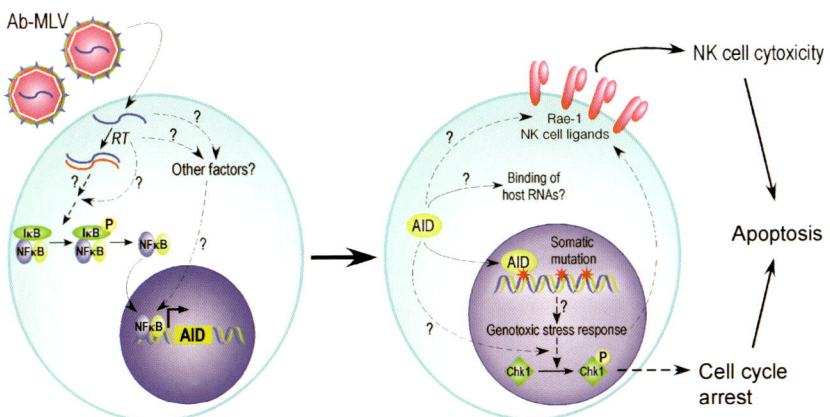

Plate 9

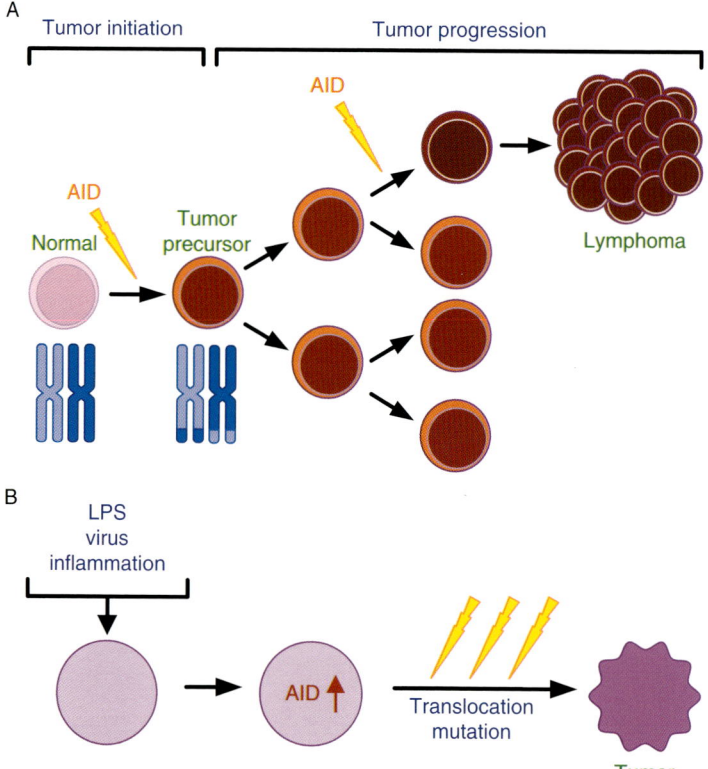

Plate 10